Chu...
Hypne
780

MW00855703

Hara Diagnosis:
Reflections on the Sea

Hara Diagnosis: Reflections on the Sea

— *by* —

Kiiko Matsumoto & Stephen Birch

Paradigm Publications • *Brookline, Massachusetts*

— *1988* —

Published by

Paradigm Publications
44 Linden Street
Brookline, Massachusetts, 02146 U.S.A.

ISBN 0-912111-13-5

Copyright © 1988 Kiiko Matsumoto and Stephen Birch

All rights reserved. No part of this publication may be reproduced, stored in a retrieval system or transmitted in any form by any means, electronic, mechanical, photocopying, recording, or otherwise, without the prior written permission of the publisher.

Library of Congress Cataloging in Publication Data:

Matsumoto, Kiiko.
Hara diagnosis.

Bibliography: p.
Includes index.
1. Medicine, Chinese. 2. Medicine, Chinese--Japan.
3. Abdomen--Examination. 4. Palpation. I. Birch,
Stephen. II. Title. [DNLM: 1. Abdomen. 2. Diagnosis.
3. Medicine Oriental Traditional. 4. Palpation--
methods. WB 275 M434h]
R602.M36 1988   616.07'54   88-17955
ISBN 0-912111-13-5

Paradigm Publications

Publisher: Robert L. Felt
Editor: Martha Lee Fielding
Cover Illustration: Yoshio Manaka
Text Illustration & Cover Design: Herb Rich III
Formatting Supervisor: T. Diane Putt

Typesetting Software:
Textware International, Cambridge, Massachusetts

Chinese Character Typesetting:
Linguistic Systems, Cambridge, Massachusetts

Additional Software & World Distribution
provided by
Redwing Book Company, Brookline, Massachusetts

Acid free, archive-quality papers have been used
in the production of this text to insure longevity.

Cover illustration from a scroll
by Yoshio Manaka, depicting
Shen Nung, the father of Chinese medicine.

Acknowledgements

I wish to extend my deepest gratitutde to Sensei Kuzome, for teaching me the essence of his style of abdominal diagnosis; and to Sensei Yoshio Manaka, for his generous sharing of his great knowledge and research, and for his boundless inspiration.

My deepest gratitude is extended to Soshichiro Tobe and Yuichiro Tobe, of Ido No Nippon Sha, for their unflagging assistance and encouragement given to me over the many years of my friendship with them.

I also thank my colleague, Stephen Birch, for his unremitting efforts and exhaustive research, without which this book might not have been completed.

I dedicate this book to the memory of my dear father, Tojiro Matsumoto.

Kiiko Matsumoto

Natick, Massachusetts.

Acknowledgements

* * *

The work involved in translating, compiling, researching, writing, and rewriting this book has been considerable. It would have been much slower and more difficult or perhaps impossible without the kind help and contributions of many people.

First and foremost are my teachers and friends Dr. Jim Oschman and Dr. Yoshio Manaka. Dr. Oschman provided considerable support and enthusiasm, with numerous articles, references, ideas, and brainstorms. His knowledge and wisdom is quite something to encounter. Dr. Manaka shared his knowledge and clinical experiences with me by hosting my study-visit to his clinic in Japan. His papers, books, questions, answers, discussions, experiments, clinical demonstrations, and great kindness have profoundly influenced my work and much of my contribution to this book. It has been my heartfelt pleasure to facilitate a greater promulgation of the ideas of these two remarkable individuals throughout the pages of this work. My debt to both of them is considerable.

My family and close friends provided much-needed emotional support; I thank them for "putting up" with me, especially my parents, my sister Helen, and friends such as Junko, Rick, Marty, April, Natalie, and Tim. Bob Felt, Martha Fielding, Diane Putt, and Herb Rich showed great patience and perseverance working on this text; their advice and our exchanges always proved fruitful.

I would like to thank Dr. Victor Penzer and Dr. Robert Sampson for their useful feedback; and Dr. Paul Zmiewski for his technical and translational assistance with the bibliography. My students and patients issued numerous challenges for which I am also grateful as a learning experience. I cannot begin to mention everyone by name without leaving some out, the support I have had and found has been extensive, I am indebted to many more than mentioned above.

Kiiko Matsumoto's tireless dedication and committment to the materials presented in this book provided the essential foundation for our work. It has been my great pleasure to expand and build upon that foundation.

Perhaps the most continuous debt I have is to my inspirational teachers, the great masters of the past, Johann Sebastian, Wolfgang Amadeus, George Frideric, Franz Joseph, Antonio, Georg Philipp et al. Their works have helped generate the focus necessary for this book.

Last but not least, the debt we have to the geniuses of ancient China and the generations of practitioners and scholars from China and Japan can never be forgotten.

Stephen Birch

Cambridge, Massachusetts

☐

Table of Contents

□

Introduction

Introduction

Whoever first said that the shortest distance between two points need not be a straight line could very well have been a classical Oriental medical theorist. Where we are going, the goal of our text, is the presentation of several extremely successful treatment systems that depend on, or are derived from, information gathered by the simple act of palpating the abdomen. It should be noted that it is the practical value of these systems that recommends their study; often the fact that a procedure works provides all the justification necessary for its instigation. There are examples in every medicine of treatments that lack a satisfactory theory. Where evidence of successful treatment is plentiful, the lack of a good explanation is easily forgotten.

Thus, we could simply begin with the numerous tables of correspondences and treatments with which we will end. However, the systems presented are the work of classicists, individuals who have approached Oriental medicine in its broadest sense. Manaka, Kuzome, and the others whose work we describe, begin with a full appreciation of the theories and observations from which Oriental medicine has been created. Abdominal diagnosis, the discovery of patterns that confirm or treat human conditions, is an extension of an extensive complex of systems and theories. Without an adequate understanding of these systems our practices will be unable to adapt to the challenges of new information and new conditions. As is sometimes said in the Orient, theory without practice is useless and practice without theory is stupid.

Practically, the most difficult concept to learn, or perhaps unlearn, is the habit we have of thinking of biophysical events as the primary diagnostic signs — a flushed face, for example, as a sign of counterflow qi. Many diagnoses in both Oriental and Western medicine are the result of a composite image. The predominance of information pointing toward a particular condition justifies a diagnosis and a corresponding treatment strategy. Pressure pain and abdominal confirmations in general are not, in the same way, signs; they are a direct manifestation of the disease. By overstatement, we can say that the abdominal confirmation is the disease, whether or not any symptoms accompany the findings. The path from diagnosis to treatment is extremely short; in effect we treat the abdomen. In the case of practitioners who use massage, or structural manipulation, diagnosis and treatment may be identical. We are not exploring classifications of disease, an element of consensual reality, but disease itself, an element of our living relationship to a macrocosmic model of reality.

The difference is subtle, but worthy of attention. When diagnosis is accomplished by the collection and classification of signs, treatment is dependent on the presentation of a sufficient quantity of data. Further, the data must conform. If there are either insufficient signs, or contradictory signs, the practitioner must, at best, depend on their qualitative sense, experience, or intuition. When what we seek is a direct manifestation of a condition, even the most subtle and asymptomatic finding is valuable evidence. When this is supported by a clear comprehension of why such a condition might exist, experience and intuition are enhanced.

It is this, the advanced asymptomatic nature of hara diagnosis, that has given the treatments derived from it such exceptional power. Explaining why the abdomen is so clearly reflective of energetic condition requires a considerable body of often complex material: internal pathways, bioelectric phenomena, anatomical and energetic structure. However, using the information is often simpler than in any other treatment system. While exploring the most abstruse aspects of Oriental medical thought may occasionally demand bewildering complexity, the struggle is more than repaid by the simplicity and directness of treatment. Rather, for example, than attempting to remedy a discordant variety of presenting complaints with complex structures of "point = effect," we are able to treat a single structural imbalance that is the root of all. This is, of course, why the greatest practitioners and proponents of these systems are indeed famous. They have successfully treated problems where others have failed.

Abdominal palpation is sometimes difficult to understand because it is among the most subtle and powerful diagnostic approaches available to us. It is able to direct the diagnosis and treatment of extremely recalcitrant problems that are the result of complex patterns of disharmony, subtle conditions that have not as yet manifest as either diseases or syndromes, and highly individual conditions. Further, it provides us information that will help to integrate a variety of treatment styles, or to apply therapeutic principles to culture-bound psycho-emotional problems never defined in the cultures from which we have borrowed Oriental medicine.

The fee for this information, however, requires learning a specific and technical vocabulary. Many Oriental medical principles exist in the realm of consensual reality. We are all able to relate the cooling refreshment of a cold glass of water on a summer day to the principle that hot is treated with cold. Again, the experience that a fever "breaks" when we sweat is not so very rare. Yet abdominal palpation does not share with many Oriental medical concepts the nearly intuitive perceptibility that comes from the use of layman's terms and experiences in the technical language of the medicine. Abdominal palpation belongs to a higher order of observation wherein few of us participate in our daily lives. Who, as naturally and simply, will relate to ideas such as reflex zones, signaling, and formless potential energies? This is the practice of the specialist, replete with its own theoretical, technical, and manual skills. Again, there are rewards for complex preparation: broad adaptability, powerful logical tools, and efficient treatment — the markings of diagnostic and therapeutic precision.

The concepts that form the basis of abdominal palpation have existed within Oriental medical theory for a long time. Its essential nature as an advanced and specialized body of knowledge has not changed, though complex technical skills in all disciplines acquire greater and greater import when the clinical observations of the most successful practitioners are carefully studied. Yet the historical development of the ideas and techniques that form a specialized discipline is often ignored. We must remember that no concept, not the simplest nor the most abstruse, leaps fully formed into practice. Not even the fantastically fertile cultural ground of the Oriental classical age could germinate the seed, grow the plant, and bring forth its flower in an instant. Even the most basic information — point location, meridian system description, disease states and treatments — evolved throughout the generations of thinkers and practitioners who created Oriental medicine. History provides us with the benefit of insight into the processes that have guided the greatest practitioners of any skill in their quest for facility.

Along with history, psychological and emotional symptoms and conditions are also frequently ignored. Is the difference between thought expressed verbally and thought expressed as action sufficient to demand our attention? What subtlety is valuable and what is no more than the nicety of translators, scholars, and intellectual critics? In some cases, distinctions of this type are only important because of the nature of palpation. If you do not palpate the body, then the difference between "subjective reactions" — physical and emotional sensations experienced by the patient — and "objective reactions" — sensations of fullness, hardness, emptiness, palpated by the practitioner — are easy to ignore. In other cases, where the signs we use to distinguish a condition have already developed to the point where they may be labeled as patterns and diseases, a more general psycho-emotional symptomology may suffice. The diagnostic predominance will be obvious. However, in those instances where we must deal with the slight, subtle variances that are not yet diseases, a supposedly abstruse distinction between thought and will may provide a telling clue.

The same informational gradation applies to even basic data. In many cases in the daily life of a practitioner, the meridian system reduces to no more than the coordinates by which we label or locate the points chosen through the intellectual process of diagnosis. It is simply a tool, and like many tools in many disciplines, more used than considered. We doubt, for example, that many allopaths think deeply of the bonds and valences that create the molecules of the drug they are about to prescribe. In some portion of cases, meridian theories are no more than another clue to the problem itself. Again, there are elements of palpation that demand an attention to the meridian system that would be unnecessary if the body were not touched. Further, there are times when a simple, superficial "wiring diagram" is insufficient and we must consider the interior pathways, the extraordinary vessels, or the nature of meridians and the energy they transfer.

Energy in Oriental medicine is a highly specialized concept that is not always given detailed consideration in clinical application. In truth, there are illnesses that can be cured without the slightest consideration of the Chinese concepts of "source," or the multi-dimensional concept of qi. It is not always necessary to enter into the theoretical realm to fix a pain in the elbow. The triple burner may be nothing more than lines on chart when a common pattern is clear. However, both in understanding the function of abdominal diagnosis and the development of the systems derived from it, the fascial sheaths of the interior body, the collagen electrical properties, the concept of "no form," and the abstruse energetics of the triple warmer are important. Like the pulse, the techniques are simple. Most beginners can recite the modern positions and correspondences, given an hour of

□

study, but the theoretical background is various, and essential to advanced application. It should not be forgotten that abdominal palpation is a powerful tool, and not the least of its powers is its ability to enhance the practical application of many profound ideas that have developed in the genesis of Oriental medicine.

In preparing this text we have been forced to grapple with what we have found to be among the most perplexing issues in the research and presentation of Oriental medicine. The stark reality is that it is not possible to present information that is divorced from interpretation. The attempt to do so is illusion at best and commercial pandering at least. Even a list of acupoints and corresponding functions imposes an interpretation on the data, implied in the compilation from the source material and the choice of terminology. All texts, in this or any field, are necessarily the result of the authors' choices and selections. In the field of Oriental medicine, this holds true not only for English-language authors, but for the generations of Oriental writers from whom the material derives.

Abdominal diagnosis has its deepest roots in the concepts of circulation that, as Paul Unschuld has noted, are the domain of the *Nan Jing*. Thus, our readers will discover a clear emphasis on the *Nan Jing* concepts and on subsequent works that share an emphasis on system-circulation. Indeed, these ideas find their most sophisticated modern expression in the works of Manaka and others of the Japanese "meridian school" that Matsumoto and Birch have helped introduce to the West. This fundamental emphasis is followed through the array of Chinese and Japanese sources for the text.

There is an additional layer of decisions to which the reader must attend. This text does not share with many of the Western works in the field the assumption that Oriental medical thought is bound by its chronology. There is a clear prejudice among Western authors that ancient Oriental ideas must be discussed via Western concepts that are themselves premodern. In the preparation of this text it became increasingly more apparent that this presumption was flawed. Simply, the material did not fit, in structure or application, an approach that presumed the Chinese ideas to be unrelated, non-technical, and absolute.

Practically, this discovery lead to a complete rewriting of the text after its initial completion. Editorially, this lead to the inclusion of Stephen Birch's considerable research in the areas of biological fields, systems, and biological information theory. For the reader what is important is a clear understanding that the text assumes that conceptual and logical structures that are only recently becoming part of the general Western awareness are appropriately and profitably applicable to the observations of Oriental medicine. This decision, one that is explicit as well in Dr. Manaka's work, finds expression not only in the inclusion of information derived from, and dependent on, modern techniques of inquiry, but in the ordering of the text as related systems and sub-systems.

With this understanding we welcome you to what we have found to be one of the most fascinating and useful creations of the Oriental medical approach. We hope you too will be captivated by the brilliance of those who have contributed the theories and techniques of hara diagnosis to the healing professions of the world.

☐

Chapter

- 1 -

The

Hara

The Hara

The importance of the abdomen to Oriental thought and medicine causes puzzlement to Westerners unfamiliar with the Oriental notion of hara. What is it about the abdomen or the hara that echoes with such fundamental resonance in Chinese and Japanese tradition? Why make such a fuss over the belly? After all, the abdomen is just the physical center of the body; fat, flat, beer belly, or tightly muscled as the "washboard" of an athlete; no more than a muscled cage. The important stuff is all inside, the organs of digestion, excretion, and reproduction. Yet what are these but anatomical pieces of flesh with a certain physiological importance, more or less necessary to our overall function? We can remove the gallbladder, spleen, parts of the stomach, small and large intestines. People live on one lung. We can get by, impaired but active, with one kidney and for a limited time with none at all. We can easily fix up something to replace the bladder. People even have their hearts and livers repaired and replaced. The brain is the singularly most vital organ, and by its failure we define death. The abdomen is positioned at the bottom of Western physiological hierarchy. Why then does not Oriental tradition concur?

An examination of this Western attitude toward the abdomen can provide the context for understanding the Oriental idea. Since Western theory believes that health is the absence of disease, rather than a recognizable state of being, concern focuses on disease and the disease process. Indeed, we rarely speak of health in any other way. Even Western "preventive medicine" concentrates on the avoidance of certain specific diseases. We vaccinate, measure and supplement nutritional values, test for the biological precursors of disease, and hope to decipher our own genetic code so well that we may predict pathological predispositions. Our statistical definitions of health, minimum nutritional requirements, expected lifespans, and survivability rates are neither ideas nor goals. These are simply mathematical assessments of "normal" as defined by averages.

Even the most superficial look at the Western ideas of health shows that we are disease-centered. This, however, is not absolute or unchanging. At the fringe of medicine, the layman's venue, individuals have preceded their professional healers in creating a concept of health. We have begun to "run for life" and "eat for health." Lifestyles that promise longevity are getting more than a cursory look. Modern cultural experience is replicating the achievement of traditional Oriental thought where we have begun to view what we do, feel, think, and how we live as the primary causes of health or distress. Our idea of health now includes capacity and ability, and other positive states measured by how they contribute to our lives, our "well-being." In the recent past we have begun to talk about the ability to

□

stay focussed from the center of one's being, to be "centered." Perhaps influenced by the gradual introduction of Oriental thought, we have begun to ascribe this physically to the abdomen, the center of the body.

We commonly use the term "centeredness" as a way of describing a state of being. Often it is an ideal, a description of optimal behavior or reaction that avoids extremes of emotion or intellect when dealing with certain situations. Yet, this idea has not developed the robust generality of the Oriental connotation of a "vital center." We continue to see the mind and body as distinct entities. Again, it is the brain that is seen to be most important, that we most closely associate with our "self." Arthur Koestler has neatly and poetically named this pervasive concept "the ghost in the machine." While it is clear that Western culture has begun to struggle with its own organizing concepts, the Oriental ideas of health, disease, and centeredness evince no such duality.

In Oriental thought and medicine, health is the sine qua non, the first principle without which disease itself may not be defined. Disease is an "out-of-balance" state and an aberration of the harmony of life. From this primary definition of health, Oriental theorists have constructed a homeostatic medicine that aims to restore harmony when it is lost through internal or external influences. To practitioners of Oriental medicine, health is the normal and natural function of the body and the goal of ideal treatment. Within the idea of health are the concepts of natural resistance to diseases and an inherent healing power. To help restore harmonious function is to bring about the state where healing may optimally occur. This is the primary objective of the practitioner of Oriental medicine and the central reason why Oriental medicine has come to include such a broad range of modes — exercise, diet, meditation, and the minutiae of daily life that each contribute to health.

This conceptual unity is reflected in the tradition of Oriental behavior and thought. Mind and body are viewed as different manifestations of the same phenomenon. The Japanese idea of hara expresses this unity well. The hara is accepted as an energetic center as well as a physical center. Not only is it an important concept in Oriental martial arts, healing arts, and contemplative practice, it is also important in many aspects of daily life. Often a Japanese person will speak of "thinking with the hara," or "feeling with the hara."[1]

Although we too have folk ideas that express similar perceptions, the energetic focus inherent in the concept of hara is not obvious, at least to Westerners. We often talk about having a "gut feeling," as a way of staking a claim to truth where fact and reason are not available. One of the most ironic examples of this usage occurs in a short documentary film concerning the philosophical school known as "Logical Positivism." This group was logically nihilistic, and quick to describe the fallacy of truths or beliefs without a rational base.[2] Yet, in the film's final dialogue about the school's demise, its founder, A.J. Ayers, cites his "gut feelings" in support of the essential truth of the system. While this example is more humorous than most, many instances of this expression are known to us all. The West has concepts for these phenomena, but they are not very well developed. It is

□

as if we were out of touch, or only vaguely remembered the ideas. Ordinarily when we talk about our feelings we point to our heart as the seat of these experiences. When we talk of our thoughts, we point to our head.

In the Orient the relationship is clear. A few examples from everyday Japanese usage should suffice. If one were to say, *hara ga ookii*, this would translate literally to mean "big hara." Colloquially it means "to have an open mind." Interestingly, receptivity and openness are qualities expected from the practice of deep, meditative breathing. Similarly, to say *hara ga chiisai* would literally translate as "small hara," but colloquially carries the meaning of having a small or narrow mind. These expressions impart the sense of mind as indistinct from the physical and energetic body, a perception also reflected in emotions and attitudes. *Hara ga tatsu* literally means "the hara stands up." The Japanese, however, use it to identify anger. Its correspondence to the Oriental medical model is direct.

Anger is associated with the liver and the wood phase. Frequently it is said that the upflow of liver qi causes anger or conversely that anger causes liver qi to upflow *(SW 39:p).*[3] Anger can also come from a general condition of counterflow qi where the qi in the hara rises upward creating a lack of qi below and relative plethora of qi above. Thus, the "hara stands up." The opposite expression, *hara ga suwaru* literally means, "the hara is sitting." This expression is used to indicate that someone's focus does not change, or is not disrupted by their surroundings. One maintains their focus and determination. This is an important concept in Japanese culture.

As a last example, consider the expression used perhaps by a coach to his athletes, *hara ga nattanai.* Literally this states that the hara is not centered or grounded and is a warning to the athlete that movement or action is not coming from the hara, the center. By offsetting the center of gravity, balance, coordination, and resolve are lost. To be balanced and yet without resolve is an impossible juxtaposition for the Japanese individual, as the two states are considered the same. Posture and movement are an important part in this concept, not just attitude. Again the idea extends into the realm of Oriental medicine. An example of this extension is Sotai exercise, a system of simple movements devised by Keizo Hashimoto of Japan to restore and maintain balanced posture and movement. [4]

In Japan the concept of hara is much larger than the simple idea of abdomen or belly. It is part of a pervasive social and cultural concept, rooted in the Chinese classics and the practice of meditation. In meditation, breathing techniques are very important and certain experiences occur, not in the mind, but in the hara. As we have suggested in a previous work *(Five Elements and Ten Stems)*, the energetic centrality of the hara was at least implied by some of the premedical classics. For example, in the *Dao De Jing* it is said:

> Therefore the Chinese sage becomes the abdomen [puts his consciousness in his abdomen]. He doesn't become his eyes [put his consciousness in his sense perceptions].[5]

In the classics of Oriental medicine, the *Huang Di Nei Jing Su Wen*, the *Huang Di Nei Jing Ling Shu*, and the *Nan Jing,* the authors presented the essential description of health on which Oriental medicine flourished and

□

developed. Since all these texts were written before the end of the Han dynasty, circa 200 A.D., and in part by the end of the Zhou dynasty, circa 300 B.C., they share with the great religious documents of mankind the veneration we reserve for ancient wisdom that holds meaning for us today. Among the great accomplishments of these unknown authors is the description of the principles of normal and balanced operation of the body and the basic patterns and developmental stages of various pathological occurences.

In places these descriptions were painted in broad strokes, in others the picture is drawn with fine, detailed lines. Often, the description of the person's intimate relationship with the macrocosm and microcosm is interwoven with the basic therapeutic principles that would, when correctly applied, restore the original balanced state. The older texts, the *Su Wen* and *Ling Shu,* were very clear in places and quite unclear in others. The *Nan Jing (Canon of Perplexities)* was created to clarify difficult ideas of the two earlier books. It explained in more detail some of the fundamental diagnostic and therapeutic principles, systematizing many of the ideas from the *Su Wen* and *Ling Shu,* along with newer ideas. Today, many of these principles are still applied in the daily practice of Oriental medicine, particularly in the practice of acupuncture.[6]

It is in these texts that we first find the hara described as the vital energetic center. In the *Nan Jing,* we learn the function of the abdomen or hara in treatment, in diagnosis, and in the natural function of the body. In one passage, we are told clearly of the hara's energetic function:

> The Yellow Emperor asked, "The pulse can be normal, yet sometimes people die, why is this?"
> Qi Bo answered, "Each of the twelve meridians has a relationship to the source of the vital energies [the living qi]. The source of the vital energies is the root origin of the twelve meridians, it is the moving qi between the kidneys. This means that the source of the vital energies is fundamental to the five yin and six yang organs, the root of the twelve meridians, the gate of breathing. It is the source [origin] of the triple warmer. Another name for it is the shen which protects against evil; therefore, qi is the root of the person. This is why if the root is dying, the stems and branches [meridians and organs] will be drying [drying-out], yet appear normal. The vital qi is dying on the inside, but it is still there on the outside" *(NJ 8(1):11).*[7]

Here the source of the body's qi or energies is described as being in the area of the "moving qi between the kidneys," which is located in the abdomen. The idea of source is not only philosophical, the relationship to the meridians is direct, the moving qi is their origin. If the source is drying-up, like the source of streams or rivers, there may be flow in the branches, but it will soon end. Thus, the abdomen is more than the physical center, the cavity in which the organs reside. It is the residence of the source of the body's energies, the energetic center from which life springs. Understanding this, understanding the condition of the center, is central to promoting the wellbeing of the person. Even the pulse and its indications are "downstream" from the hara. Thus, diagnosing and treating the hara is central to the practice of Oriental medicine.

□

This centrality is demonstrated in a variety of ways. The *Nan Jing* theory states the basic energetics well and the earlier texts present ideas that serve to connect a number of energetic theories. The specific energetic models of the *Ling Shu* and *Nan Jing*, and their respective source theories, each contribute to a picture of the energetics of hara which are important and extensible. Further, the internal trajectories of each of the twelve meridians and the pathways of the eight extraordinary vessels are rooted in the hara. An analysis of the more significant points used for diagnosis of the abdomen by palpation and their relationships to distal acupoints reveals that these points are named to emphasize their central location and function. We also find the energetic centrality of the hara when we examine the basic energetics of the abdomen and study the Chinese concepts of mind and spirit.

Chapter

- 2 -

Palpation

Palpation

Most English translations of Oriental medical literature say very little about palpation as a diagnostic tool. In some schools of thought, palpation is supposed to concern only the pulses of the radial arteries. There are styles of acupuncture practice where patients are touched only when the pulses are evaluated. While this absence of interaction is often the result of a clinical reality that must contend with vast numbers of patients in short periods of time, there is nonetheless a noticeable lack of considered emphasis on the tactile arts in the basic teaching literature available in the West. Of course, this does not apply to those who use massage as their basic therapeutic modality. Yet even in most massage literature, a systematic diagnostic system or even a broad understanding of point reactiveness cannot be found. Judged by the contents of our current texts, palpation has become a neglected art. There are exceptions. In Japan the educational curricula of acupuncture, moxibustion, and internal medicine teach palpatory programs that provide information relevant to both diagnosis and treatment.

There are reasons why palpation has been neglected in Western training. Nowhere, however, are there reasons sufficient to conclude that the practice of palpation is redundant or inadvisable. Certainly the classical texts did not ignore palpation, recognizing the importance of palpation as a means of expanding the practitioner's diagnostic and therapeutic repertory. Traditionally, when diagnosis was presented as a system, palpation was discussed as one of the four observations (LS 4; NJ 61:p).[1] As a diagnostic tool, it was taken in relationship to the other three observations — looking, listening and smelling, and questioning. In these discussions of the four observations, palpation was mentioned specifically in reference to pulse diagnosis. Pulse diagnosis gained a special place in the overall diagnosis of the patient. Using this single palpatory technique, practitioners and theorists were able to determine information regarding almost all the conditions to which the patient's meridians, organs, warmers, phases, yin, yang, blood, and qi were subject. As a consequence, the Chinese often went no further in their own palpatory investigations. The desire for a single, absolute investigatory mechanism is strongly attractive in any discipline.

While recognizing the importance and centrality of pulse diagnosis, as is delineated by the essential medical texts themselves, we must also acknowledge that the absolute reliability and effectiveness of this diagnostic tool is only true in a general sense. We must be careful that the centrality of the pulse in acupuncture theory does not devolve into an exclusivity never intended by the classical theorists and unsupportable in practice.

□

Chapter 8 of the *Nan Jing* warns us about placing all our emphasis on the pulse, cautioning that diagnosis of the abdomen or hara is also important. In his commentary on the first chapter of the *Nan Jing*, Wang Shu He tells us, "The origin of the pulse is at the moving qi between the kidneys."[2] The moving qi between the kidneys is the central focus of the hara, and thus of the whole body. Diagnosing the hara by palpation directly diagnoses the condition of the body at its most central point. This is an exciting concept, one that has inspired a body of brilliant and useful work throughout the history of Oriental medicine.

Because this present work addresses the void of available English-language information about palpation, there is little detail of pulse diagnosis available in the pages of clinical information to be found in this text. Please be aware that it is not our intention to detract from the value of the pulse, or any other technique, to dispute relative importance, or to provoke some imaginary "contest" between the exploits of "pulse masters" and "belly pokers." It is clear that the living masters of hara diagnosis are themselves expert in the use of the pulse. Thus, where we present palpation as the main diagnostic tool, relegating other diagnostic techniques to a confirmatory role, we intend only to direct your attention to the subject at hand, and convincingly demonstrate how useful palpation may be.

The Uses of Palpation

Palpation of areas of the body, of the meridians, and of the acupoints is of diagnostic utility, providing clues to the patient's condition, and in particular to the general condition of the meridians and organs. Palpation simultaneously extends into the realm of treatment. It may tell us exactly which acupoints should be selected. For example, simply treating reactive acupoints is sometimes advisable. Treating the acupoints that directly reflect the disharmonies often resolves these disharmonies, probably as a reversal of the mechanism by which those disharmonies reflect in the acupoints. In certain cases, palpation provides us with a preliminary diagnosis of the phases, meridians, extraordinary vessels, or organs affected. We can also learn whether corrective exercises are appropriate from the structural or physical problems we discover with our eyes and hands. This preliminary diagnosis is subsequently differentiated by more palpation, pulse diagnosis, looking, listening and smelling, and asking.

Another use of palpation is the preparation of the acupoints for treatment. This is important when using either needles or moxa, though particularly when using needles. Palpatory techniques are used to protect certain types of qi and to draw qi to the points where it may be manipulated by the needles. This is one technique that allows the practice of acupuncture to become a fine art. The way that acupoints are touched and prepared and the techniques of needle manipulation are important skills that determine exactly how the qi will be affected. It is at this level of practice and skill that the importance of touch becomes most evident. The energetic exchange between the practitioner and patient in palpatory technique is one factor that determines why one acupuncturist may gain far more positive results than another, even when both have selected the same points for treatment.

□

Palpation may also be expedient as a guidepost for treatments that minister harmonizing and preventive effects. To perform subtle diagnoses of diseases before they manifest pathologically has long been considered the highest expression of the art of acupuncture. Treating the subtle precursors of disease has been referred to as the work of the "great person" or the "skilled artisan." Palpation is a major tool used to achieve this goal. Dr. Yoshio Manaka, a truly inspiring acupuncturist, has offered some useful and interesting comments on the subject of palpation.[3] In his experience pressure pain elicited by palpation does not necessarily reflect diseases or problems that have a Western name, or even problems that have advanced to the state where they may be labeled with a specific Oriental medical term or syndrome. Both Eastern and Western concepts of disease imply a measurable pathology — tuberculosis or hepatitis; liver qi stagnation or splenic transformation failure. However, pressure pain is a sign of imbalance that may not have progressed to the point of manifestation on the symptomatic level. They are, in Manaka's words, "biases" or the tendencies and probabilities that precede some more specific pathological state. Thus, treating distal acupoints to eliminate the pain found on palpation, or treating the reactive acupoints themselves, may change these subtle influences. With experience and understanding, one can treat problems before they develop to named diseases or specific syndromes. In these cases, the acupuncturist is truly performing preventive treatment.

The implications of this concept are spectacular. If palpation is able to cue us to the existence of pre-disease tendencies or states that have some probability of developing into specific pathologies, it thereby achieves a unique place in the diagnostic tool chest of Oriental medicine. By objectifying and confirming the existence of conditions of extreme subtlety, palpation serves us as the major methodology when the pulse, tongue, and symptomatic data may be "normal" or extremely difficult to evaluate. If we can develop treatments based on the information derived from palpation, using methods that reduce or eliminate pressure pain in reactive acupoints, we can begin to treat less symptomatically.

In tracing the history and development of palpation theory using the classical texts as our source material, we can begin to acquire a sense of the importance of touch in energetic exchange. Importantly, we can also see that the theoretical background of palpation is particularly subtle. This, indeed, may be one reason that palpatory discussions have not become part of the basic student literature of acupuncture. It is also true that information gained from palpation is often not evaluated in a linear fashion, that is, *if A, then B*. Frequently, palpation presents us with multi-dimensional decisions: *if A, then B in the presence of C, or D in the presence of E*. However, the use of palpation itself is not so obscure nor difficult that it is limited to some few particular specialists. It is the objective nature of the information gained — swelling, pressure pain, coloration, texture — that makes palpation such a usable tool. Since these qualities are more easily recorded and observed, learning may be effectively realized through the clinical experience of top practitioners whose oral or written records are available.

□

Acupoints and Body Landscape

Energetic exchange is deeply set within the concept of an acupoint. Some interesting implications for the diagnosis and selection of acupoints are provided by the etymology of the original Chinese term. The character *xue* 穴, commonly translated as "point" or "acupoint," literally means "hole." In Chinese medical texts the term *qi xue* 氣穴, literally "qi hole," is used to signify "acupoint." *Gong xue* 孔穴, which also carries the literal meaning of "hole," is another frequently used term. Although it is common practice to translate the characters xue, qi xue, or gong xue as "point" or "acupoint," the English word leaves us with the idea that the xue are little more than their anatomical locations, i.e., points on the surface of the body.

The true connotations that accompany the Chinese character need to be associated with the English translation. The character xue itself has more the meaning of a hole, a pit, than the more geometrical concept of a point or position. Classically it meant a cave. The *Shuo Wen Jie Zi* says the xue refers to a "chamber below the earth" *(Mor)*.[4] Several other classical texts report that the term refers specifically to a grave or gravesite.[5]

There is an historical context to the term xue that has an implied meaning when used in the medical texts. This connotation also relates to the practice of palpation in the medicine of classic times. Most particularly, the term was used by pre-Han geomancers, particularly the school known as the *Feng-Shui* 風水.[6] The xue were locations on the surface of the earth, divined using the relationships of symbolized principles. Many of these principles are shared with acupuncture theory. The choice of these xue, or locations in the landscape, was determined by many factors, including locations of mountains, rivers, and nearby streams. Once found, these locations were used as gravesites. Here, the energies of the earth were in harmony with the energies of heaven. These places represented propitious spots to bury the dead, since the harmonious geomantic relationship would ease the passage of a corpse's energies into heaven and into earth.

The energies concerned were probably the *hun* 魂 and the *po* 魄 familiar to acupuncture theory. The *Huai Nan Zi* tells us, "Heaven's qi becomes hun, earth's qi becomes po" *(Mor)*. The hun and the po are important energetic entities vital to life. They are stored respectively in the liver and lungs *(SW 23:p)* and are described in the *Li Ji* as leaving the body at death: "The hun, qi, returns to heaven; the form, po, returns to earth" *(Mor)*.

It is worth noting that the use of the term xue in relation to the acupoints of the body was not haphazard or coincidental. These xue have much the same connotation as the geomantic xue. The body too has a certain landscape. At certain places on this landscape the qi has a particular function and movement. This is one of the obvious implications of the yin — yang divisions of the body, the meridian classifications, and the chronobiological circulation of the meridian qi. It is an idea reflected even in the names of points, which reference streams, wells, holes, and hills. Not only is this an important factor in the choice of the particular names of each of the body's xue, but it is also potentially important for the selection of points to treat. Point selection itself becomes almost a geomantic process.

□

According to how the internal and external landscapes of the body change, certain xue are chosen for treatment. There are a number of ways to determine which xue to use, not the least of which is palpation.

The xue are generally said to have fixed locations and these are what we find in the acupoint location texts. However, as the qi flows and as the landscape of the body changes, so too do the locations of the xue. Since these changes are usually quite subtle, so are the changes in location. Certainly, the positional changes are far more subtle than can be detected by reference to two-dimensional acupuncture charts or verbal descriptions. The practitioner must find the xue to administer treatment. Palpation is probably the most direct way. It is curious and indicative that as researchers have responded to the Western urge for precise measurement, it has not been a sophisticated three-dimensional charting that has satisfied our itch for precision. It is instead an electronically assisted palpation, electrical measurement of skin resistance, that has been chosen. This indirectly recognizes that points are not fixed or precisely locatable in the sense of a mapped position. (Perhaps the researcher's "gut feelings" were at work.)

Whether fixed or mobile, acupoints project a quality that reflects the bodily landscape. This is why palpation is so important. Not only does it help us find the acupoints we want to treat, but these acupoints project certain qualities relative to the nature of the problems we seek to cure: pressure pain, tension, tightness, swelling, indentation, thickness and suppleness of the skin, temperature variation. Through palpation we are able simultaneously to gain diagnostic information and find the xue. Based on the patterns of reactivity found and the records of many years of research and practice, we are able to interpret this information and to understand the body landscape.

Simply stated, this is one main reason why palpation has such widespread use in Japan. Practitioners there generally recognize that the acupoints always move and that treating the location at which a reaction is found is more therapeutically valuable. It is perhaps a cultural tendency of the Japanese (their reticence to discuss their condition or their social conventions that discourage the admission of pain or discomfort) that has produced this clinical emphasis on palpation. In practice the location of even theoretically "fixed" points is often palpatory. The geography that describes the locations — the edges of muscles, bones, or tendons — serve as the starting point. The results that indicate correct location, for instance, the strongest needle stimulation, or a specific direction or extent of the stimulation, are also variable within the confines of the descriptions by which they are recognized. In short, whether we consider the points fixed or movable, precise location is often best achieved through touch.

Palpation in Classical Literature

Examining some of the important medical texts from Han to modern times, one may find many places where palpation is discussed, often in a clinical context. Palpation was a common practice at certain times in classical China, yet there are not frequent theoretical discussions of palpation in the classical texts. An understanding of the etymological background of the xue or acupoints can help us to see that palpation was incorporated in the

□

practical discussions of classical acupuncture and was frequently implied by the very nature of the terms used to explain medical procedures, most frequently for specific techniques of diagnosis and treatment.

We know with certainty that practitioners of the Han dynasty used palpation as part of the diagnostic process. When Han Chinese culture was imported to Japan, Chinese medicine arrived along with the entirety of the Chinese cultural and philosophical systems. The practitioners of that era found it easiest to understand the medical classics by using palpation, and as a result major trends of palpatory diagnosis developed in Japan. However, palpation was not a practice unique to Japan; as with any human activity that proves useful and adaptable, Chinese medicine has become Oriental medicine through the contribution of the many cultures in which it developed. Palpation arrived at a sophisticated level of refinement in Japan as a function of their interpretation and adaptation of the Chinese medical system, and perhaps as well as a consquence of cultural predisposition.

One other facet of palpation worthy of note in regard to its place in the medical classics is the probable role touch played in the development of the meridian and acupoint theories. According to Joseph Needham, this was a significant role, a major tool by which the meridians and acupoints were found and systematized:

> There can be little doubt that visceral malfunction of many kinds can be reflected in all sorts of phenomena ascertainable on palpation.[7]

It is probable that after such early developments, the medical classics themselves were compiled to detail the theories and treatment principles derived from earlier observations. Certainly, there is documentary evidence that the meridian system concept developed from earlier descriptions of fewer and less detailed lines and points. While shrouded in prehistory, countless experimentations no doubt preceded the theory and practice of Chinese medicine.

On examining the classical texts, among them the *Su Wen* and *Ling Shu*, we find numerous passages that relate to palpation. The *Su Wen* does not discuss palpation in depth; it was mostly a text of theories and principles, rather than practice. However, within general discussions of classical needle technique, palpation was noted. In the *Ling Shu* there are several chapters that posit general diagnostic principles and techniques, as well as general therapeutic principles. Point palpation frequently figures in these discussions. This is also true of later texts through the Ming dynasty.

Despite the inherent obscurity of passages from these early texts, they become intellectually and practically comprehensible when understood as describing palpation. Often the only clear interpretation assumes some palpatory process. For example, while discussing the luo meridians, the author of the *Ling Shu* tells us to look for signs of vacancy or repletion, such as a pulsing or an indentation around the luo acupoint. If one cannot see anything, we are told, "ask above and below the point, because each person's meridians are not the same" *(LS 10:145).*[8] This "asking" only makes sense if it is palpatory.

When discussing the back shu points, the *Ling Shu* tells us about location and selection:

> If you want to get the points or examine them, you have to rub
> them. Inside [the point], there will be some reaction or pain;
> this is the shu point (LS 51:381).

This is an explicit description of point selection and diagnosis by palpation. The points that are painful are the shu points. The *Ling Shu* also tells us a little about the treatment of the back shu points when there is a pathogenic invasion of the lungs. To treat the problem, "rub [the point] with one's hands. Then, if the patient feels comfortable, the needle can be inserted" (LS 20:208). Here again, palpation is part of the treatment.

More general palpatory diagnostic principles are derived from and presented in the *Ling Shu*. These are important and particularly useful in modern practice. It is often stated that if palpation of a point or area elicits pain, repletion is indicated. If palpation elicits a comfortable sensation, vacancy is indicated.

> [After] researching and palpating the painful points on the left
> and right, the upper and lower parts, and diagnosing the tem-
> perature of the body, to see if it is uniform, [after this] one can
> diagnose the meridians that have the problems (LS 73:513).

These principles of diagnosis are important and particularly useful in modern practice. Pain or lack of pain on points, the comparison of left, right, upper, and lower relationships as pressure pain or temperature variations, are the fundamental aspects of several important palpatory systems.

In discussing the use of needling techniques, the *Ling Shu* tells us:

> First, attentively observe and differentiate the repletion or
> vacancy of the meridians by pressing with the fingers, using
> sliding techniques, and also rubbing and flicking the points.
> Then, very attentively, watch the response and reactiveness of
> the point (LS 75:544).

In short, observe, analyze, and treat to decrease the reactiveness, whatever it may be.

Clearly then, palpation played a significant role in the diagnostic and treatment procedures of the *Ling Shu*. These procedures remain open to interpretation and further research. Throughout the progression of medical history, many practitioners and authors have taken these vague references and sketchy techniques as the starting point of their research. Two further passages from the *Ling Shu* point us to possible interpretations that may be used to develop our understanding of palpation:

> If there is abdominal pain, insert the needle to the moving
> [pulse] place at both sides of the umbilicus.[9] After removing
> the needle, rub the place, it can immediately cure the problem.
> But, if it doesn't cure the problem, needle qichong [ST-30].
> Then rub the place when the needle has been removed. This
> can immediately cure the problem (LS 26:249).

Understanding what is the "moving place at both sides of the umbilicus," and how to observe this pulse is at once clear if one considers this passage a description of an event observed by abdominal palpation. Rarely in clinical practice is a pulse visually observed in a simple case of abdominal pain. However, a pulse in the location described is a frequent palpatory finding.

In the same manner Chao Yu, one of the famed figures of the *Ling Shu,* discusses different types of lumps in the intestines:

> If the skin is thin and dry, the flesh not hard [elastic], but muddy [weak and soft], this is a sign of bad intestines and stomach (*LS 48:347*).

There are times when the flesh will lose its elasticity, becoming weak and soft to such an extent that the condition will be visibly obvious. However, this condition is more easily confirmed with palpation.

The *Nan Jing* has several comments to make about palpation as a diagnostic and treatment technique:

> Palpation below the sternum conveys the condition of heart/fire. Palpation around the umbilicus conveys the condition of spleen/earth. Palpation below the umbilicus conveys the condition of kidneys/water. Palpation on the right side below the ribs conveys the condition of lungs/metal. Palpation on the left side below the ribs conveys the condition of liver/wood (*NJ 16; NJ 56*).

There are several ways we may interpret these correspondences, and more possible interpretations will be discussed in a later chapter; the correspondences are obviously important and have remained so in later developments of five-phase theory. The *Nan Jing* also talks about palpating the skin of the forearm as a way of confirming the quality one finds in the pulse (*NJ 13*). In effect, it recommends parallel qualities as confirmation. Thus, when one finds a tight pulse, the skin of the forearm should feel tight. For a slippery pulse, the skin of the forearm should feel slippery.

As the major medical text that detailed and explained ideas introduced only randomly or discursively in other texts, the *Nan Jing* is an essential resource. In regard to palpation, the *Nan Jing* most intruiguingly details the importance of the abdomen, correct breathing, and diagnosis and treatment of the source qi, each a concept central to the understanding of an advanced use of palpation. If we compare, for example, the *Su Wen* discussion of needle techniques with the *Nan Jing* interpretation of the same concept, we can see how the later authors systematized the idea.

The earlier *Su Wen* described the needling technique for tonification:

> When the point has been chosen, rub it lightly, then harder. Then flick or tap the point with your finger to stimulate the point. With your fingernail, press the point slightly, then with the finger and thumb, pinch the skin slightly. All this serves to close the shen . . . [Upon removing the needle] rub the point; this will protect and preserve the shen qi (*SW 27:170*).[10]

The later *Nan Jing* explanation demonstrates a systematic development of this concept:

> When putting the needle into the yang [wei qi area], angle the needle and then insert. When putting the needle into the ying [qi area], use the left hand, rub the point to disperse the qi [wei qi], then insert the needle *(NJ 76(4):19)*.

The *Nan Jing* contains further discussions of the treatment technique that describe the importance of feeling the qi with the left hand while inserting and manipulating the needle with the right hand *(NJ 78(4):20-21)*. In effect, the *Nan Jing* outlines a technique for the preparation of the acupoints that protects the various qi circulating throughout the body.[11]

The *Ling Shu* succinctly states the most vital facet of needle technique:

> The important part of tonification and dispersion techniques when using the nine needles lies in the subtle sensitivity of the fingers *(LS 1:6)*.

Extrapolating from the Classical Texts

As is often the case in Oriental medicine, the discussions from the earliest texts, the *Su Wen, Ling Shu,* and *Nan Jing,* comprise the foundation for further studies. This holds true for what has been said about palpation.

Expanding on the *Ling Shu* ideas, the *Jin Gui Yao Lue Fang Lun (Essential Prescriptions from the Golden Chest),* one of the very earliest internal medicine texts from approximately 200-300 B.C., states:

> When one palpates an abdomen that is swollen and full, and the patient does not feel pain, this indicates vacancy. If the patient feels pain, this indicates repletion. Therefore with replete patients, one must address and eliminate the repletion.[12]

The author of this text was Zhang Zhong-Jing, who also wrote the *Shang Han Lun (Treatise of Injury by Cold),* probably the earliest systematic text of herbal medicine. In this text are other references to abdominal palpation, including tension felt in the upper part of the abdomen below the ribs and sternum. As a primary abdominal confirmation, tension in that area is usually indicative of a disease progression at the shao yang stage. However, the condition is also noted in regard to the yang ming state.

> When there is a lump or tightness below the heart, the patient feels stagnation in this area, and the healer feels tightness when touching.[13]

Medications are prescribed for this abdominal conformation.

The *Shang Han Lun* also describes a feeling of subcostal fullness, in reference to a shao yang disease.[14]

> The patient feels the presence of stagnation, and when one touches [in the subcostal region], it feels like a knot or is tight. The patient feels uncomfortable or full in the subcostal region, and there is resistance or pressure pain when one touches.[15]

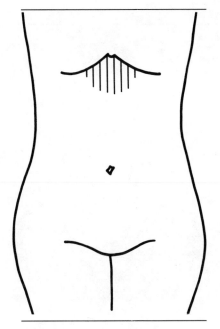

Figure 2.1 Shao yang substernal tightness

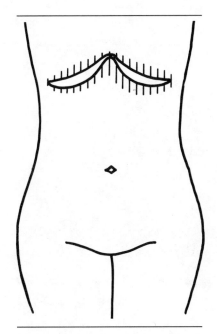

Figure 2.2 Shao yang subcostal discomfort

These passages, and others from the *Shang Han Lun,* have stimulated considerable work and research on abdominal palpation in herbal diagnosis, both in China and Japan. In Japan, where abdominal diagnosis is routinely used in the *Kanpo Yaku* diagnosis for the prescription of herbal formulae, this research has yielded a recognized system of drug prescription that has penetrated Western medical practice. The accompanying two illustrations are taken from *Fuku Sho Kiran* by Inaba Bunrei, an herbal text compiled at the beginning of the nineteenth century. These are representative of the degree of sophistication achieved with the use of abdominal diagnosis for determining herbal prescriptions.

Palpation Systems

Several systems of palpatory diagnosis have arisen in both China and Japan over the years. Sorei Yanagiya discusses a number of these in his text, *Kanmei Humon Shinsatsu Ho (Diagnosis of the Body Without Asking Questions).* This book is among the best in presentation of these systems in synopsis. At the heart of the book are presentations of correspondences that detail the areas of the abdomen that have been found to correspond to different diagnoses by different practitioners.[16] As might be expected, there are many different interpretations, each based on the work and experience of the practitioner who has formulated each idea. These ideas are important since they help expand our perspective of palpation and because they are historically interesting. However, many concentrate on the practice of internal medicine and thus will not be described or explained in detail in this text. In each of the following diagrams the correspondences are noted as abdominal positions. These are keyed to an associated diagram that details the areas of the abdomen and their correspondences.

In the following diagram, positions one and two are from the work of Todo Yoshimasu and positions three through eight are from Mr. Tokaku. The types of lumps that may be palpated on the abdomen are:

Position	Correspondence
1	qi lump
2	food lump
3	wind lump
4	dry stool lump
5	pregnancy
6	water lump
7	blood lump
8	blood lump

Yanagiya also presents diagrams from Dr. Tai Zhou. In this example the findings at each of the positions are various. The first diagram gives general indications, the second greater detail:

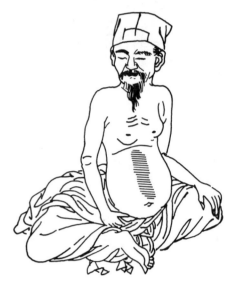

Figure 2.3 Jujube combination sho

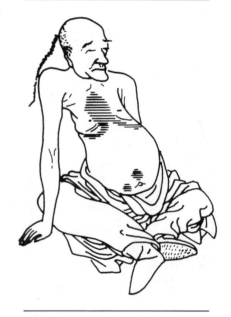

Figure 2.4 Major bupleurum sho

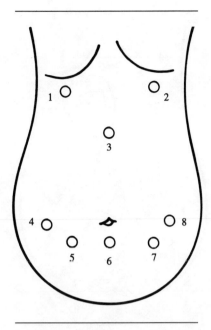

Position	Correspondence
1	stagnation from drinking
2	pulsing below the heart
3	digestate accumulation
4 (around CV-10)	pulsing of an empty stomach
5	blood lump
6	dry stool lump
7	blood lump
8	blood lump or dry stool lump
9	dry stool lump

Figure 2.5 Abdominal Lumps - Yoshimasu & Tokaku.

In an infectious disease, position 1 and position 2 (Figure 2.7) will feel hot. If there is a pulsing at position 2 that is becoming larger, it means ascendant vacant yang, or ascendant *gu qi* 穀氣. At position 3, if one feels accumulating qi (fullness) below the sternum, press hard with the thumb while the fingers rest on the sternum and the discomfort will be relieved. If you hear water rumbling while rubbing or tapping at position 4, it is a sign of fluid accumulation. Something felt at position 5 is a sign of digestate accumulation. If this stagnation becomes worse, the indication will grow to reach positions 3 and 4. It will feel hard and tight like a stone. Dietary changes are recommended. At position 6, if there is pain when the skin and flesh are pinched, this means a vacant middle warmer. Position 7 is the place of blood lumps. Occasionally a lump may be felt here that stretches down to position 9. Position 8 is the place of dry stools, it is often painful with slight pressure. When the fingers seem to press through into a valley at position 9 — that is, the muscle walls are soft and seem to separate — this indicates vacant kidney. If it is very soft at this position, like cotton, the condition will be hard to treat. If you find an area that feels like a bar at positions 10 and 11, this is a hernia. Positions 12 and 13 are the spleen mu points. If these feel like cotton, there is a vacant qi condition.

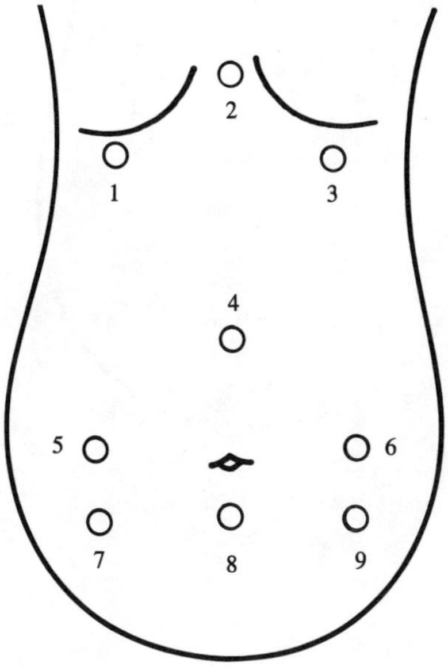

The following schema comes from from Dr. Wu Chao:

Position	Correspondence
1	spleen (reflex) zone
2	qi (reflex) zone
3	(reflex) zone of the right kidney and small intestine.
4	(reflex) zone of the left kidney and large intestine.

Figure 2.6 Tai Zhou's abdominal diagnosis.

Todo Yoshimasu, an important herbalist in Japan in the 1700's, based his research on the work of the Kohotta Herbal Medical Group, which during the preceding century had researched the use of herbal medicines according to the classics. He makes two interesting comments about abdominal palpation:

□

The hara is the basic place of the living energy. Therefore, the roots of all diseases are here. When you diagnose the disease, you must diagnose the hara.

Before touching the pulse, one has to diagnose the symptoms. Before diagnosing the symptoms, one has to touch the hara.[17]

China's great medical sage, Li Shi Zhen, is another famous herbalist who referenced palpating the abdomen. In his study of the eight extraordinary vessels, the *Qi Jing Ba Mai Kao,* he said:

To the right and left, above and below the umbilicus, if the qi is stabbing [a sensation as if being stuck by something], and when pressing hard, a [prison] strong pulsing or pain can be felt, we can think that it might be the chong mai, the ren mai, the leg shao yin or leg tai yin. . . .

To the left is the liver, to the right is the lungs, above is the heart, and below is the kidneys.[18]

Li Shi Zhen was obviously well studied in *Nan Jing* five-phase diagnosis, as well as the eight extraordinary vessels. It is likely that this comment is what has led some modern practitioners to confirm the same or similar diagnoses for the area around the umbilicus. In modern practice the idea has been extended to incorporate different acupuncture treatments and not only the herbal formulae that Li Shi Zhen would have prescribed.

One of the earliest acupuncture texts, the *Zhen Jiu Jia Yi Jing (Systematic Classic of Acupuncture and Moxibustion),* of 282 A.D., makes numerous references to certain acupoints that are able to treat tension or tightness in certain areas of the body, particularly the abdomen. For instance:

Qugu [CV-2] can treat tightness of the small abdomen [lower abdomen].[19]

Shuifen [CV-9] can treat tension of the spine and lining, and twitching, tense, acute pain in the abdomen.[20]

Zhongwan [CV-12], zhongting [CV-16], zigong [CV-19], and huagai [CV-20] treat tension and pain below the ribs.[21]

Tiantu [CV-22] treats a full condition of the chest, with abdominal skin that feels hot when touched.[22]

These references are similar to the quotes from the *Ling Shu.* While each may be interpreted as referring to symptoms reported by patients, these are diagnostic signs often ascertained by palpation.

Sun Si-Mo, an herbalist and acupuncturist of the seventh century famous for his contributions to the Daoist treatise, the *Dao Zang,* as well as the internal medicine text *Qian Jin Yao Fang (Priceless Prescriptions),* and its supplement, *Qian Jin Yi Fang (Supplemental Priceless Prescriptions),* wrote in his discussion "for the protection of one's health,"

After eating, massage [or rub] the hara; one can take away all diseases.[23]

Gao Wu, whose work from 1537 A.D., the *Zhen Jiu Ju Ying (Gathering of Eminent Acupuncturists),* compiled information from many different sources, summarized his understanding of *Nan Jing* five-phase diagnosis

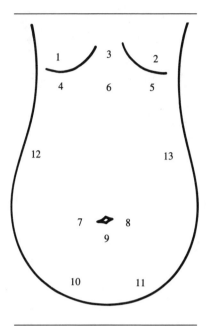

Figure 2.7 Tai Zhou's abdominal diagnosis

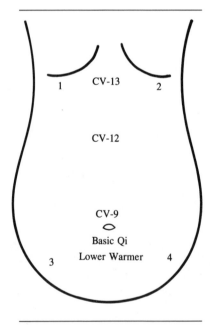

Figure 2.8 Wu Chao's reflex positions

and treatment by presenting abdominal correspondences. Although his ideas are simple, they have useful clinical merit. His synopsis retains the *Nan Jing* emphasis on abdominal palpation, at least with respect to the five yin organs:

> For the liver, there will be a pulsing, lump, tightness or pain on the left side of the umbilicus. . . .
>
> . . . For the heart . . . above the umbilicus. . . .
>
> . . . For the spleen . . . around the umbilicus. . . .
>
> . . . For the lungs . . . to the right side of the umbilicus. . . .
>
> . . . For the kidneys . . . a sudden pain in the area below the umbilicus.

One last historical example comes from the work of Yoshio Manaka.[24] In his considerable work with Oriental medical literature, he has researched and explained many theories and styles. One of these is the Mubunryu style of hara or abdominal diagnosis, created in the late sixteenth century by a Japanese acupuncturist, Isai Misonou. Using exclusively abdominal diagnosis and treatment, Misonou achieved phenomenal results with problems occurring anywhere in the body. He identified conditions that he treated using gold needles and special insertion techniques. According to Manaka's research on this style of diagnosis and treatment, Misonou's pattern of abdominal diagnosis made noticeably distinct assignments of areas to internal organs.

Abdominal diagnosis is an idea that has appeared in the famous texts of internal medicine and acupuncture through the entire history of Oriental medicine. It has played a greater or lesser role in the systems of diagnosis used at different times by different practitioners, gaining or losing prestige and acceptance based on a variety of trends and cultural conditions, few of which have been clearly identified or studied. Abdominal diagnosis by palpation was used in the Ming dynasty in China, but does not seem to have played a large role in the practice of internal medicine or acupuncture of the time. However, in Japan at the same time, the classics had been absorbed and were being applied in practice. The art and practice of palpation was beginning to become generally known. Todo Yoshimasu's work concerning abdominal palpation had become very important. In the field of acupuncture, Waichi Sugiyama refined and developed palpation to a very fine art. Sugiyama, a blind acupuncturist who lived from 1610-1695, was the inventor of the insertion tube. In Japan, he is often seen as the father of acupuncture. Developing extraordinary sensitivity and skill with his hands, he became a great healer, and contributed a significant body of information regarding palpation.

The core of information that Sugiyama taught is still of great utility, providing an excellent theoretical foundation for much of modern practice. In addition, much of what Li Shi Zhen said about the area around the umbilicus is used today, as is the *Nan Jing* theory. All offer basic extensible and eminently useful information. Here we quote Sugiyama's eight principles of abdominal or hara diagnosis from his book, *Sugiyama Ryu Sanbusho (Sugiyama's Style of Treatment in Three Parts).*[25]

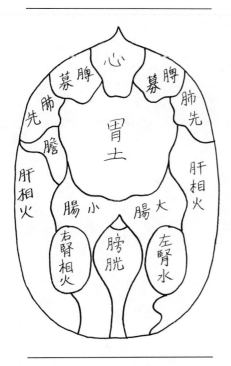

Figure 2.9 Mubunryu hara diagnosis

The Essentials of Hara Diagnosis	
Principle 1:	Press below the rib cage, to see if one side is harder, tighter, or has a lump.
Principle 2:	Touch CV-12 and move it slightly; if you feel a slight lump, it is a sign of a problem.
Principle 3:	Feel below the navel, if you feel a pulse that goes up to the chest, it is a sign of a problem.
Principle 4:	Feel around the navel, if the muscle feels like it is separating slightly, it is a sign of a weak hara.
Principle 5:	Feel from inside the navel down to CV-6, if you feel a lump, it is a sign of a problem.
Principle 6:	If on palpation around the hara, you feel many small lumps like beans in a bag, this is a sign of problems of the hara.
Principle 7:	If you feel a lump like a brush around CV-6, it is a sign of a problem.
Principle 8:	Press SP-15, GB-27, and LV-14. If there is a depression on slight pressure and on greater pressure it is loose or slippery without elasticity, it is a sign of a weak hara.

What we learn with certainty from an overview of the variety and extent of the historical systems of palpation is that there have been periods of attention and inattention, development and decline. Some systems contradict other systems, even to the extent that they seem to represent a different diagnostic paradigm. We must approach the subject of palpation with an open mind and with caution. It is all too easy to become confused.

For the theoretical framework of palpation, we must delve again into the past, into classic times and texts. While it is remarkable that after the *Nan Jing*, little seems to have been said about palpation other than palpation of the abdomen or hara, this is the direction we must take. This is the historical emphasis in the realm of palpation. It is then appropriate to shift our concerns to a closer examination of the hara; to look deeply into its energetics and theories. Fortunately, most of the historical information has been tested by a number of excellent modern practitioners during many years of practice. In modern practice, at least in Japan, the treatment of what what one finds on the hara, either directly or indirectly, has proven to have profound effects on the patient's health and wellbeing. Thus, we are able to use the experience of these clinicians to gain an understanding of how palpation may be successfully applied. The emphasis of the diagnostic and therapeutic chapters of this book will be on the work of these modern masters.

Chapter

- 3 -

Spiritual, Mental,

& Emotional Aspects

of

Chinese Medicine

The Spiritual, Mental, and Emotional Aspects of Chinese Medicine

One pronounced trend of Western medical thought has been the separation of mind and body. This tendency has a long history and has particular dramatic expression in the famous 1637 statement of Rene Descartes, "Cogito ergo sum" — I think therefore I am [1] This single dualism is one of the major stumbling blocks for understanding Oriental thought and philosophy. This, and several other major cultural differences, give rise to numerous natural, conceptual, and translational difficulties. For the Western mind, that mental and emotional phenomena can be distinguished from physical phenomena is a sine qua non. In Oriental medicine no such distinction is recognized. The Chinese sage does put his mind in his abdomen and the Japanese youth's hara does "stand up" when he is angry. To think of these as colorful aphorisms and no more is a critical error. When we render this last expression, *"hara ga tatsu,"* as "he is angry" our words really don't capture the sense of the original. This indeed, is the fascinating question — can we render the expression in English without the shared experience that creates meaning in natural languages?

This problem exists for many important concepts in Oriental thought and medicine. For instance, the character that is often translated as "joy" in the medical literature, the emotion of the heart, is *xi* 喜. Etymological study yields the meaning of "joy or pleasure derived from eating." *(Fuj)*[2] In a medical context, xi accurately refers more to the notion of problems caused by overeating than to "joie de vivre" or the pleasure of astute and attractive company. It is really overeating that causes the problem, the pleasure or joy derived from overeating is what animates the difficulty. In English texts, xi is rendered as "joy." Practitioners say with assurance that this emotion may injure the heart. How much greater is our comprehension when we understand the literal derivation of this term!

There are many other examples that actually exhibit greater translational problems. Terms like *qi, jing,* and *shen* are not renderable into English and are best left untranslated. We do not have concepts for these technical terms, and those words that most closely fit the characters carry connotations deeply colored by our cultural experience. Until we do master the concepts, from our absorption of the ideas and practices, whatever words we choose will inevitably carry the flavors of our early misconceptions. Mental and emotional states are particularly subject to these translational problems. Although we will be translating terms in this text that describe mental and emotional life, we will do so as approximations, as clues that will help us relate our own experiences to those of the authors quoted. The etymological context of many terms precisely demonstrates this point.

□

The spiritual, mental, and emotional states that are studied by Chinese medicine are often simply stated but profoundly implicated in the process of disease. These ideas were almost universally understood to relate to qi rooting in the hara. If the correct interactions of qi, jing, and shen in the hara do not occur, problems begin to manifest in all the "non-physical" arenas of human life — spiritual, mental, emotional. This is why counter-flow qi is a pathological entity of such profound clinical importance. It is more than the signs that we translate as its indications. Due to vacancy in the lower warmer the root is not nourished sufficiently, the qi cannot root itself; it becomes entrapped and replete in the upper parts of the body. This condition, in turn, disturbs the yin organ functions of storing and regulating the jing, shen, qi, hun, po, yi, and zhi, creating disturbances of the spiritual, mental, and emotional elements of human life.

However, these disturbances are not "emotional problems;" this Cartesian separation is neither implied nor justified. As the condition of counterflow qi is established as a lasting pattern, spiritual, mental, and emotional states become disturbed. There are often energy blocks in the body, particularly in the diaphragm. If the diaphragm is overtense and rigid, it restricts the flow toward correct balance. This is not a "physical problem," it too is counterflow qi.

Breathing into the abdomen, simple diaphragmatic breathing, is the single most powerful correction of such an imbalance. Abdominal breathing cures neither mental difficulties, nor a blocked diaphragm; rather, it helps ameliorate counterflow qi.[3]

Adequate circulation among the various energy centers of the body is essential to the Oriental concept of a dynamic homeostasis. Indeed, this is most clearly implied by the pulse diagnosis of the *Su Wen* where palpation of the deep positions reveals not the condition of the yin organs, but the condition of the energetic centers and the diaphragm *(SW 17)*. Clearly, there are profound implications inherent in a diagnostic system that reflects the *Su Wen* idea of the "great sage" who treats disease before it manifests. Attention to the diaphragm and energetic center are means by which this may be accomplished. In the *Nan Jing,* the same pulse positions and depths relate to the yin and yang meridians *(NJ 18)*. Again, the organ level, the most physical, is less important since "the great artisan treats disease before it happens." The differences between the artisan and the sage are many and various. There is a wealth of research, argument, and discovery in just the differences of pulse positions.

Some specific passages in the *Ling Shu* and *Su Wen* can focus our research most directly. In one interesting and perplexing passage from the *Ling Shu,* the Yellow Emperor asked:

> When we study the technique of needle insertion, the basic [most important] part is always the shen. The blood, the vessels, the ying, the qi, the jing, the shen, are each stored in the five yin organs. Excessive dissoluteness [will cause them to] leave the organs. This means one will lose the jing; the hun and po will jump up [become unsettled]; the zhi [will] and yi [ideas] will become unclear. Intelligence will leave the body.

> What causes this? Is it a punishment from heaven or a mistake
> by the person? What are de 德, qi 氣, zhi 志, jing 精, shen 神,
> hun 魂, po 魄, and yi 意? *(LS 8:84-85); (TS 70)*[4]

These are questions Oriental philosophers have attempted to answer in all
times. Today it is no more possible to give totally satisfactory answers than
it has ever been. But in Qi Bo's answer there are important clues to the
solutions the Chinese practitioners provided for themselves:

> The heaven in one is de. The earth in one is qi. The de
> streams down and the qi reaches up to it, subsequently there is
> life. Therefore, the coming of life is called jing. Both jing beat
> [meet] together; this is called shen. Following shen, going and
> returning, this is hun. Paralleling jing, going-out and coming-in,
> this is called po *(LS 8:85)*.

The two jing beating together becoming shen refers to the physical expression of the male and female jing sperm and ovum — that unite during conception. Of the last two lines, the *Tai Su* comments:

> Hun is a different ling [spirit] of shen; therefore it follows
> shen; going and returning, it is stored in the liver, it is called
> hun. Po is also a different ling of shen, it parallels jing; going
> out and coming in, it is called po *(TS 70-71)*.

Of these same lines Xie Lin of the late Qing dynasty makes an interesting comment:

> The liver stores the hun. The hun is the jing of the yang, the
> ling of qi. The qi of the person is yang, the blood is yin. The
> liver controls the blood and inside it is the yang qi, this is called
> the hun. [On] researching the root of hun [we can say that] it is
> created at the one yang of ☵ water. [Thus] we can infer that
> the actions of the hun begin at and are the basic [fundamental]
> qi of ☰ metal. [The *Ling Shu* says] the hun follows the shen
> coming and going; this is ling's manifestation in the senses.
> The lung stores the po, the po is the jing of yin, the ling of the
> form. The liver controls the blood, basically it is yin and stores
> the yang hun, the yang is hidden in the yin. The lung controls
> the qi, basically it is yang and stores the yin po; yin is created
> in the yang. After labor, the ears, eyes, heart/mind, the hands
> and feet move, the baby's cries are the voice, all are the ling of
> po. [The *Ling Shu* says] that which parallels the jing and comes
> out and goes in is the po. This is the capacity of movement.[5]

As is often the case with the circular logic of Chinese medicine, each basic
term is referenced to and defined by the other. To explain Qi Bo's answer,
we need to enter the spiralling metaphor and attempt to define some of the
basic terminology. What are the jing, shen, hun, po, de, zhi, yi, xin and
ling?

Such answers cannot, and will not, come quickly or simply. In each
area of human energetics that we will explore in this text, we will meet
these essential terms. In each exploration greater detail will appear, and
more will become clear about each idea. To begin, there are the basic

☐

translational clues. Jing, shen, and qi are general terms referring to various forms of energy and energetic function. The jing is akin to "vital energies," the kinetic processes intimately involved in life itself. It is an energetic precursor of matter. Shen is a more rarified form of energy; defining it in English brings to mind superlatives such as "most pure" or "most vital." It is a functionally activating energy. Qi is energy almost in the sense of modern quantum physics. It is in everything, both animate and inanimate. It is involved in and composes all things and all processes. It is the kinetic aspect of matter, the functional quality of phenomenae.

Hun and po are more specific energetic entities. Of all the Chinese concepts, hun is most like the Christian idea of soul. It differs most explicitly as it recycles, rather than belonging to a specific being for all time, entering the body at conception and leaving at death to return in another conception. It comes from and returns to heaven. Po is like the hun except that it is more material, coming from earth and returning to earth. Ling is another general term, similar to shen. It too is a more spiritual energy, even more strongly associated with the energy of heaven than is shen. De is more a state of being, developing with self cultivation yet bestowed on us by heaven; it is often translated as "virtue" or "power," and is seen as part of character or personality. As healers it is part of what we must cultivate to become good practitioners.

While none of the isolated translations of these elemental concepts are sufficient, and no one quotation describes their qualities completely, there is a consistency from which we may gain a more complete idea, even something of a feeling for the words as they were used by the Chinese. The quote from the *Ling Shu*, for example, speaks of the de streaming down from heaven to meet with the qi that is reaching up to it. This is echoed by the *Su Wen* discussion of the idea of *ming* 命 that comes down from heaven to create the living being. In the Wang Bing commentary on this passage, from *Su Wen 25:158*, the *Ling Shu* idea of de and qi is footnoted as an explanation of the idea of ming.

The concepts with which we are here most concerned are *zhi* 志, *yi* 意, and *xin* 心. Xin is both "heart" and "mind." Etymologically it is derived from a picture of a heart *(Fuj)*. It is almost impossible to say for sure that the classical Chinese scholars and practitioners made an explicit distinction between the heart and mind, or if, depending on context, they understood implicit differences between them. It is probable that for them, the heart and mind were inextricably linked. Thought of one necessarily involved some reference to the other. In an interesting allegorical story from the *Lie Zi*,[6] the famed physician Bian Que, whose name was used by the author of the *Nan Jing*, but who actually lived several centuries before the *Nan Jing* was written, was presented with two male patients. He designed a radical treatment for the two which illustrates these relationships. Diagnosing one patient as having weak will and strong qi and the other as having strong will but weak qi, he suggested to the two that the best therapy would be to transfer their hearts from one to the other. The two agreed. Bian Que performed the surgery and sent the patients home.

□

The patients returned complaining that their wives and family no longer recognized them. Bian Que found that the men had returned to what they considered home, but no one recognized their physical appearance, because each had taken on the physical appearance of the other. The personality associated with a particular family now had the physical appearance of the other. This allegorical tale demonstrates dramatically that the conceptual associations of what we call the "mind" and "heart" are far more intimate than we would suppose by thinking only that the "heart stores the shen," as if it were some prized jewel packed away in a treasure trove. In the context of the *Ling Shu* passage, the Yellow Emperor's question about xin does seem to refer more to the concept we call "mind," but we should not forget the reference to the heart.

Both zhi and yi are also related to xin, "mind." This can be seen in the characters themselves, both have the xin radical 心. This connection is also stated in the *Ling Shu*:

> The controller of the body is xin [the mind]. The unexpressed thoughts [of the mind] are called yi [ideas]. The place at which the ideas exist is zhi [the will] *(LS 8:85)*.

Ideas and will are seen in direct relationship to the mind, xin.

The *Shuo Wen Jie Zi* says of yi, ideas: "The yi is the same as the zhi, will" *(Mor)*. Etymologically, The character yi is comprised of two basic component parts, 音 which means "verbally expressed thoughts," and 心, which means heart—mind *(Fuj)*. The yi itself seems to refer to putting the mind into the verbally expressed thoughts. Hence the common translation as thoughts, ideas.

The character *zhi* 志 which means "will" approximates this meaning: 士 refers to a foot; 心 refers to the heart/mind *(Fuj)*.

The mind controls the feet to bring about movement and ultimately action. This capacity for instigating actions with what we call will is expressive of the mind's fixed purpose.

The yi, "ideas," relates to the intention someone expresses with words or sounds. Zhi are the actions that express the mind, the verbal expressions of the mind. The *Ling Shu* concept is thus more simply seen as an expression of the interrelation of the mind and ideas, that manifest through both thought and action.

The energetic and medical implications are also found in the *Ling Shu*:

> Zhi and yi [will and ideas] are therefore the controller [harmonizer] of jing and shen, the secure place of the hun and po, the regulator of the temperature. They harmonize joy and anger . . .
> When the will and ideas are harmonized, the jing and shen become straight [fluid]. The hun and po don't disperse. One doesn't become too regretful or too angry. The five yin organs don't accept evil qi *(LS 47:349); (TS 76)*.

When thought, expression, and action are in harmony, everything works well and the body remains healthy.

□

Problems of too much or not enough, too weak or too strong of will, can engender serious consequences. This particular passage is very important to remember when we examine the concept of counterflow qi in greater detail. Having come so far in this metaphoric spiral, it is perhaps hard to remember that the discussions from which the *Ling Shu* comment derived was a discussion of needle technique. The important aspect of needle technique is the shen. For the classical practitioners these ideas had many practical consequences for how we should approach our patients and with what states of mind we can best work.

The *Zhen Jiu Da Cheng,* from 1601 A.D., discusses a "shen needle technique" that reflects the *Ling Shu* discussion:

> The shen needle, eight techniques:
> In the mind of the physician there should be no desires, only a receptive and accepting attitude, then the mind can become shen. The mind of the physician and the mind of the patient should be level, in harmony, following the movements of the needle. First, focus on protecting the needle. Place the tip of the needle in the mouth to keep it warm. With the left hand rub the point where one will insert the needle. When rubbing, be very attentive and careful, as though one were holding a tiger by the tail. With the right hand, insert and rotate the needle, but with no power. Do not be tense, keep one's hand relaxed.[7]

Though modern sterilization procedure requires that we never place the tip of the needle in the mouth, the crux of the idea remains to warm the needle so as to not disturb the patient with a cold needle. Most important are the instructions regarding the physician's attitude. This passage stresses the importance of remaining calm and not emotional, both for the patient and practitioner. Emotional, mental, or attitudinal states were seen as both causes and effects and the barriers between one individual's mental and spiritual condition and that of another individual were experienced as far more permeable than they are in the West. Not only were touch and technique required to protect the patients' vital energies, but as importantly the spirit of the physician was a necessary and important consideration. Little wonder that there was such great emphasis on the development of character for the "great artisan."

The *Ling Shu,* in the same chapter as the discussion of needle techniques, presents a brief discussion of the five yin organs, concerning general energetics:

> The liver stores the blood. The blood stores the hun. When liver qi becomes vacant, the emotions are of fear. When liver qi is replete, anger and irritability result. The heart stores the vessels. The vessels store the shen. When heart qi becomes vacant, grief results. When heart qi becomes replete, there is laughter that never stops. The spleen stores the ying. The ying stores the ideas. When spleen qi becomes vacant, the four limbs lose their normal motion and the five yin organs become insecure. When spleen qi becomes replete, the body becomes swollen and the urine and menses lose their smoothness. The lung stores the qi, the qi stores the po. When lung qi becomes

vacant, shortness of breath will develop. When lung qi becomes replete, panting, a feeling of fullness and discomfort in the chest, and difficulty breathing will develop. The kidney stores the jing; the jing stores the zhi. When kidney qi becomes vacant, it means counterflow. When kidney qi becomes replete, there will be swelling and the five yin organs become insecure. Pay attention to the form of the disease of the five yin organs, the emptiness and fullness of the qi, and then carefully control this (LS 8:88-89).

Aside from the emotional and energetic characteristics of yin organ problems, it is important to note that if the spleen qi becomes vacant or the kidney qi becomes replete, insecurity of the five yin organs will result. This echoes the other discussion from the *Ling Shu* regarding the harmony of the zhi and yi, will and ideas. Harmony results in protection of the five yin organs from evil qi. Note too that the author of the *Tai Su* comments that the swelling produced by spleen qi repletion is a swollen abdomen and that the swelling produced by kidney qi repletion is edema (TS 75).

The description of heart qi vacancy resulting in grief and heart qi repletion resulting in laughter that never stops is paralleled in the *Su Wen*:

> The Yellow Emperor asked, "Is there replete shen or vacant shen?"
> Qi Bo answered, "Replete shen is laughter that doesn't stop; vacant shen is grief" (SW 62:335).

The function of the heart qi is synonymous or similar to shen. Problems of the heart ultimately are problems of the shen, or at least the heart's capacity for storing shen. As the *Su Wen* tells us, when the shen is impaired in any way it is more difficult to treat the patient (SW 14:87). This is one reason why some practitioners see the heart as incapable of being diseased or as the root of its own disease. Problems of the heart come from other sources, other organs and meridians.

The relationships of emotional and mental states and diseases are by no means simplistic. The mechanisms are not linear causes and effects, rather they are simultaneous occurrences. Energetic and emotional problems are bidirectional. The yin organs can become imbalanced resulting in emotional manifestations, which in turn can lead to further energetic disharmonies. Emotional disharmonies can lead to organ imbalances. It is not that one causes the other, although we do tend to perceive the relationship in that way. There is only one energetic pattern and it manifests both internal organ problems and emotional states. The nature of our perceptions leads us to see one or the other and rarely the two together, and we presume a causal relationship. It may be a useful attitude, but is definitely a questionable explanation. To see these Chinese medical discussions as implying the same causal relationships that we are culturally conditioned to see can lead to neglect or overemphasis of one part of the pattern or another. This is even true for the Chinese themselves, for whom the emotional and mental aspects have become increasingly understated as their own cultural tendency toward a reduced emphasis on personal mental states has been accelerated and exacerbated by their recent social history.

□

Returning to the pattern of counterflow qi, for example, we find that the general category of counterflow qi is most commonly a repletion in the upper body that results from a vacancy below. Many of the symptoms associated with the condition are emotional or mental, yet emotional and mental states themselves can engender a pattern of counterflow qi. The following passage from the *Su Wen* is representative of its various discussions on the nature and causes of counterflow qi, and demonstrates the relationship of the various types of counterflow qi and the paired yin-yang meridians.

> To diagnose the beginning of diseases, there are the principles of the five decisions. To know the beginning of the disease, first find the mother [origin]. The five decisions are the five vessels. If there is headache and epilepsy, this is vacancy below and repletion above. The disease is in the leg shao yin [kidney] and ju yang [vast yang - probably tai yang—bladder]. If the disease gets worse it comes into the kidneys.
>
> If there is vertigo, a loss of the sense of a center of gravity, if the eyes are unclear and there is hardness of hearing, this is repletion below and vacancy above. The disease is in leg shao yang [gallbladder] and jue yin [liver]. If the disease becomes serious it goes to the liver.
>
> If the abdomen is swollen and tense, if the diaphragm and lower edges of the sides of the ribs feel stagnant, this is counterflow. This passes through at leg tai yin [spleen] and yang ming [stomach].
>
> If there is panting, coughing and rising qi [like a forced, harsh exhalation], the counterflow is inside the chest. The disease is in arm yang ming [large intestine] and tai yin [lung].
>
> If there is [physical and/or mental] suffering of the heart and headache, the disease is in the diaphragm. The disease is at arm ju yang [small intestine] and shao yin [heart] *(SW 10:73-74)*.

This notable passage categorizes five kinds of counterflow qi according to the five pairs of yin and yang meridians. Each is referenced in the context of seeking the origin of disease, finding the precursors of morbidity prior to its more serious symptomatic expression. The third and fifth passages, associated with the spleen—stomach and heart—small intestine, are directly related to problems of the diaphragm, an area that commonly becomes tight or blocked in mental or emotional disturbances. For instance, the yin wei mai in modern acupuncture practice is diagnosed by palpating the subcostal area in the upper abdomen. Tension here is often related to the yin wei mai. The yin wei mai, because of its connection through PC-6 to the heart, has powerful effects on emotional and mental states. "Inside the chest" is a category that relates many energetic, emotional, and mental states. Several meridians pass through to the inside of the chest — the kidney, pericardium, gallbladder, pericardium luo, and the chong mai. The inside of the chest is associated with or comprises the "upper qihai" where zong qi is stored:

> That which does not follow the stream of ying and wei piles up at the inside of the chest. It is called qihai *(LS 56:402)*.

☐

Pulse diagnosis in the *Su Wen* subtly reflects the discussion of the various forms of counterflow qi *(SW 17:106-107).* The left pulse at the inch position superficially reflects the heart. Deeper it reflects CV-17. At the left bar position, the surface reflects the liver, the deeper pulse the diaphragm. At the left foot position, the superficial pulse is the kidney, the deeper pulse is inside the abdomen. In the right pulse, at the inch position, the lungs are reflected at the surface, deeper we are told that the inside of the chest may be diagnosed. At the right bar position, the superficial pulse is the stomach; the deeper pulse is the spleen. Both bar positions reflect the rib cage. In the right foot position, the kidneys are reflected at the surface, deeper we find the inside of the abdomen.

Except for the right bar position, the deeper radial pulses reflect general areas or specific locations, as opposed to organs. Included here is the diaphragm, thus interpreted as being at a deeper or more fundamental energetic level. Although it is possible that "inside the abdomen" is a literal reference, it is more likely that it refers to the energetic centers in the abdomen, qihai and dantian.

In the clinical practice of many renowned acupuncture and moxibustion therapists in Japan, certain areas of the body are commonly found to be reactive when patients have mental or emotional problems. These areas include: on the sternum, around CV-17, on the spine (T2-T10), on the du mai, around GV-20, around qihai—dantian. The areas in the upper parts are seen to become reactive because of a repletion of energy above. Qihai dantian is often found to be weak and empty, indicating a vacancy below. This is the pattern of counterflow qi.

In the *Su Wen,* different emotional states were seen in relation to different manifestations of qi.

> The Yellow Emperor asked, "I heard all diseases are created by qi. [With] anger the qi rises; [with] joy the qi becomes loose or moderate; [with] grief the qi disappears, [with] fear the qi descends; [with] cold the qi shrinks; [with] heat the qi leaks; [with] fright the qi is disordered. [With] tiredness, the qi wilts; [with] thinking the qi knots [becomes stagnant]. These nine qi are not the same. What causes these diseases?"
>
> Qi Bo answered, "[With] anger the qi becomes counterflow; if it gets worse, one will vomit blood and there will be diarrhea with undigested food. Therefore, this is qi rising up. [With] joy the qi becomes harmonized and the will becomes stronger. The ying and wei are able to flow through; therefore, the qi is loose or moderate. [With] grief the supporter of the heart becomes tense; the lungs become swollen and weak; the upper warmer does not pass through; the ying and wei cannot disperse; there is hot qi in it; therefore, the qi disappears. [With] fear then the jing returns; the upper warmer closes; then the qi circles and returns. Upon circling or returning the lower warmer becomes swollen. Therefore the qi doesn't move. [With] cold the skin tissues close, the qi doesn't move; therefore the qi contracts. [With] heat, the skin tissues open, the ying and wei pass through, there is a great sweating. Therefore,

the qi leaks. [With] fright the heart cannot perform its regal tasks. The shen cannot return. The thoughts and consciousness are not stable; therefore, the qi becomes disordered. [With] tiredness there is panting and sweating; the inside and outside are overcome; therefore, the qi wilts. [With] thoughts the mind—heart has a focal point. The shen has a place of return [focus]; the correct qi becomes stagnant and doesn't move; therefore, the qi becomes stagnant" *(SW 39:221-222).*

This passage details the relationships among emotional and mental states and the various qi manifestations and pathologies. The "supporter of the heart" is the series of blood vessels coming out of the heart — the aorta, vena cava, pulmonary arteries and veins. It is interesting that grief was seen to create tension at this location and to affect the lungs. Perhaps this explains how vacancy of the heart qi or shen results in grief. The heart meridian does not "belong to" or "permeate" the heart itself, rather the supporter of the heart. (See next chapter.)

Fear causes the ascending jing from the kidneys and dantian to return. This in turn causes the upper warmer to close; meaning perhaps that the diaphragm becomes blocked. As the upper warmer closes, the qi in the lower warmer becomes stuck, and circles in the lower warmer. This could also be seen as relating to both the ascension of qi from qihai dantian and the ascension of breath on exhalation causing stagnation of the qi in the lower warmer.

Fright or shock disturbs the heart causing it to lose its ability to store the shen. This creates instability in the mental states resulting in disordered qi. With tiredness or fatigue, the outside is overcome by the sweating and the inside by the panting. The character we translate as "thoughts" is si 思, another very interesting character much like zhi and yi. It refers more to the interior thoughts that are neither verbally nor actively expressed. The *Shuo Wen Jie Zi* says of si: "Thought is capacity, it is the expressed words of the brain-mind" *(Mor)*. That is, si refers more to the mental process that results from the interaction of the mind with the brain, what we now call mental activity. We can distinguish between zhi, yi and si thus:

> Yi refers to verbally expressed thoughts.
> Zhi refers to actively expressed thoughts.
> Si refers to thoughts that manifest in the process
> of the interaction between the mind and brain.

All three terms describe facets of the mind, functional properties. How these functions work together, in and out of harmony, has various influences on overall health.

The yi and zhi, when balanced, harmonize the jing and shen, secure the hun and po, regulate the temperature, and prevent excessive emotions such as regret or anger. Si, thought, carries a slightly different connotation. Yi and zhi help regulate and harmonize. Si, from the quote above, seems to cause problems by its very nature. Mental thought, si, is a focal point of the mind. It represents a place for shen to return to, coalesce, causing stagnation of the correct qi and thus stagnation of qi in general. It is unclear whether this is true of all thought, but it is rather a startling idea. Too much mentation causes stagnation of qi. Perhaps this is part of the reason for the aphorism "thinking with the hara."

Mental and emotional states are at once the result of energetic imbalances and the cause of energetic imbalances. It is easiest to see many of these disorders as a parallel to the condition of counterflow qi. The qi is not rooted at its source; it is too actively engaged elsewhere in the body, causing problems in the organs and meridians, and manifesting as mental and emotional disturbances.

Treating the conditions when they manifest as tension, tightness, or pressure pain at specifically reflective areas found by palpation is particularly advantageous. Not only will such treatments address the underlying problems, they will do so prior to the obvious manifestation of the mental or emotional symptoms or the simultaneous physical correlates. As mentioned, some therapists see mental problems as coming from vacancy of the dantian. Dantian functions to store the jing and shen. If it is weak, the jing and shen are not well retained. Since the yi and zhi harmonize and balance the jing and shen, it is not unreasonable to suspect that imbalanced thinking (which may cause or result from disharmony of the yi and zhi), also causes this dispersion of jing and shen. Since the yi is stored by the spleen and the zhi by the kidney, disharmonies of the spleen and kidney may be the root of this problem.

That dantian should show vacancy in mental or emotional problems correlates to its palpatory description as the area on the abdomen where the spleen and kidney reflex positions overlap. Is dantian's ability to store the jing and shen related to mental and emotional stability and the balance of the spleen and kidney? Certainly underlying and resulting vacancies can be seen in emotional disorders. This is indicated in several passages from the *Su Wen*. Very commonly, the five emotions are seen to cause vacancy of the corresponding yin organs by injuring *shang* 傷, the yin organs. This injury is usually described as something that weakens function.

> Anger injures the liver . . . joy injures the heart . . . depression injures the lung . . . fear, shock injures the kidney . . . thinking injures the spleen (SW 5:37-42).

Here the emotions injure the organs. Whatever the cause of a certain emotion, expressing the emotion too much (or possibly even at all) can weaken an organ. One cause of the emotional expression can be a weakness or vacancy of the organs. It is almost a spiral, a vicious circle. In the classical descriptions of the relationship of emotions to organ weakness, the one gives rise to the other, which in turn can give rise to the first again. English language and cultural conditioning do not express well the simultaneity of these manifestations; rather our tendency to assume one-way, causal relationships is emphasized.

The *Su Wen* discussions of organ weakness and emotional states is quite complex. It involves the reverse process of the "controlling cycle" among the five yin organs. When there is weakness or vacancy of the organ that should transmit jing qi to any of the five yin organs, the result is that the jing qi will unite with the transmitting organ, producing a certain correspondent emotional state.

□

It is useful to remember that the Chinese almost never distinguished mind, energy, emotion, and body. These were viewed as a continuum. Indeed, considering how cyclical the psyche—soma relationship was in Chinese thought, we can conclude that dwelling mentally or emotionally on an element of the psyche that has caused problems makes little sense at all. The "cure" might cause the "problem." Contrary to modern urges in acupuncture practice in the West, the emotive and mental correspondences of Oriental medicine were not the basis of a form of counseling. While the adoption of counseling techniques into the practice of acupuncture may be an outcome of the cross-cultural journey, its creation and development cannot be based on simplistic "translations" of Oriental spirit-affect concepts. This is a translation the Orientals never implied.

Individuals from an Oriental culture do not customarily discuss their problems. Their attitudes toward such issues are more likely to reject even the idea of a psychological counselor. Even today, Orientals tend to express their emotional concerns in terms of their work group, family, or social environment rather than in personal emotive conditions. Indeed, much of what is the realm of the counselor in Western therapies are issues that are decided in Oriental societies as familial or social processes. One need study very little of cultural anthropology to understand that Oriental peoples have many very different means, Zen Buddhism for example, for dealing with the psyche. These methods have been uniquely successful for their cultures. We cannot assume from our cultural perspective that what they do is similar to what we do in the West.

From the medical perspective, the very act of focusing on mental or emotional states is a logic that presumes a dualistic framework. Looking for an underlying emotional trauma requires the assumption that the emotion really is distinct from the body and its symptoms. For the Oriental practitioner this is really approaching the problem backward, since the dualism itself is neither seen nor acceptable. The underlying trauma and the symptoms are two ends of the same stick, indeed, there is no need to emphasize or recall the trauma, the symptoms are quite obviously doing so already.

We have seen some of the interdependent relationships between mental, emotional, energetic, and physiological function. These are all expressions of the same human reality. Recognizing this, the Oriental practitioner does not focus on the emotional or mental states, but perceives these as more input to the diagnostic process. For example, in the Japanese tradition, were the practitioner to hear a statement such as, "he has a psychological problem," what would come immediately to the practitioner's mind would be the tightness of the patient's neck, shoulders and back. How the patient's structure was imbalanced might be the focus of exploration.

It is a necessary part of learning of Oriental medicine that students enjoy a focus on the simpler aspects of the medicine before progressing to a more sophisticated understanding and practice. Certainly, a review of the famed Oriental apprenticeship demonstrates that it supplies ample periods of just such a concentration. Thus, it is practical that students of medicine in the West should focus on the simpler aspects, the correspondences of pathological syndromes, as a means of grasping the initial concepts.

□

However, as in the Orient, this understanding should mature, and the early focus should give way to a more sophisticated understanding. One synchronistic model we can use to develop a deeper understanding of the inseparability of mental, emotive, energetic, and physical states, is natural adaptation.

Any organism, whether "diseased" or "healthy," manifests a continuous adaptation to changing internal and external environments. The pathologies of Oriental medicine are adaptive responses to either internally or externally generated pressures on the organism. No distinction need be made between mental, emotive, energetic, or bodily sources of adaptive stress. Each is a stress on the individual's condition to which the person must adapt or suffer some degradation of capacity. The homeostatic functions work at all levels, from the biochemical to the energetic. The fact that we label those states we consider undesirable as disease or pathology does not make the condition any less adaptive. In the Oriental tradition, where the relativistic nature of energy, the continuum of what we call mind, emotion, energy, and body, is more strongly reinforced by the intellectual environment, there is less temptation to separate the adaptations of mind and body. For us, with our longstanding Cartesian prejudices, difficult conceptual problems arise, not because the models are inherently difficult, but because we must maintain a constant vigilance for our own habits of mind.

Using our adaptive model there is no need to differentiate mind, body, emotions, energetics. Since the pathology is the result of an adaptive response to environmental pressures, the person will exhibit natural homeostatic responses. It is likely that if these responses are desirable for the person, they will not seek a cure, there being no perceived need to change the condition. Those for whom the adaptations are undesirable will seek help at some individually and culturally determined threshold of pain, discomfort, or even some perceived departure from an ideal or norm. Since the patient is already in an adapted, homeostatic state, any disruption of that state, the insertion of needles for instance, can initiate a further adaptive response. Healing results from influencing the natural, adaptive homeostasis.

□

Chapter

- 4 -

Internal Trajectories

of the

Twelve Meridians

The Internal Trajectories of the Twelve Meridians

Although definitive statements about the internal trajectories of the twelve meridians, and the relationships these internal pathways have with the internal organs, can be made only presumptuously, interesting and noteworthy energetic connections between the organs and meridians are commonly described. To understand these relationships it is helpful to examine the language with which these pathways are classically described. When the internal trajectory of a meridian goes to its own organ — for example, when the liver meridian arrives at the liver organ — it is said to "permeate" or "belong to" that organ. Here the character used, *shu* 屬, has the connotation of a complete permeation of the organ by the meridian. Rather than just passing through or arriving at the organ, it roots into it completely. This use also seems to imply a concept of mutual ownership: the organ owns the meridian and vice versa. It is a complete, total relationship, as if the distinction between the meridian and the organ were only a matter of degree. Thus, the liver and the liver meridian are a whole, just as a river and the lakes that it forms are separately named, yet inseparable.

This is not the case for the relationship between a meridian and its coupled organ. When an internal trajectory goes to a coupled organ — for example, the liver to the gallbladder — the internal trajectory is said to "spirally wrap" (*luo* 絡) the organ. This implies a less physical and less total energetic connection than is expressed by the term "permeate." The meridian encloses or wraps rather than permeates. Continuing the metaphor, the river passes around a boulder in its stream.

The physical or energetic analogs of these ideas are speculative. Based on other discussions regarding the nature of the relationship of the meridians in anatomical structures, which we will pursue in greater detail later in the text, we propose that these connections are effected through the fascia and connective tissues of the organs. In the instance of a meridian permeating the organ, the connection would be created through the organ tissues themselves. "Spiral wrapping" would be a connection through the fascial envelopes of the organs.

However, the general sense of these relationships is not easily formed as an absolute rule. The model is more complex. There are some interesting exceptions to the general concept, namely, the internal trajectories of the heart and the kidney meridians. Further, the internal trajectories at times go to or through other organs, not just those with which they are associated or coupled. These energetic connections are of another order. Indeed, the kidney internal trajectory, the triple warmer, and "master of the heart" (pericardium) internal trajectories, are of a very different nature than all the others, as we shall see as we pursue our inquiry.

□

While it is the external trajectories of the twelve meridians that are the subject of most meridian theories or discussions, it is the internal trajectories that were classically thought to be the "main" meridians. The superficial aspects, on which are located the acupoints, were seen as the "branches." This implies a less significant role in the energetics of the body. Again, there are exceptions to this rule — the heart, stomach, and bladder meridians. The main information to be derived from this idea is that the more important energetic exchanges and interactions occur within the internal meridians; the superficial extensions of the meridians describe the movement of energy through the rest of the body. It is also interesting to note that some of the body's most important points, including those that are important for diagnostic palpation and treatment, lie on the "main" meridians that are the exceptions to the rule, i.e., the stomach and bladder meridians.

Again, we are learning by inference more of what the idea of "main meridians" means. The overall importance of understanding the internal trajectories, at least in this context, is two-fold. First, a detailed understanding and knowledge of the internal pathways plainly demonstrates the energetic centrality and importance of the hara. Second, a close scrutiny of the acupoints on these trajectories through the abdomen, particularly those that are on main pathways, gives us a basic working knowledge of acupoint, meridian, and organ correspondences. These are extremely useful in diagnosis.

To help provide an accurate image of the internal trajectories, we have assembled information from several respected sources. These sources include the *Ling Shu (LS 10:104-135);* also the *Shisi Jing Fa Hui (Elucidation of the Fourteen Meridians)* from the Ming dynasty in 1341 A.D..[1] The author, Hua Shou, includes the internal trajectories of the meridians, and also gives detailed descriptions of the earlier *Ling Shu* information. From modern China, the *Nei Jing Jie Po Sheng Li Xue (Anatomy and Physiology of the Yellow Emperor's Internal Classic),* a useful compilation of theoretical materials from a broad range of classical sources, provided us with significant information.[2] A modern Japanese researcher, Shinji Imamura, M.D. PhD., in his article, *Zofu Keiraku Oyobi Chukankeiraku no Ruchu Ni Tsuite (Pathways of the Internal Meridians),*[3] provided us with remarkable internal meridian descriptions. These are the results of his careful and detailed research of all the old texts coupled with the data of modern anatomy and physiology.

For each meridian, the *Ling Shu* description provides the basic information. This is supplemented by the detailed explanations and diagrams derived from other sources and commentaries. Generally, the yin meridians are more complex and detailed than the yang meridians, reflecting their relatively greater importance.

□

Internal Trajectories of the Lung Meridian

The *Ling Shu* describes the internal trajectories of the lung meridian thus:

> The vessel 脈 of the lungs, hand tai yin, starts at the middle warmer. It comes down and then spirally wraps the large intestine. It then returns to and circles the entrance of the stomach, coming up, and permeates the lungs, then going to and coming out at the sides *(LS 10)*.

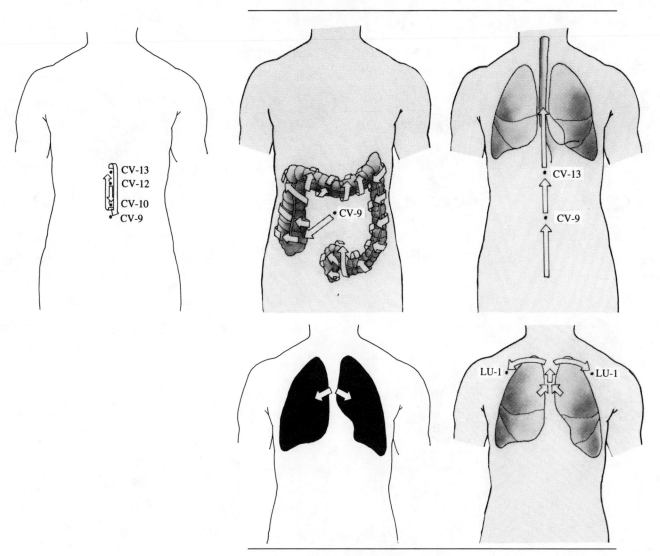

Figure 4.1 - 4.5 Lung meridian trajectory

We may interpret this description in the following manner: The starting place is seen as CV-12 (middle of the stomach); from here it passes to CV-10 (exit of the stomach), then up to CV-13 (entrance of the stomach), then down to CV-9 (dividing place of water) *(Shisi)*. Next it traverses the lower part of the large intestine, by way of the greater omentum or possibly the mesenterial folds, following the length of the large intestine and spirally wrapping it until it reaches the rectum *(Ima)*. From here it returns to CV-13, then passes up to the lungs, permeating the lungs *(Ima)*. It then follows the "supporter of the lungs" *(Shisi)*, the bronchii and trachea *(Ima)*, to pass out to the surface at LU-1 *(Shisi)*.

We can also view the first stages of the meridian as a spiral from a three-dimensional perspective:

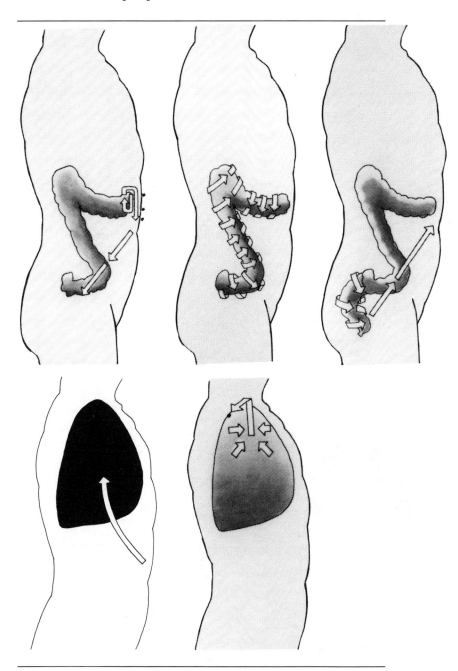

Figure 4.6 - 4.10 Side view of lung meridian trajectory

Internal Trajectories of the Large Intestine Meridian

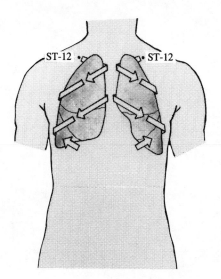

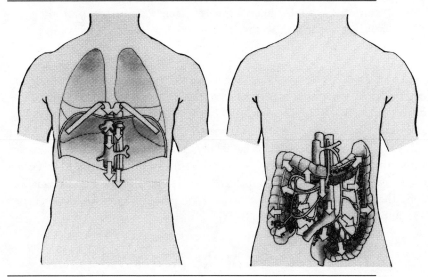

Figure 4.11 - 4.13 Large intestine meridian

The *Ling Shu* describes the main internal trajectory of the large intestine meridian thus:

> [It] comes into ST-12, down to and spirally wrapping the lungs, then down to the diaphragm, and then permeates the large intestine *(LS 10)*.

We may interpret this description in the following manner: From ST-12 the trajectory passes to and spirally wraps the lungs; then, following the aorta, it passes downward through the diaphragm. Here it splits to permeate the large intestine *(Shisi)*. Several commentators, including Hua Shuo, think that this trajectory involves ST-25 *(Li Xue)*.

Internal Trajectories of the Stomach Meridian

The *Ling Shu* tells us that at ST-12, the "main" meridian passes down along the chest and abdomen to ST-30, while the branch:

> . . . passes down to the diaphragm (from ST-12), permeates the stomach, and spirally wraps the spleen. Another branch starting at the exit of the stomach passes down through the lining of the abdomen to ST-30 *(LS 10)*.

Most commentaries agree with this simple trajectory, the one notable exception being the *Lei Jing (The Classic of Categories)*, which tells us that the branch that comes down through the lining of the abdomen to ST-30, comes down slightly lateral to the kidney meridian, starting at the same level as KI-16 *(Li Xue)*.

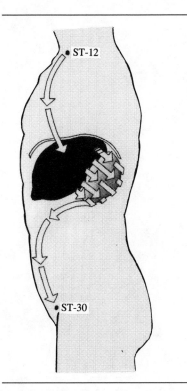

Figure 4.14 Stomach meridian trajectory

Internal Trajectories of the Spleen Meridian

The spleen vessel comes into the abdomen, permeates the spleen, and spirally wraps the stomach, comes up past the diaphragm, surrounds the throat, makes contact with and disperses into the base of the tongue *(LS 10)*.

This passage is interpeted to mean that the spleen meridian rises up the leg to SP-12 on the abdomen, thence to SP-13, to CV-3, to CV-4, to SP-14, to SP-15, to CV-10, to SP-16, to GB-24 to LV-14, to CV-12. There is also some suggestion of a downward connection to CV-10 from here, which would create a cyclic pattern. Generally, however, the internal trajectory starts from CV-12, passes inside to and permeates the spleen, then comes to and spirally wraps the stomach *(Shisi)*. There it comes up through or along the esophagus to the base of the tongue *(Ima)*. From this trajectory a branch passes to the heart *(Ima) (Shisi)*.

Internal Trajectories of the Heart Meridian

The heart, hand shao yin vessel, starts at the center of the heart, comes out and permeates the supporter of the heart, goes down to and spirally wraps the small intestine. A branch following the supporter of the heart surrounds the throat and passes up to and makes contact with the supporter of the eye. The main meridian following the supporter of the heart goes up to the lungs, comes out below the armpit, and then starts at HT-1 *(LS 10)*.

The heart meridian has its origin in the heart itself, but does not permeate the heart, rather it permeates the "supporter of the heart," probably the aorta and other major blood vessels entering and exiting the heart *(Ima)*. Following the descending abdominal aorta, the descending part of the "supporter of the heart," it passes down to the mesenteric artery and to the small intestine, spirally wrapping the small intestine *(Ima)*. The branch that passes upwards, surrounding the throat, and going to the "supporter of the eyes" (the optic nerve), probably follows the blood vessels passing up into the head, i.e., the carotid artery *(Ima)*. The main meridian passes from the "supporter of the heart," probably along the pulmonary artery, to the lungs and thence to the side of the body, exiting at HT-1 *(Ima)*. A passage from the *Su Wen* tells us how the heart and uterus are related:

> When the menstruation doesn't come, it means that the blood vessel of the uterus is stagnant. The vessel of the uterus, belonging to the heart [meridian], spirally wraps the inside of the uterus. In this case, qi rises up and presses the lungs from the lower parts. The heart qi cannot pass down smoothly, therefore the menses do not come *(SW 33:197)*.

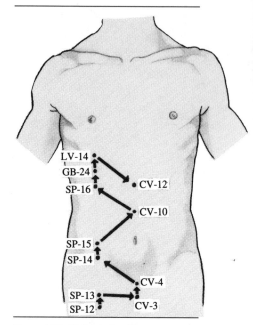

Figure 4.15 Abdominal pathway of the spleen meridian

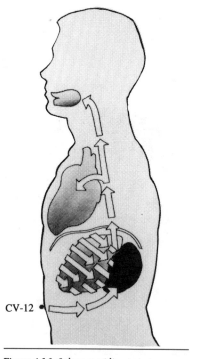

Figure 4.16 Spleen meridian trajectory

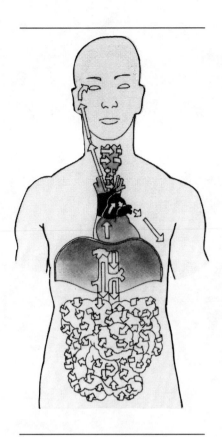

Figure 4.17 Heart meridian trajectory

There are several important distinctions regarding the heart meridian trajectory. The heart meridian does not permeate the heart itself, rather it permeates the "supporter of the heart," which becomes the descending abdominal aorta. This vessel is palpable as the moving qi between the kidneys. The energetic consequences of this distinction are enormously important. We feel that this is making a very direct statement about the energetic nature of the heart, especially about the relation of the heart to the blood and to the shen. As we shall see later in this text, this has a major influence on how we understand the nature of the source 原, the source qi 原氣, the moving qi between the kidneys 腎間動氣, and ultimately the way in which the authors of the *Ling Shu* understood the origins of life. The relationship between the heart and the uterus is very significant. Some authors see the uterus as the place where the moving qi between the kidneys resides. This tends to reinforce the energetic connections that the heart has to this source. Further, it is the superficial trajectory of the supporter of the heart that is the main meridian. This is possibly one reason why many great practitioners have consistently refused to treat the heart meridian directly.

Internal Trajectories of the Small Intestine Meridian

After rising up the arm from SI-1, a trajectory passes to ST-12:

> . . . then it enters ST-12, [passes down to] and spirally wraps the heart. It circles down and around the throat [and esophagus], passes through the diaphragm to the stomach, then permeates the small intestine (*LS 10*).

This trajectory is generally accepted and uncomplicated. The *Lei Jing* author comments that CV-10 is the "place of the small intestine" (*Li Xue*). Thus, it may be reflective of the small intestine.

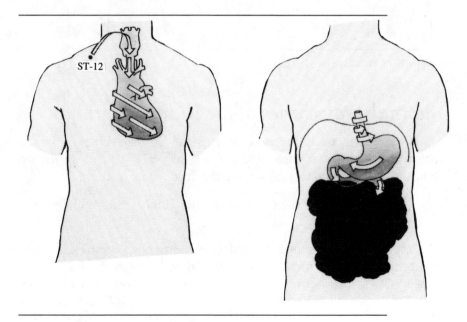

Figure 4.18 - 4.19 Small intestine meridian trajectory

Internal Trajectories of the Bladder Meridian

The vessel of the bladder, foot tai yang, starts at BL-1 and passes over the head. The main meridian is the first line on the back, the shu points line. It then:

> . . . comes down the shu line to the lumbar area and goes into the body, spirally wraps the kidneys, then passes down to and permeates the bladder *(LS 10).*

This quotation is usually understood to mean that after spirally wrapping the kidneys, the trajectory descends through or with the ureter to the bladder, to permeate the bladder *(Ima).* It is possible that in passing from the lumbar area to spirally wrap the kidneys it passes through the renal artery.

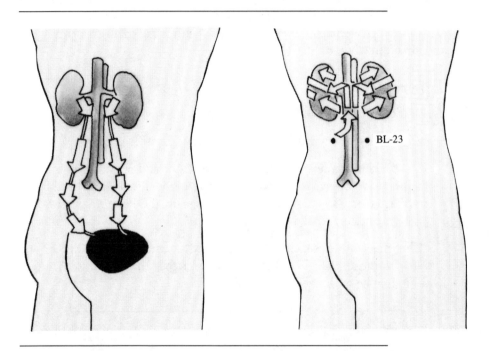

Figure 4.20 - 4.21 Bladder meridian trajectory

Internal Trajectories of the Kidney Meridian

The kidney meridian begins below the small toe, then comes across the foot to the "heart of the sole" (near KI-1), then to KI-2, and up the leg along the kidney meridian pathway. At the thigh it goes interior:

> [It] passes up the spine, permeates the kidneys, and spirally wraps the bladder *(LS 10).*

According to most sources the kidney meridian has a complex series of trajectories. Once the meridian goes internal at the thigh, it passes to the spine at GV-1, then up the spine (an indefinite distance), back down the spine and out to KI-11 *(Shisi).* From KI-11 it superficially passes up to KI-16.

□

At KI-16 an internal trajectory circles backward between the skin and the peritoneum *(Ima)*, almost following the dai mai trajectory. The meridian then enters and permeates the kidneys *(Shisi)*. Then, passing downward through the ureter *(Ima)* to the bladder, it spirally wraps the bladder. This path also passes out to CV-3 and CV-4 *(Li Xue)*.

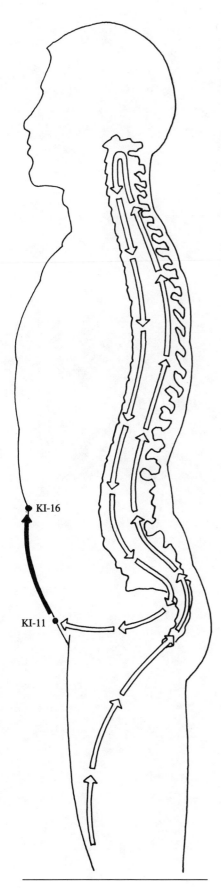

Figure 4.23 Spinal trajectory of the kidney meridian

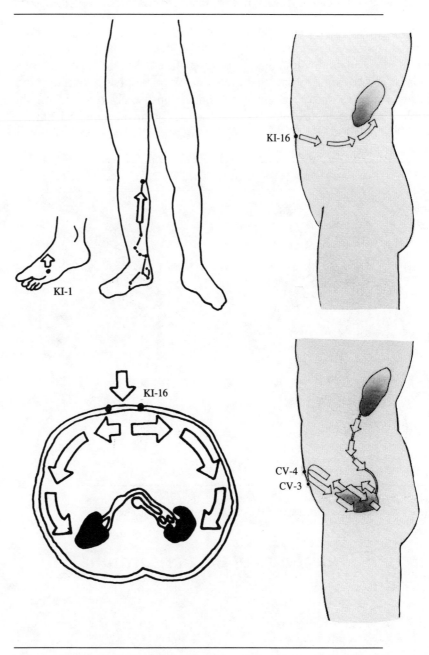

Figure 4.22 Beginnings of the kidney meridian.
Figure 4.24 - 4.25 (Peritoneal) kidney meridian trajectory.
Figure 4.26 Kidney meridian trajectory passing to the bladder.

From KI-16 the external meridian passes up to KI-21. Here, another trajectory goes internally to and through the liver and up through the diaphragm into the lungs *(Shisi)*. There are two main interpretations of the trajectory after it reaches the lungs. The first posits that from the lungs the meridian passes along the pulmonary vein to the heart and spirally wraps

☐

the heart. It further travels to the "inside of the chest," usually seen as CV-17. CV-17 is the reflex point of the "inside of the chest" and may be a synonym for upper qihai *(Ima)*. A second interpretation proposes that the internal trajectory ends at the lungs and that from KI-21 the external meridian passes up to KI-25. From this point a trajectory passes inward to spirally wrap the heart and reach to the "inside of the chest," CV-17 *(Ima)*.

Since Yoshio Manaka's research suggests that KI-25 is a better reflex point, or mu point, for the heart than the traditional point, CV-14,[4] the second interpretation would thus be better justified. Regardless of interpretation, it is interesting to note that the kidney meridian has a trajectory that spirally wraps the heart, an energetic connection usually reserved for the coupled yin-yang meridians. These kidney meridian deviations from the usual relationships have major energetic consequences and ramifications.

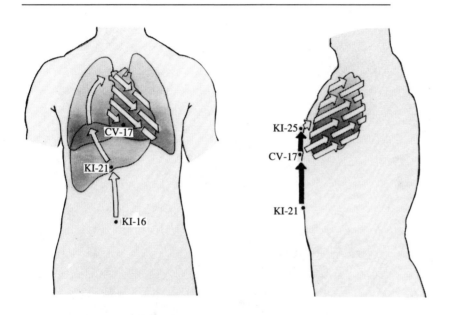
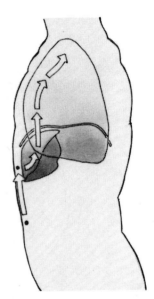

Figure 4.27 Kidney meridian trajectory passes through the liver and lungs to the heart.
Figure 4.28 - 4.29 Alternative interpretation of the kidney meridian trajectory.

Internal Trajectories of the Pericardium Meridian

> The vessel of the master of the heart, hand jue yin, heart-wrapping luo [pericardium], starts at the inside of the chest, comes out and permeates the heart-wrapping luo, passes down through the diaphragm, then timelessly spirals down through the triple warmers *(LS 10)*.

The "inside of the chest" is commonly viewed as CV-17 *(Shisi)*. The internal trajectory starts at CV-17, then passes to the pericardium. From here it passes downwards, probably along the aorta or the esophagus *(Ima)*, through the diaphragm, then "timelessly" spirally wraps the triple warmers.

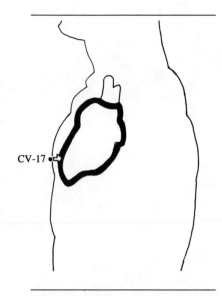

CV-17

Figure 4.30 Pericardium meridian trajectory

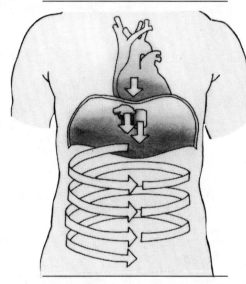

Figure 4.31 Pericardium meridian trajectory

The idea of timelessness offers fascinating insights into the nature of the triple warmers. The character we translate as "timeless," is *li* 歷. This character has a number of different meanings, including "to pass through" and "successively." Our selection of "timeless" is based on the *Nan Jing* and *Zhuang Zi.* We propose that this interpretation ameliorates commonly misinterpreted ideas about the triple warmer and the master of the heart by emphasizing the absolute energetic nature of these concepts. In a discussion relating to the reasons why there are five yin organs and six yang organs, the *Nan Jing* comments:

> The triple warmer has the function of dividing the source qi 原氣 and controlling each of these qi. This has a name but has no form *(NJ 38:3,3).*

Another passage discusses the same problem:

> The master of the heart with the triple warmer are the outside and lining of the body. They have a name but they have no form *(NJ 25:2,12).*

This idea of "no form," in this context, is usually seen to refer to the absence of a physical organ in the body for the set of functions which we identify as the triple warmer. It actually has much deeper implications than the absence of physical substance.

The term "no form," 無形, *wu xing,* is used by *Zhuang Zi.* We feel that the *Nan Jing* references the idea of no form from *Zhuang Zi.*

> Absolute jing 微精 has no form. The jing is tinier than the small [the concept of smallness]. Rough jing has form. No form means that it cannot be divided further.[5]

The idea of no form does not simply refer to absence of material substance. It refers to the essential change of state between matter and energy, to the basic underlying substrate of material substance. Much like the concept of the atom in pre-relativistic physics, or quarks and the multitudinous sub-atomic particles of current physics, it is the theoretical smallest particle of matter. The "absolute jing" is the precursor of matter or form. While it is always delightful to find an idea of such sophistication in an ancient medical text which Western scientific prejudice has overlooked, this is not such a rare idea. Other classical texts have referred to the concept of no form in similar terms and we will meet this idea again in our studies. For now, however, the essential information that we must relate to the interior energetics from classical description is the sense that rather than the attachments of so many imaginary wires, the connections indicated are the confluence of quintessential forces. What occurs at this intersection is not completely described by a terminology that allows us to think of the connection of simple electrical currents. It is more like the opposed coils of a generator or transformer where the currents create a change of state, or a cyclotron where matter becomes energy.

While admitting that the "passing through" translation of the character *li* 歷 is sufficient for the description of the body's interior "wiring diagram," and certainly less subject to the criticism of orthodox translation, it lacks the recognition of the profound relativism of the classical idea of energy. It is not just that the trajectory of the pericardium intersects the triple warmer. The pericardium and triple warmer intertwine and become identical. It is not just that both the triple warmer and pericardium have no material organ. Both are gateways to an energetic environment that is not limited by the boundaries of form. Space, matter, and time are not descriptions that suit the "tiny absolute jing." These are the dimensions of form, not the boundaries of energy.

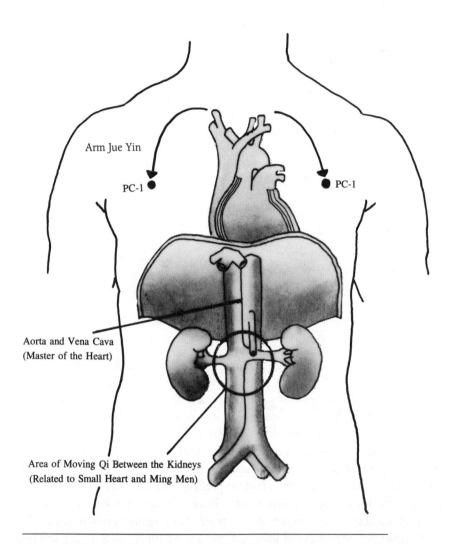

Figure 4.32 The pericardium meridian trajectory comprises three parts, the meridian branches - arm jue yin - the pericardium proper (the protector of the heart) and the master of the heart. Notice the relationships with the "moving qi between the kidneys," the "small heart/ming men," and the kidneys.

We feel at least poetically justified to allow the concept of timelessness to indicate that this deep, interior connection represented for the classical authors a boundary where the particular human energies of the body meet and become the more absolute energies of cosmology.

Regardless of our reader's willingness to accept our feelings that there is a tremendous relativism in the ideas, the fact remains that the master of the heart, the heart-wrapping luo (pericardium) is intimately connected to the triple warmer. It carries out similar functions. There are effectively three distinct aspects of this meridian. The first is the branch, arm jue yin, which emerges at PC-1 and passes down the arms to PC-9. The second is the heart-wrapping luo which is a trajectory that passes only around the heart, in normal usage, the pericardium. The third is the master of the heart. There are many places (for instance *Ling Shu,* chapter 10) where these three names are used in reference to the one meridian.

Diagrammatically these three aspects can be seen as follows: The master of the heart most logically relates to the aorta. It is an extension of the heart; branching from this is the heart-wrapping luo and the arm jue yin.[6] That arm jue yin branches from the master of the heart is something we can derive by inference from an understanding of how the other meridians branch from their main pathways, and from the text of the *Ling Shu:*

> The heart-wrapping luo is the vessel of the master of the heart
> (LS 71:494).

The master of the heart is likely the main pathway, with both arm jue yin and the heart-wrapping luo as branches.

The master of the heart carries out the functions of the shen;[7] the heart stores the shen (SW 23:153). The pericardium, heart-wrapping luo, functions to protect the heart from all types of disturbance (LS 71:494). If the heart is injured, the shen will be disturbed and this will result in death or an incurable disease (SW 14:87); (LS 71:494). The master of the heart functions energetically as a communicative pathway for the shen between the heart and the moving qi between the kidneys.[8] In conceptualizing these pathways and functions, it is even possible to see this pathway as the meridian of the "small heart" or ming men:

> The *Su Wen* says, "At the sides of the seventh vertebra on the inside, is the small heart." Mr. Yang, the writer of the *Tai Su,* says, "There are twenty-one vertebrae in the person. Counting upwards from the lower parts, to the sides of the seventh vertebra, on the left is the kidney, on the right is ming men. Ming men is the small heart." The *Nan Jing* says, "The source of the heart comes out at PC-7; thus PC-7 belongs to arm jue yin. Wrapping luo, helping fire, this is the meridian of the small heart."[9]

This particular passage from Liu Wan Su gives us a significant description of the pericardium meridian, as it is commonly called, and its various internal trajectories. This significance will become clearer in later chapters. For now, however, we may expand our diagrammatic representation of the internal trajectories to the kidney (see last figure).

Internal Trajectories of the Triple Warmer Meridian

Having passed up the lateral aspect of the arm from the ring finger, the triple warmer meridian passes to ST-12:

> [It] comes in at ST-12, then passes down to CV-17, disperses [into the chest], and drops down into the pericardium. It then passes down through the diaphragm, circles down through and permeates the triple warmers. A branch starting at CV-17 passes back up to ST-12 *(LS 10)*.

When the meridian "disperses" into the chest it is like a pervasive spray. The stream widens and becomes less dense, the picture is one of rain covering and moistening rather than a river passing through. Notice also that it does not spirally wrap the pericardium. Rather, it "drops down" as if it filtered through after dispersing from CV-17 into the chest.

This idea helps us see the relationship of the triple warmer to the breathing process. Perhaps this relationship to breath and the movement of breath downward to below the umbilicus is related to the action of "dispersion into the chest." Air is drawn into the lungs upon inhalation; once inside the lungs (inside the chest), it then mingles with the triple warmer pathway which is dispersing into the chest. Then, it filters down to the pericardium. From there it may circle downward through the triple warmers. This downward movement through the triple warmers may well be the means by which the qi of breathing arrives below the umbilicus where it is an important ingredient in the formation of the source qi and the nourishment of the source.

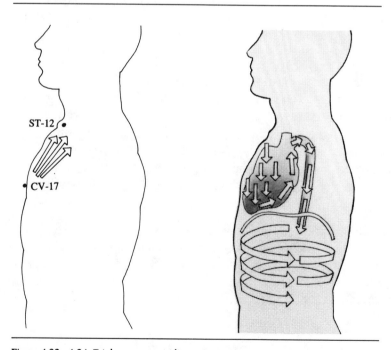

Figure 4.33 - 4.34 Triple warmer meridian trajectory.

Internal Trajectories of the Gallbladder Meridian

Having come down from the head, a trajectory passes to ST-12.

[Thence] it passes to the inside of the chest and then down. It passes through the diaphragm, spirally wraps the liver and permeates the gallbladder. Then it circles round the inside of the lining of the ribs and the side of the body, and comes down to ST-30 *(LS 10)*.

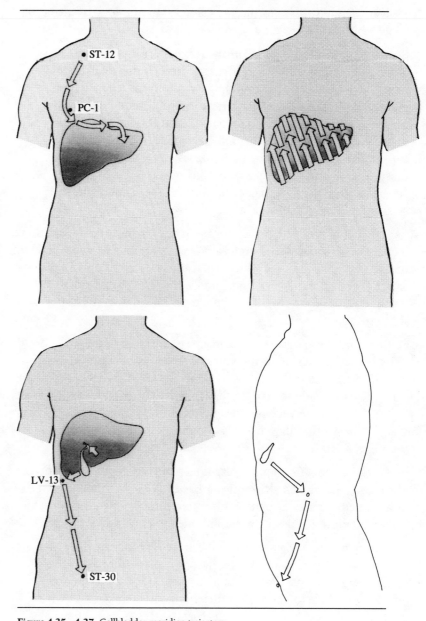

Figure 4.35 - 4.37 Gallbladder meridian trajectory.
Figure 4.38 Side view of the gallbladder meridian trajectory to ST-30.

In this case, "the inside of the chest" is seen as the sides of the chest, around PC-1 *(Shisi)*. In general, we should be aware that the inside of the chest has a wider meaning which depends on context. It can be inside the chest, CV-17, the sides of the chest, as well as some other less common referents. In coming down through the diaphragm it probably passes through the esophagus and then the stomach, before it passes to and spirally wraps the liver *(Ima)*. After this, it permeates the gallbladder. In circling around on the inside of the lining of the ribs and the sides of the body it passes out to LV-13, and then to ST-30 *(Shisi)*.

Internal Trajectories of the Liver Meridian

The liver meridian rises up the medial sides of the legs from the big toes.

> [It then] comes into the yin organs [sexual organs] and circles around the yin organs. Then it passes through the small abdomen; then up to and surrounding the stomach; then it permeates the liver, and spirally wraps the gallbladder. It comes up and passes through the diaphragm, up the sides of the ribs, up behind the trachea, to behind the throat. Then it rises up the cheeks, comes into the eyes, passes up the forehead and meets the du mai at the top of the head. . . . A branch separates from the liver, passes up through the diaphragm, and goes to the lungs *(LS 10)*.

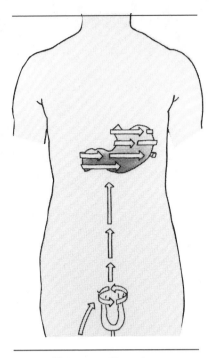

Figure 4.39 Liver meridian trajectory

After circling around the sexual organs it passes into the small abdomen, the kidney reflex area, and an area below the umbilicus described by, or including CV-2, CV-3, CV-4 *(Shisi)*. Then it passes up to and surrounds the stomach, permeates the liver, and spirally wraps the gallbladder. When it passes up and out to the sides, it surfaces at LV-13 and re-enters internally at LV-14 *(Shisi)*.

The trajectory that passes up to and meets the du mai joins at GV-20 *(Shisi)*. The branch passes up to the lungs, then comes down to the middle warmer and "surrounds CV-12" *(Shisi)*. Once at CV-12, the cycle of the twelve meridians is ready to start again, as the lung meridian has its origin at CV-12. This interpretation of the meridians beginning at CV-12 and ending at CV-12 so that they make a complete circuit is one that comes from the *Shisi Jing Fa Hui*.

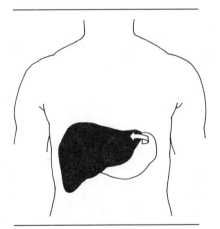

Figure 4.40 Liver meridian trajectory

The *Ling Shu* contains another very different idea about the pathways of the liver meridian which also brings it back full circle to the lung meridian. This interpretation is particularly interesting in that the trajectory includes the du mai and passes up the abdomen to enter the chest at ST-12.

> The liver meridian passes up to the liver. [From the liver] it passes up through to the lungs, rises up to the throat, to the nasal pharynx, to the nose. A branch splits and rises to the top of the forehead, to the top of the head. It then goes down around the spine into the sacrum-coccyx; this is the du mai. [It passes inside and] spirally wraps the yin organs. It passes up to the pubic hairs, [goes up to and] enters the umbilicus, rises up the lining of the abdomen, enters at ST-12, passes down into the lungs and comes out at tai yin [the lung meridian] *(LS 16:186)*.

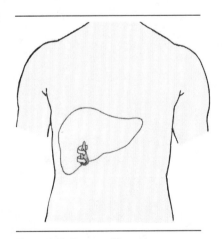

Figure 4.41 Liver meridian trajectory

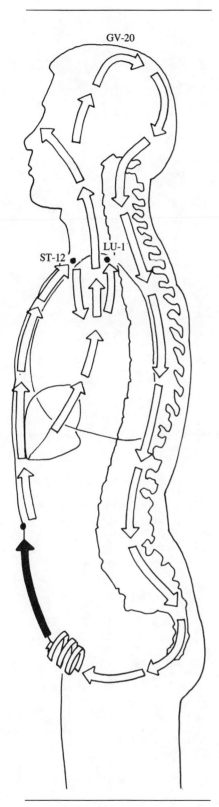

This trajectory is paralleled in complexity only by the kidney meridian, and seems to be even more inclusive, as the du mai is seen as its branch. It is seen to spirally wrap all the yin organs. It definitely provides an alternate route by which the qi passes from the liver to the lung meridian to complete the circuit. Whichever interpretation we accept, we can see that the internal connections of the meridians play an important role in the circulation of the qi through the twelve meridians, beginning at CV-12 and ending at CV-12, or beginning and ending at the lung meridian ready to circle again.

These descriptions from the *Ling Shu* also describe some energetic pathways and connections among the internal organs that are very important if we are to understand in any detail many of the energetic concepts of Oriental medicine. This is particularly true of symptom-sign pictures which are derived from such precise understanding, but which do not usually present such detail. For example, if the "clear qi" derived from the "turbid qi" of the stomach, is to rise to the lungs, an action it is ascribed in modern Chinese medicine, there must be some functional medium by which this occurs. The same is true for all the other internal energetic interactions. The internal meridian pathways are a principal medium for these relations. These sets of connections through internal pathways, which are often the "main" pathways to the branch pathways and the acupoints, are also the source of the energetic relationships we generally describe as the "actions and effects" of acupoints. Thus, the internal meridian pathways are part of the essential knowledge necessary for a theoretical understanding of concepts that have become central to the teaching of acupuncture.

These connections are not, however, the exclusive source of connection or of theoretical understanding. As we shall see later in greater detail, the relationship of the source qi and the source points of the twelve meridians through the triple warmer is also profoundly important.

Figure 4.44 Alternate description of the liver meridian trajectory. Note its relationships to the du mai and possibly the ren mai.

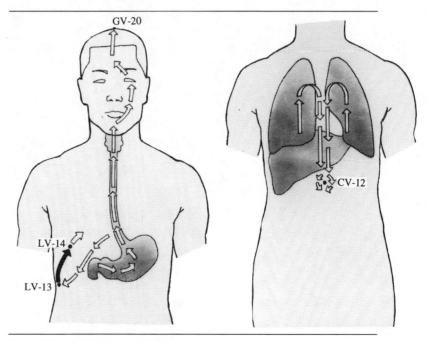

Figure 4.42 and 4.43 Liver meridian trajectory

Chapter

- 5 -

Origins

and

Energetics

Origins and Energetics

In Chinese thought, the concept of an origin or source is very common. It is important to the systems of Chinese astronomy and is mirrored on a smaller scale in the human body. This source is known by many names, but is always essentially the same concept. Since the language in which the source is described is difficult in many ways, the interpretation of the source concept tends to be specialized. Cultural anthropologists find descriptions of cultural trends, students of religion find religious ideas, and practitioners of the meditative arts discover descriptions of meditative experiences. In translated Oriental medical literature the idea of source is often either ignored or left as a vague generalization. Modern medical language in particular finds interpretation of such ideas speculative, and in many ways prefers more precise, if smaller, ideas.

Again we meet with the difficulty of translating a character language where borrowing or re-defining, and the loss of the context necessary to understand the characters as they were used in a particular time and place, complicates the understanding of any passage. Finally, we are faced with the admission that any discussion attempting to interpret very central ideas must be speculative. However, the reasons to shy away from speculation — opposing criticism or interpretation — are not sufficient to vitiate the benefits of speculative discussion. From our efforts to understand the ideas most important to the Chinese who helped create Oriental medicine we may gain broader perspectives, deeper insights, new applications, and increased sensitivity to the refinements of the medicine.

One of the first sciences in which the idea of an ultimate source was developed and discussed was astronomy. In a very early age, as happened in most civilizations, the Chinese recognized that the stars moved in regular patterns. They learned to measure these movements, to make accurate calendars, and to predict seasonal variances that were helpful to an agrarian society. Indeed their records remain today as a source for modern astronomers seeking historic data.

As the earth rotates, the stars are seen to describe near circular patterns around an axis. This axis corresponds to a line that coincides with the axis of the earth's rotation, at about twenty three and a half degrees from the vertical.[1] If we were to stand on the terrestrial north pole and look directly upward for a period of time, we would notice that all the stars revolve around one star that doesn't appear to move. This star is the north pole star and lies almost exactly on the axis of the earth's rotation. Today this star is Polaris, which can be found in the Little Dipper (Ursa Minor) constellation. The south pole star presents the same illusion of centrality in the southern hemisphere.

Polaris was not always the north pole star, nor will it always be. Because the earth is not a perfect sphere, its axis wobbles through a period of approximately 26,500 years, describing an imaginary circle through the heavens. This imaginary circle is what is called the ecliptic. The process is known as the precession of the equinoxes. What results over this period of time is a series of different stars becoming the pole star. For instance, from around 1000-500 B.C. the star Kochab, which is at the the end of the Ursa Minor constellation opposite the star Polaris, was the north pole star around which the heavens were seen to turn. By approximately 13,000 A.D., the star Vega will become the north pole star *(S&C 3:259)*.[2] The Chinese were aware of this precession at least as early as 3000 B.C. .

Needham's research recounts that many other stars were once pole stars and that this function is reflected in their names:

> It is therefore a fact of the greatest interest that we find, along the whole length of the path which it [the pole] has traversed since that date (about 3000 B.C.), stars which have preserved Chinese names indicating that they were at various times pole stars, but later ceased to be so *(S&C 3:259)*.

One of these stars, for example, is *tian shu* 天樞, the pole star in 350 A.D. *(S&C 3:278,281)*. Tian shu lies within the *si fu*, four supports constellation. This was the pole star of the Han dynasty *(S&C 3:260-261)*. Tian shu is also the name of the first star in the big dipper. In fact, several of the stars of the big dipper have relevance for us *(S&C 3:232-233)*.

Thus, we have two stars named tian shu, one of which was once a pole star, and one of which has significance with reference to the pole star. The name tian shu seems to have been a general synonym for the north pole star. It was accorded much significance in the systems of Chinese astronomy.

The *Shi Ming* says that tian shu is "the master of heaven, the north star" *(Mor)*. The *Guan Xiang Wan Zhan* says:

> The first is tian shu; the first is the north constellation. This is the most respectable star of heaven; this string star is the shu [pivot] of heaven *(Mor)*.

Another pole star, or synonym for the pole star, was *zhong ji* 中極, which was thus described by the *Yun Ji Qi Qian*:

> [Zhong ji is] the center of heaven, the highest star. This star is in the best place in the heavens. This is the highest and most respectable; it is the master of many stars *(Mor)*.

Zhong ji doesn't seem to refer to a specific star, it is more a general synonym for the pole star.

Another name commonly associated with the pole star is *tai yi* 太乙. The star tai yi was also a former pole star *(S&C 3:260)*. This name is of particular interest since *tai yi* 太乙 is synonymous with *tai yi* 太一.[3] "The great one," tai yi is also synonymous with *tai ji* 太極 the great, ultimate pole *(Fuj)*. Tai yi, the great one, is another general synonym for the pole star. The *Shi Ji* tells us:

> The middle palace, heaven's ultimate star, the one which is
> bright, is the great one. The position of it is always the same
> (Mor).

The middle palace is the area around the pole star that was seen as the
center of the heavens. The *Shi Ji* informs us that it is synonymous with *zi
gong* 紫宮, the purple palace (Mor).

The *Sou Shen Ji* says that zi gong is "the place where the shen xien
dwell" (Mor). The shen xien are the immortals of Daoist mythology. The
general significance of the great one can be seen in the following quotes
from the *Shi Ji* and the *Lu Shi Chun Qiu*.

> The noble heaven, shen, is the great one (Mor). The myriad
> things emerge and are created in the great one, the alchemical
> changing of yin and yang (Mor).

As the heavens turn around the pole star, the creation of yin and yang was
seen to occur, for the pole star is the very center and thus the origin of all
movement and process in the universe. It is the only place in the heavens
whose "position is always the same."

The one, *yi* 一 is often synonymous with the tai yi; the *Huai Nan Zi* says
of the one:

> The Dao begins at the one.
> The one itself does not create.
> The one divides and then becomes yin and yang.
> Yin and yang unite harmoniously,
> subsequently everything is created (HNZ 3:167).[4]

Tai ji can be seen in a similar vein:

> In tai ji the basic qi is still blending before heaven and earth
> divide.[5]

This idea is very similar to the concept of tai yi as that from which everything emerges and is created, since the basic qi is like the primordial qi
from which all else comes.

The tai yi, the great one, and tai ji, the great ultimate, are nearly
synonymous with one another. The *Yi Jing* references tai ji to the creation
of yin and yang, the dual nature: "The yi has tai ji; this creates the dual
nature."[6]

As the reader has undoubtedly recognized, tian shu is the name of the
acupoint ST-25 found to either side of the umbilicus. Zhong ji is the acupoint CV-3 and tai yi is the name of ST-23. Thus, we have at least three
points on the abdomen which are named after the north pole star or a previous pole star. Zi gong, the purple palace, an area around the pole star, is
also the name of an acupoint, CV-19. Tian shu, tai yi, and zhong ji are
important philosophical concepts as well. They represent the original
movement, the "one" from which spring yin and yang and all else. What
the names of these acupoints indicate is that the Chinese chose to relate an
area in the abdomen to the polar region of the heavens. In some fashion,
they considered this area as a microcosmic reflection of the center of the
heavens. The Chinese envisioned a microcosmic universe in the body that
mirrored the universe itself.

□

This parallel is consistent in the medical context. ST-25 is described as having a pivotal role in the body; metaphorically it is equivalent to tian shu's pivotal role in the heavens:

> Above tian shu is controlled by heaven qi.
> Below tian shu is controlled by earth qi (*SW 68:397*).

In this quotation, tian shu is very probably ST-25, which would accord great significance to this acupoint.

The same parallels exist for tai yi and tai ji. In the eleventh century, the *Tong Ren Shu Xue Zhen Jiu Tu Jing (Bronze Statue Textbook of Acupuncture)* named ST-23 *tai yi* 太一 rather than *tai yi* 太乙.[7] Tai yi, in its known relationship to tai yi the great one, can be seen in the following passage from the famous twelfth century herbalist Liu Wan Su, who quite clearly expresses the importance of tai yi in the body:

> Tai yi is the heavenly true basic qi. It is not yin; it is not yang.
> It is not cold; it is not hot. Inside the jing, qi is created. Inside
> the qi, shen is created. Shen is able to control the form. There-
> fore, jing is the root of the shen qi.[8]

Tai yi as the "heavenly true basic qi" is seen in the same vein as tai ji, the great ultimate. Both ideas attempt to express the ultimate point where the basic qi acts before heaven and earth, yin and yang, divide. Before the qualities of hot and cold, yin and yang exist, there is a single unity and this unity is named and philosophically related to the polar region of the heavens.

The north pole star has many other interesting names and connotations, one of which relates to the emperor and his family. The Chinese emperor was the heavenly child, *tian zi*. He inhabited the middle palace; he was the mediator of heavenly and human affairs. Certain stars around the pole star or found within the middle palace carry the names of the emperor and his family (*S&C 3:260-261*). The Big Dipper, Ursa Major, held something of a similar significance (*S&C 3:241*). Needham describes this figure in the ladle as a "celestial bureaucrat" (*S&C 3:241*).

The big dipper and the pole star were symbolically significant in many ways. Consider Henri Maspero's description of a vision of certain entities in the body as experienced through a particular Daoist meditation.

> On the day of the establishing of spring, at the midnight hour, I
> sit down facing the east; I breathe the breath nine times, I swal-
> low saliva thirty five times. That done, I concentrate upon the
> seven stars of the great bear; little by little they come down
> onto the top of my head. Then, I turn toward heaven, in the
> direction of the handle [of the great bear] . . .[9]

Maspero comments on the whole passage describing this vision:

> We see that the gods come down from the great bear for the
> adept. This is because man and heaven are in fact alike. These
> gods that the adept sees through meditation, sitting upon
> thrones within him, are also the gods who are enthroned in
> heaven and govern the world.[10]

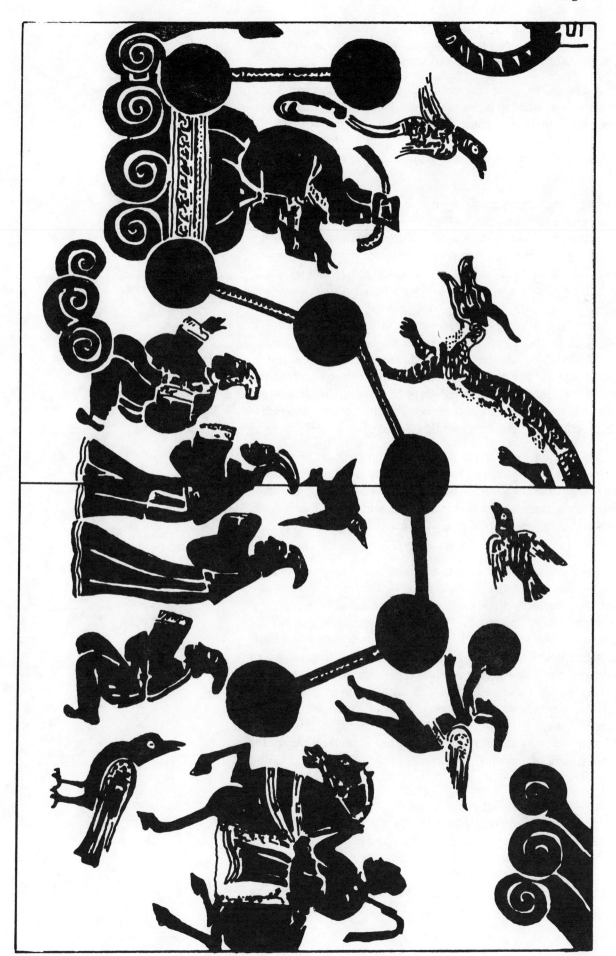

There are other passages that have analagous correspondences and ideas. In describing the "three ones, supreme divinities of the three sections of the body," Maspero quotes a Daoist work:

> The perfect man, the great one, in his left hand holds the handle of the bushel [the big dipper, great bear]; in his right hand the first net of the boreal constellation; that is, the star which does not move [the pole star]. This perfect man dwells within the mysterious cinnabar field that is associated with upper dantian.[11]

These passages describe symbolic figures, but what is most interesting is that phenomena in the heavens had analogous phenomena in people, since we are mirrors of heaven. The details of these correspondences are complicated by the fact that many authors at different times, and even in different areas of China, used a host of different names for the same phenomena. Though compounding the problems of scholarship, the system of correspondences is sufficiently documented to be understood. What then is the crucial importance and significance of the pole star? It represents a fixed center in a moving heaven; thus, it provided a fixed point from which to make observations and measurements. For example, the twenty-eight *xiu,* or twenty-eight mansions, are centered around the pole star (*S&C 3:261*). These mansions represent fixed points relative to the pole star by which the movements of the moon could be gauged and measured. Needham calls these "lunar mansions" (*S&C 3:239*).

We understand these mansions as a system of star boundaries or coordinates by which the moon's relative movements may be measured and as the means by which the twelve branches are delineated. In fact, the temporal sequence of the trigrams, the twelve branches and the four directions, were all seen in relation to the twenty-eight lunar mansions and the pole star (*S&C 3:248*).

The twelve-year cycle of the branches is related to the nearly twelve-year cycle of Jupiter (*S&C 3:402*). The daily cycle of the branches in twelve bihourly periods is related to the division of the day and thus the rotation of the earth around its own axis (*S&C 3:398*). Some scholars propose that the ten stems are also centered around the pole star, with the fifth and sixth stems at the center near the pole star itself.[12] The stems are thus related to the movements of the earth around the sun.[13] The sixty years of the stem-branch cycle appear to be correlated to the conjunction of Jupiter and Saturn (*S&C 3:408*). Aside from the correspondences of the twelve branches to the twelve meridians (*LS 10; NJ 1*), and the ten stems to the five-phase points and organs (*NJ 64; NJ 33*). They were important in medical theory for calibrating and describing rhythmic occurrences in the body, such as the cycling of the wei qi and ying qi (*LS 15; LS 76; NJ 1*).

What is important in the uses of the stems and branches as circumpolar systems is that the astronomical phenomena they reference produce cyclic rhythms on the earth, in particular in the geomagnetic field directly (or through the earth's gravitational field). As such it is possible to see the stem-branch cycles as describing geometrical coordinates within space and time, or within the "space-time continuum." These coordinates, using the north pole star as the most fixed reference point, then used the regular and repeated movements of other celestial bodies, the Sun, Moon, and Jupiter, as further reference points. At any particular time within this geometrical system, specific changes and phenomena were described as occurring in the body. If the geomagnetic field is seen as the main medium for these phenomena, we can find much support in modern literature.[14]

The north pole star, as the central coordinate in this geometrical system, was thus extremely significant. Indeed, many of the important systems or ideas that influenced much of Chinese life and medicine are centered around or based on the pole star. It is probably because of these relationships that the emperor, who was symbolically the center of Chinese culture, was compared to the pole star (*S&C 3:240*). We feel that the deliberate selection of names for acupoints or areas of the body from the vocabulary of astronomy, and the particular symbolism of the pole star, was designed to create symbolic analogies. This is especially true in the relation of tian shu and the pivotal nature of the pole star to the moving qi between the kidneys. This, the central energetic focus of the body, has a pivotal role as the yin-yang, water-fire poles are centered here. We can also think of this as being the "great one."

These relationships are more significant as they are neither partial, nor occasional, but consistent and complete. Several of the big dipper stars are significant as they complete the pole star analogy found in the names of important points in the hara. In particular the second and third stars, (tian) xuan and (tian) ji are important.[15] Xuan ji is the name of an astronomical sighting tube used by classical Chinese astronomers. It was pointed at the pole star, then observations and measurements were made.[16] Also, xuan ji is used to refer to the second and third stars of the big dipper, and is thus a synonym for the big dipper itself (*Mor*). Xuan ji is also the name of the acupoint CV-21. The relationship of CV-21 to zhong ji, CV-3, for example, is speculative, but fascinating. One practitioner in Japan, Naoichi Kuzome, notes that tension of the rectus abdominis muscles (on which lie ST-25 and ST-23, and between which lies CV-3) stresses the rib cage, resulting in a palpable pain around CV-21. Thus, pain found around CV-21 is indicative of tension in these areas and a particular shiatsu technique that relieves this tension.

The fourth and fifth stars of the big dipper are also important. If we examine the etymology of the name of the fifth star, yu heng, we note that *heng* 衡 refers to an astronomical machine used to calibrate the movement of the stars.[17] Heng is associated with another important concept, chuan heng, pivot. Chuan is part of the name of the fourth star of the big dipper, tian chuan. The *Su Wen* explains,

> The qi goes back to chuan heng [the pivot]. If the pivot is normal, the pulse will be normal (*SW 21:139*).

The characters we translate as "pivot" are the same characters used to refer to the fourth and fifth stars of the big dipper. Chuan also refers to the weight on a bar scale; heng also refers to the bar of a bar scale (*Fuj*). The pivot refers to the kidneys or the moving qi between the kidneys.[18] At the least, this concept pertains to a balance of fundamental energies. The relative balance (healthiness) of the qihai dantian area of the hara is the pivot, the relative balance of water-fire, yin-yang in the moving qi between the kidneys.

□

The big dipper was generally called the *bei tou qi xing* 北斗七星 and at times called simply *bei tou*, north constellation *(Mor)*. The *Huai Nan Zi* says of the bei tou:

> The shen of the north constellation has female and male [parts]. The male goes to the left side, the female to the right *(HNZ 3:190)*.

In medical literature, the left side of the body was seen as more yang (male) and the right side of the body more yin, (female) *(SW 5)*. This idea is probably based in part on the quote from the *Huai Nan Zi*.

We can see that not only the specific areas of the abdomen, below and around the umbilicus, were named after highly significant stars and constellations, but also the general nature of the body was reflected in the analogy thus created. Again, these relationships are neither unusual nor isolated, but appear in medical and non-medical literature alike.

There are other energetic considerations that represent extensions of this cosmological model. The umbilicus itself was considered a central focus for the body. This idea also specifically references the north pole star acupoints on the abdomen as well as other important philosophical and energetic concepts that appear as the names of acupoints. The *Yun-Ji Qi Jian* says:

> The umbilicus is the life of the person [represents the living energies of the person].
> One name [for it] is zhong ji.
> One name [for it] is tai yuan.
> One name [for it] is kun lun.
> One name [for it] is te shu.
> One name [for it] is wu cheng *(Mor)*.

Zhong ji is CV-3, tai yuan is LU-9, kun lun is BL-60. Te shu probably refers to tian shu and wu cheng refers to the five mansions on the top of kun lun mountain. Bao Pu Zi says: "On the top of the kun lun mountains, there are the five mansions" *(Mor)*.

In Daoist mythology, the Kun Lun mountain or mountain range was imagined to be at the western end of China in Tibet. This was the origin of the Yellow River and was seen as the origin of the center of early Chinese civilization. It is now given a certain location and said to be a specific mountain range, but there are no ancient maps that show any particular location. Morohashi notes that kunlun is often thought of as kuntun; the two can be seen as synonymous partly because their pronunciation is very similar and partly from etymological considerations. In Daoist mythology kuntun is also very important, as the origin of everything, as a precursor of qi. The *Yun Ji Qi Qian*, apparently quoting the *Tai Su*, states:

> The great origin of nature's qi [before the basic qi divides] are the big rains. It is like the condition of the child of a chicken [an egg]. It is called kuntun. [It is] dark yellow; [it has] no light, no form, no sounds, no voice, no beginning,[19] no roots. Inside this [place] dark [and] deep inside, there is jing. This jing is for certain. [With] the great threads [there is] no longer an exterior, [it is] wide, slow and empty. At the center [of this] deep and dark origin, the one qi is created *(Mor)*.

This is an extremely difficult passage. It is helpful to know that in Daoist mythology the earth was seen as suspended and cocooned within a vast network or web of threads hanging down from heaven that controlled terrestrial events. If we try to analyze this passage completely, we become lost in speculation. However, it is clear that the idea of kuntun and thus kunlun is, like the idea of the pole star, an idea of the origin of everything. Kunlun is the earthly equivalent of the pole star.

The *Huai Nan Zi* supports the interpretation of kunlun as kuntun.

> Everything is madly, hurriedly created; subsequently, there is
> no origin. The river has nine curves and streams to the ocean.
> Subsequently (it) streams without end, because of the transpor-
> tation of kun lun (HNZ 6:3-4).

This is a strong parallel to the idea of kun tun. Kun lun, as the mythical mountain range on which the Daoist immortals dwelled, has tai yuan as a synonym. Morohashi describes tai yuan as the place where the realized person or sage dwells. The *Huang Di Wai Jing Jing* makes reference to it as the place where the sages obtain their sustenance, a symbolic place in heaven where the sage lives, "riding on the dragon's back to travel the five oceans (Mor). The *Can Dong Qi* describes the peculiar qualities of tai yuan:

> The realized person [sage] attains the unusual; it is like some-
> thing; it is like nothing. Wandering at tai yuan, sometimes
> sinking, sometimes floating (Mor).

Tai yuan, as LU-9, is particularly important for us as it is the place of the pulse.

The *Nan Jing* begins with discussions of pulse diagnosis. Initially it seems to be explaining and expanding an earlier discussion from the *Ling Shu*. Here again, we reference the north pole star and the Chinese system of astronomy.

> The Yellow Emperor asked, "What does 'fifty ying' mean?"
> Qi Bo answered, "Heaven has twenty-eight xiu [mansions].
> One xiu equals thirty-six measurements. Thirty-six parts to the
> twenty-eight yields one thousand and eight. During one day [it
> circles through] the twenty-eight mansions. The person's meri-
> dians, pulses are above and below, right and left, front and
> back [totaling] twenty-eight vessels. They circle the body
> [through] 1,620 divisions. Therefore when the person per-
> forms one exhalation, the pulse moves [beats] twice and the qi
> moves three divisions. In one inhalation and one exhalation of
> regular breathing, the qi moves six divisions. In ten breaths the
> qi moves sixty divisions and the day moves two [tenths of a
> degree]. In 270 breaths, the qi moves 1,620 divisions [one
> complete circulation of all the meridians]" (LS 15:182).

As is evident, there is a definite need for some clarification, which the *Nan Jing* author tried to supply. Many of the numbers here have interesting numerological correspondences. At the least, we may determine that the Chinese understood and used a definite parallel of the movements and qualities of the heavens and the movements and qualities of the energies that structured the human body. The pulse reflects these energies as their movements are regular, measured and named through an analogy to the heavens. The *Nan Jing* tell us:

> All the twelve meridians have moving pulses. Using only the division mouth [radial pulse] we can decide the death or life, getting better or worse, of the five yin and six yang organs. How can we do this? Exactly [because] the division mouth is the great meeting place of the pulses, vessels. This is the moving pulse of hand tai yin. Inhaling and exhaling two hundred seventy breaths makes the pulse move sixteen zhang and two forearm divisions. This makes one circulation [of the meridians]. Fifty times a day as thirteen thousand five hundred breaths, the pulse moves eight hundred ten zhang. It starts at [the time of] the tiger [third branch], then comes back and starts again. When the person does one inhalation, the pulse moves three divisions [and with] one exhalation the pulse moves three divisions. With one inhalation and one exhalation, breathed regularly, the pulse moves six divisions; in one day and one night, the person breathes about thirteen thousand five hundred times. The pulse moves fifty circulations through the body. The clepsydra water drips one hundred times; the ying and wei go through the yang [areas] twenty-five times. The ying and wei [move] according to the pulse and go [through the] yin also twenty five times, and then [this] is one circulation. Therefore [they go] fifty times [and] meet again at hand tai yin. Division mouth [the radial pulse] is the beginning and ending place of the five yin and six yang organs *(NJ 1:1-2)*.

This all serves to expand upon the earlier *Ling Shu* discussion. Knowing that one forearm division is ten divisions and that the clepsydra water is a reference to a Han dynasty water clock is interesting, but none of this helps us understand pulse diagnosis very well. The fact that the *Nan Jing* author accorded this strange passage the priority of the first chapter tends to suggest that this is extremely important material. Fortunately, Wang Shu He in his wonderful commentary on the *Nan Jing* is much more explicit in explaining the energetics.

> The meridian is [like] a vertical street [way]. The twelve meridians are the hand and foot three yin and three yang. The three hand yang run from the hands [to] the head; the three leg yang run from the head [to] the feet. The three leg yin run from the feet [to] the chest. The three arm yin run from the chest [to] the hands. The pulse, vessel's origin [root, beginning] is at the moving qi between the kidneys. A source of the moving qi between the kidneys is created inside the stomach [from food]. Gu qi passes [to] the twelve meridians. All twelve meridians have moving pulses; [of these] hand tai yin, foot shao yin and foot yang ming move together and never rest. Using only the division mouth of arm tai yin, we can decide the death or life, getting better or worse, of the five yin and six yang organs. The stomach is the ocean of the five yin and six yang organs. Clear qi comes up [from the stomach] into the lungs. The lung qi

starts at tai yin, [moving] next [to] hand yang ming [and] next
[to] foot yang ming, going around and circling all the meridians
day and night without stopping. In the *Nei Jing:* All [one hun-
dred] of the pulses, vessels meet at tai yuan, LU-9, the point
LU-9 is called division mouth *(NJ 1:1-2)*.

This passage quite elegantly and more clearly explains why we are able
to take the pulse at the radial artery. But, to fully explain the relationships
described in this passage we must go back to the *Ling Shu* theory of clear
and unclear qi to which Wang Shu He refers *(LS 40)*.

Foods are seen as unclear; breath, qi, as clear. The breath comes into
the yin organ part of the body. Foods come into the yang organ part of the
body. Portions of the unclear are transformed into a clear part that rises to
the lungs and exits at the throat. Part of the clear is transformed into an
unclear part that is passed downward to enter the stomach. There, since
the stomach is the ocean of the five yin and six yang organs, this qi passes
to the meridian [probably leg tai yin] and then amasses at the ocean.[20] The
remaining unclear part of the unclear passes into hand tai yang. The
remaining clear part of the clear passes into hand tai yin and then to the
acupoints.

Wang Shu He's explanation is that gu qi is passed to the twelve meridians. This probably represents the unclear part of the unclear. This nourishes the moving qi between the kidneys. This is the hai, ocean, at which
the unclear part collects. The clear qi derived from the unclear rises to the
lungs to become the meridian qi, which enters the lung meridian. This
would be carried via the internal trajectory of the lung meridian from the
acupoints, CV-10, CV-12, CV-13, often seen at the lower, middle, and
upper portions of the stomach, to the lungs:

> Hand tai yin, foot shao yin, and foot yang ming move together
> and never rest.

The constant process of refining and separating the clear and the
unclear is a permanent dynamic function of the stomach and lungs. The
relationship of the stomach and lungs to the meridians, qihai, and the moving qi between the kidneys is the interrelation that drives the pulse. Wang
Shu He seems to be saying that it is because of tai yuan's function that we
are able to measure the wellbeing of the organs. Tai yuan's relationship to
zhong ji, the root of the body, qihai dantian, is the critical connection. The
energetics of breathing and eating center in the moving qi between the kidneys.[21]

Interestingly, tai yuan also refers to the bottom of a waterfall where the
water has worn away the rock. It is a pond created by the force of a moving stream: "All the pulses, vessels meet at tai yuan" *(Fuj; Mor)*. Energetically
and symbolically, the radial pulse is a powerful diagnostic tool because the
hara is an energetic center.

This can be seen diagrammatically as:

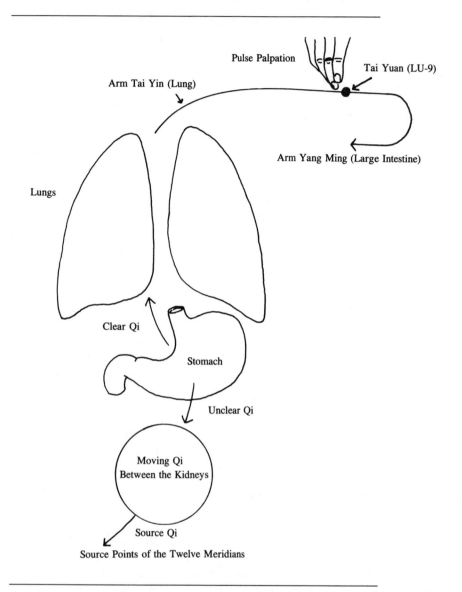

Figure 5.2 Diagrammatic representation of tai yuan - radial pulse palpation and the energetics of breathing, digestion, moving qi between the kidneys, and the source qi.

The area below the umbilicus in all its names and functions — the moving qi between the kidneys, the lower dantian, or qihai dantian — has a vitally important and central role in the body. It is as important to the body as kunlun is to the formation of qi on the earth and as the north pole star, zhong ji or tian shu, or tai yi, is to the creation of yin and yang in heaven.

This importance can also be seen in references to dantian. Classically there were three dantian in the body.[22] The lower dantian, "qihai dantian," is situated below the umbilicus near CV-6 and CV-4. Middle dantian is related to the heart and is situated on the chest, in front of, or near to the heart. Upper dantian is situated between the eyebrows. The dantian are energetic centers at which certain energies are stored, interact, and transform. They are important centers to which the breath is directed and through which it is circulated in Daoist contemplative breathing practices.[23]

Dantian is important in Chinese alchemy, both in external alchemy or early chemistry and in internal alchemy, the process of self-transformation through the pursuit of specific developmental techniques and practices.

The areas in the body more specifically related to the internal practices of alchemy are also symbolic of some of the external alchemies. The difference is not uniquely defined. Dan 丹 refers to cinnabar (HgS, Mercuric Sulphide).[24] This is a red-colored ore that has some peculiar properties. It was mined for early alchemical practices. In fact this must have been a widespread practice. The *Shuo Wen Jie Zi* defines dan thus:

> A red stone from Ba Yue [an area to the north and east of ancient China], it symbolizes digging holes [mining] *(Mor)*.

The origin of the character dan 丹 refers to a mine 丹 in which one finds cinnabar, the ` inside the character dan *(Fuj; Mor)*. The *Shuo Wen Jie Zi* tells us that an alternate form of the character refers to the actual vessel or kiln in which the cinnabar was placed by the alchemists for purification to a more potent form *(Mor)*.

Tian 田 refers to a field, specifically a field tilled to grow food *(Fuj)*. This is how the the common translation of the term dantian, "red fields" or "cinnabar fields" comes to be.

Dan is a substance that was seen to symbolize life itself. There are a number of reasons for this. Partly because of its transformative and mutable qualities, partly because the color of dan in its natural state is bright red, the substance had powerful magical qualities. At certain times in the early history of China, in particular the Zhou dynasty, red was a symbolically important color, the imperial colors *(S&C 5:5)*.

Joseph Needham notes that the practice of alchemy seems to date from before five hundred B.C. *(S&C 5:4)*. The earliest recorded reference to dan comes from the *Yu Gong* chapter of the *Shu Jing (S&C 5:5)* where it was given symbolic significance since the emperor in China during the Zhou dynasty was the heavenly child, tian zi, and held a special position in the religious practices of the people. Needham also comments that the use of red things or painting things red was a "natural piece of sympathetic magic," as red was the "colour of blood, and its ceaseless movement" *(S&C 5:3)*. In the five phases, red symbolizes the phase of fire and fire rules transformation.[25]

Most importantly for our study, jing 精 (or at least the jing qi) is stored at dantian and is distributed to the rest of the body from there. The *Huang Ting Wai Jing Jing* says:

> In the dantian is jing qi; the jing qi disperses [to the whole body] *(Mor)*.

The modern character for jing, 精, has the moon radical in the lower right corner; however, the classical character for jing, 精, had the dan character in that place *(Mor)*. This has important connotations for the nature of jing as well as dantian: 米 is the rice radical, a general term for food. 土 refers to newly germinated young grasses growing in spring. 丹 symbolizes life and living energies. The whole character refers to vital energies in living things, possibly those derived from food *(Fuj)*.

□

The *Shuo Wen Jie Zi* supports this idea, and explains the relation of this to the five phases. In talking about qing, the right part of the jing character which means blue green (cyan), it says:

> Qing is the color of the east direction.
> Wood creates fire.
> Accordingly it [jing] creates dan.
> Believe in dan's creation, this is obvious *(Mor)*.

The author of the *Shuo Wen* was firm about the creation of dan from qing and its parallel to wood creating fire. Wood relates to qing, the color cyan, and the east direction. Life was created in the east, symbolically the origin of everything (the sun rises from the east). This symbolism is stated in the *Su Wen*: "The liver creates at the left side" *(SW 52:275)*. Later the *Nan Jing* associates the east, left side as the reflex area of the liver *(NJ 16; NJ 56)*. Since dan is created from qing, east (wood) naturally symbolizes life, and all the associated symbolism carries over to jing. Needham comments:

> It can hardly be without significance that the bright red sub-
> stance, used in ancient times as what might be called a strong
> magic of resurrection, should have turned out to give rise to the
> most living of the metals, quick (living) silver, metallic mercury.
> It but a small step to see dan as symbolizing life itself *(S&C 5:3)*.

By storing this jing the three dantian take on an important energetic function as storehouses of the qi and jing. By symbolic implication and energetic function, the three dantian are centers of extreme importance. The lower dantian also lies in the same area, the hara, where the other important energetic functions are found.

There is general agreement about the exact location of lower dantian. It is said to be three divisions below the umbilicus,[26] near the acupoint CV-4. Shohaku Honma states that dantian is three divisions below the umbilicus, centered around CV-4 and extending two divisions either side of that point.[27] Passages from Henri Maspero also support the view that the lower dantian is three divisions below the umbilicus.[28] Yang's seventh-century commentary on the *Nan Jing* concurs.[29] However, when known by the name "qihai dantian" a slightly different location is suggested. Since qihai is the name of the acupoint CV-6 and is found one and a half divisions below the umbilicus, the qihai dantian is often located there. Since dantian is more an area extending to CV-6 and centered around CV-4, this location too is consistent.

Again, the implications all point to an energetic center of symbolic and functional import. In Daoist contemplative and inner alchemical practices many practical relationships are suggested. Henri Maspero summarizes the basic theory and practice:

> The human body is indeed a world (microcosm) like the exte-
> rior world, that of heaven and earth as the Chinese say (macro-
> cosm). And it too is peopled with divinities. Life enters into it
> with breath (qi). This breath descending into the belly through
> breathing, there joins the essence (jing) enclosed in the lower
> cinnabar field, and their union produces the spirit (shen) which

is the master principle of man, causing him to act well or badly, giving him his personality. This spirit, unlike what we call the soul, is temporary: formed by the union of breath which has come from the outside and essence which is contained within each man, it is destroyed when these separate at the moment of death; it is reinforced by increasing breath and essence through appropriate practices.[30]

This centrality is further demonstrated by the symbolism of the names of acupoints near dantian in the hara. Qihai, CV-6, is known as the "ocean of qi," implying an energetic reservoir. The *Shuo Wen Jie Zi* supports this interpretation, stating that qihai is "heaven's pond, to which all rivers come" *(Mor)*. Qi flows in the body just as rivers flow on the earth's surface. Qihai is the place to which all rivers flow.

More than just a center of energies, qihai dantian is the center from which the energies emanate. This can be seen, for example, in the triple warmer function of carrying source qi from the center to the extremities, the source points of the twelve meridians *(NJ 66)*. It is also the center from which healers derive their energy used for healing. Two of Japan's most famous acupuncturists, Sorei Yanagiya and Keiri Inoue, used non-insertion needle techniques, utilizing qi alone to stimulate the acupoints.[31] There are many more examples of qi gong masters, martial artists, and healers who attribute their abilities to the cultivation of this center.

Dantian is focussed around guan yuan, "the gate of basic," CV-4. The name guan yuan also has considerable significance. Bunshi Shiroda, a modern scholar and practitioner, tells us that CV-4 was seen as the "lower regulator":

> The upper regulator is wei wan [CV-12].
> The lower regulator is guan yuan [CV-4].[32]

He also notes that CV-4 is called dantian and quotes Kisei Matsui as saying "dantian is the secure place of the master of the heart."[33] The most significant aspect of the name is the relationship of yuan 元 (basic) to the basic qi, the original or fundamental qi, one of the most fundamental energies of the body, indeed of the universe itself.

According to the *Zhou Yi*, basic qi precedes the division or separation of heaven and earth:

> The great ultimate, tai ji, is where the basic qi is still blending or swirling before heaven and earth are divided.[34]

The *Shuo Wen* says of the basic qi:

> The basic qi divides.
> The light, clear, yang part becomes heaven.
> The heavy, unclear, yin part becomes earth.[35]

Heaven and earth arise from the division of the cosmic or basic qi.

There are many ideas about basic qi. It has been seen to arise from several sources and bring about a number of different effects:

The basic qi is the beginning qi of the great transformation.[36]
The dao is the basic qi.[37]
Space creates the basic qi. Basic qi has boundaries [limits].[38]

As these expressions show, basic qi is a broad concept. The great transformation probably refers to the division of yin and yang, from the primordial source, tai yi. The second quote is one of many that demonstrate the importance of the concept of basic qi in Daoism. Interestingly, we are told that basic qi arises from the void, space, but is not limitless. In this sense basic qi is an underlying qi, the division of which produces other forms of qi, yin, and yang. Classically it was related to the process of birth and death, in particular to the cycles of birth, death, and rebirth:

> All living things have qi, they are born and then they die. This is the common cycle of heaven and earth. This is nature. Death is when the basic qi leaves the body and the hun disperses, returning to the root, returning to the beginning, returning to the cycle.[39]

An examination of yuan 原, source, is also revealing. The *Chun Qiu* defines yuan as the source and *ben* 本, the root or basic part.[40] Basic qi is almost the same as source qi except that source qi is more active in the interaction of prenatal and postnatal qi. The basic qi is a somewhat more primordial concept, related to the creation of life itself. As Sugiyama says, "The basic qi of before heaven [prenatal qi] is said to be the moving qi between the kidneys"[41] Thus, basic qi is the source of the source qi. Quoting from the *Chun Qiu Wei Yuan Ming Bao*, the authors of *Ki No Shiso* tell us, "The basic has limits and is also the spring of qi."[42]

The effects of the basic qi are explained in the following passage quoted from Shinsai Ota, a late seventeenth-century practitioner of *anma*, traditional Japanese massage:

> If the basic qi of the body stagnates, disease will result. If the basic qi cannot move, it means impending death. How do we get stagnation of the basic qi? It is from of overwork of the heart and shen or just from overworking (psychological or physical stress). If one has a lot of self-serving desires, the basic qi stagnates. Overeating, drinking too much alcohol, too much sexual desire, [exposure to] too much wind, cold, heat, dampness or physical trauma, all cause the basic qi to stagnate. When the basic qi stagnates, the shen qi loses its freshness. This causes disharmony of the five yin and six yang organs; the blood and vessels become stagnant; the joints lose flexibility; the muscles become tense; the skin becomes dry or edematous.[43]

Virtually all pathologies are seen as stemming from stagnation of the basic qi. This passage expresses quite clearly the underlying, undifferentiated form of the basic qi.

That there is a point on the abdomen called guan yuan, implies for this point a very significant role or symbolic function. As with dantian and qihai, guan yuan may symbolize life. These points and areas all lie at the energetic center of the body at the moving qi between the kidneys.

Through their names and associated symbolism, they may be seen symbolically as belonging to the center where the source is located.

There are also a number of points on the back at the same level as these points on the abdomen. Qihai shu, BL-24, and guan yuan shu, BL-26, are probably related to CV-6 and CV-4. Often, these points are checked for reactions when CV-6 or CV-4 are reactive on palpation. It is possible that these two points treat the problems that create the reactiveness on CV-6 or CV-4. Ming men, GV-4, is also related to these points and this area in the abdomen. It too shares a relation to the energetic center and the origin of life:

> The person is created on the earth, the 悬 [thread that hangs
> down to hook onto the] ming, in heaven. Heaven and earth
> meet the qi; it is called the person (SW 25:159).

This is a difficult passage. The character 悬 is the modern form of 懸, which commonly means to "hang" or "suspend." Thus, the passage refers to the creation of the person and the suspension of personal life (ming) from heaven. The character 懸 specifically refers to a thread that hangs down to hook onto something (Fuj). This usage recalls the Daoist creation story that explains the relation of heaven, person, and earth. In this story, ji 機, "heaven's loom," weaves the threads, the jing (vertical threads, meridians) of the fabric of the universe (Kad).[44] This may be related to the other Chinese concepts of meridian cycles controlled by the cycles of the stars and constellations.[45]

The term ji, in other Daoist contexts, refers to the idea of a "germ." Here, germ implies the sense of "germ cell" or "germination," the source of life. The *Zhuang Zi* contains an interesting discussion that appears to be a theory of evolution. All things start at the ji, the germ, changing into larger creatures, ultimately producing man. Needham offers an excellent translation of this passage (S&C 2:78-79). Similar articles may also be found in the *Lie Zi*: "All things come out from the germ and return to the germ."[46] These ideas at least hint at the microscopic origins of life. Both these ideas of ji may well be the same. The threads may be thought of as a germ too, producing the same effects in living things.

A passage from the *Huai Nan Zi* raises more questions about our understanding of this term.

> The realized man [the sage] is able to attach or connect to tian ji
> [heaven's loom, heaven's germ] inside the body (HNZ 1:74).

This may be referring to a cultivated ability to connect with the threads from heaven, or the *Ling Shu* concept of ming. Thus, we should not think of the threads as literal threads, but as some kind of energetic connection. This is important in this context because there are two points on the back which relate specifically to this idea. Ming men, GV-4, lies below the point xuan shu, GV-5. If we take the *Su Wen* idea of the thread suspending ming from heaven, we can see this in these two points. The thread suspends the ming, life, at ming men from xuan shu. As we will see in the next chapters, ming men is intimately tied to the ideas of the water-fire interaction as the "small heart," the active aspect of water, the source, and the moving qi

□

between the kidneys. While this too is interpretive, we see once again the implication of a very significant and symbolic function in this area of the body below the umbilicus, the hara.

Transformations

The classical concept of a source is like a puzzle, each piece joins and supports the others. We see the hara as the place where many essential energetic functions occur. It is the residence of basic qi, that energy that precedes yin and yang, fire and water. It is the meditative center, the driving force of the pulse, the center of meridian circulation, and it plays a powerful role in classical nutrition theory. The hara is associated with jing, shen, qi, the essential energies; it is related to major philosophical concepts: middle palace, purple palace, heavenly child, trigrams, branches, stems, and the dantian. Some of the most important acupoints — CV-3, CV-4, CV-6, CV-12, CV-17, CV-19, CV-21, ST-23, ST-25, LU-9, BL-60, are either named as part of the philosophical concepts related to the hara, to its functions, or to both. As we have seen, the interior branches of the meridians interweave the abdomen in a fine tapestry.

While it is true that we must speculate to understand much in the classical literature, the philosophical centrality of the hara is hard to deny. Yet, if we carefully consider the work of the classical authors, we may also see that there is another consistent theme: transformation. The area below the umbilicus, qihai dantian, as well as the other dantian in front of the heart and between the eyebrows, are areas particularly associated with transformation. In regards to nutrition, energetic anatomy, and qi function, the abdomen is where essential transformations occur. This idea, though requiring some interpretation, is particularly reinforced by Daoist alchemical practices.

Transformation is a difficult cause to champion. The misconceptions and misrepresentations that have plagued the ideas of alchemy and transmutation have colored the word with derision. For many, the idea is superstitious nonsense. However, there are ways we can think of transformation that are worth our investigation. It is possible, for example, to think of transformation as simply the processes of digestion and respiration where elements of the environment are utilized by the body. It is also possible to think of transmutation as the result of the processes of nuclear fission and fusion where chemical elements are transformed by the emission of subatomic particles. However, it does not always take nuclear reactions, as we currently know them, to cause transformation.

Scientists in the last few decades have demonstrated beyond reasonable doubt that life can transform chemical elements according to need. Much of the research work done has centered on plants; however, animals and humans also demonstrate this ability. Louis Kervran, a well-known and respected French scientist, has led the field in this research.[47] He conducted much of his own research and compiled the results from a large number of other studies. These studies range from the geophysical to the microorganismic and include research on industrial accidents, agriculture, plant development, and bone mending. His conclusions provide a startling challenge to our lay understanding, demonstrating that the old chemical theories of Lavoisier are outmoded and do not apply in biological systems.

Scientists have, until quite recently, assumed that chemical elements are immutable; that is, in a chemical reaction, nothing is lost, nothing created. Instead, all the elements of the reaction are changed from one state to another, retaining the integrity and structure of the basic building blocks, the atoms. This assumption is based on the idea that atomic interaction occurs only by the exchange of electrons from the outer orbits of the atom.

Kervran has shown that in biological systems, there are other fundamental reactions involving the exchange of protons from the core or nucleus of the atom. One chemical element, for instance Sodium, can be transmuted to another element, Potassium. These changes are mediated by biological reactions and catalysts, such as enzymes, and do not require the enormous power involved in nuclear fission and fusion. Kervran postulates that this function is essential to the continued survival of living things, an essential part of life's adaptability.

Most biological transmutations occur within the first twenty elements of the periodic table and to a lesser degree with the next ten.[48] Some examples he cites are the abilities of man's physiology to transmute Nitrogen to Carbon and Oxygen, Sodium to Potassium, Sodium to Magnesium, Iron to Manganese and vice versa. Animals such as chickens are able to transmute Potassium to Calcium, and rats Calcium to Magnesium. In plants, Phosphorus to Magnesium, and Manganese to Iron transmutations occur.[49] The list of examples is large. What it evidences is that the basic building blocks of matter are not immutable and are constantly changing. As Kervran says:

> Most of the reactions studied can occur with the movement of
> an atom of Hydrogen or an atom of Oxygen, thus with the
> addition or subtraction of H or addition or subtraction of O.[50]

The greatest source of Hydrogen and Oxygen is water. Thus it would follow that water is a substance essential in these transmutations. This mirrors the nature of water in Chinese thought. The *Dao De Jing* states:

> Under heaven, nothing is more soft and yielding than water.
> Yet for attacking the solid and strong, nothing is better. It has
> no equal. The weak can overcome the strong.[51]

At times the Daoist literature expresses the mutability of water obscurely. An interesting and potentially important passage from the *Huai Nan Zi* compares the nature of heaven and earth, brightness and darkness, fire and water:

> The dao of heaven is round.
> The dao of earth is square.
> The square controls the darkness.
> The round controls the brightness.
> Brightness is like blowing qi.
> Therefore, fire is the outer shadow.
> Darkness is absorbing (containing) qi.
> Therefore, water is the internal shadow.
> The blowing qi is nourishing.
> The absorbing (containing) qi alchemically transforms.
> Therefore yang is giving,
> and yin is transforming *(HNZ 3:133)*.

The parts of the passage we want to focus on are the fifth through eighth lines. Various commentators contend that the "outer shadow" refers to the shadow that is cast by a light source, such as a fire. The energy or light from the fire emanates outwards, "blows out," casting its shadow externally. These commentators note that the "internal shadow" refers to the shadow that can be seen in water, a reflection. The light is reflected from the water and the shadow appears internally, as if floating in the water. Not only does this important reference express the classical conception of the inherent difference between the symbols water and fire, it also expresses the mutability of water.

If we can recall our own youthful playing in ponds we will remember that when different objects are placed by the water the reflection will change. If the water is disturbed, the shadow or image in the water will change. Water has, in this sense, the ability to transform the image. Thus, in terms of the passage "the absorbing qi alchemically transforms," and the nature of yin is "transformative," we see the classical idea of transformation described through the metaphor of the subtle, moving changes of a reflection. The changing image, the interior shadow, stands for the process of transmutation.

There are passages in the medical literature that state similar principles: "Water can alchemically transform everything."[52] The relationship between the great symbols fire and water and their associated functions — the kidneys, heart, master of the heart and triple warmer, the interaction of the jing, qi, and shen — are the relationships of transmutation. The Daoist alchemists utilized these elements in their techniques of internal alchemy. This concept of transmutation was the one that the medical authors most probably presupposed in their theoretical discussions. We are thus able to understand that the Chinese concept of transmutation, the result sought through their alchemies, carries none of the gross misperceptions that have come to be associated with the word. Instead, they understood that subtle processes of transformation occurred within the human body, that these processes were important to human life, and were part of the general nutritive, yin, category of events.

While we cannot say, nor expect, that the ancient Chinese medical authors were aware of biological transmutation in the sense of modern language and principles of science, we can say that their observations and theoretical principles lead them to suppose and attempt to describe in their own symbols the ability of living beings to transform. Perhaps, in the light of the accomplishments of Kervran and his associates, we can realize that the ideas of alchemical practices and transformations are not so bizarre. Kervran suggests that his ideas and findings challenge modern relativistic and quantum theory, by showing that it cannot be applied to living things or biological processes. These basic transformations at low energy levels differ from the exchanges studied in high energy physics.[53] It is not that the general laws of nuclear physics cannot be applied to biological systems, more that these laws are not the exclusive explanation of transformative events. There are definitely similarities in these processes, though fundamentally of different energetic orders.

□

That biological transmutation or transformation is a concept and phenomenon seen in Chinese thought, complements those parts of Chinese theory that parallel the modern ideas of quantum physics. Detailed examination of Daoist and medical concepts reveal ideas quite similar to concepts and ideas that are basic to our modern conception of the physical world. In the Chinese model, *bian*, change 變; *hua*, alchemical transformation 化; *xing*, form 形; *wu xing*, no form 無形; *shen*, spirit 神; *qi*, 氣 each exemplify aspects that suppose a far more sophisticated understanding of physical nature than we might expect.

Translations of most of Oriental energetic terminology into simple English equivalents is usually fruitless, an almost impossible task. Simple renditions of qi as "energy" did work to facilitate communication of the earliest understandings, and basic concepts, of a complex symbol, but should not be taken too literally. The connotations attached to the English words are sometimes subtly, sometimes grossly different than those of the concept as it was used traditionally. The idea of "no form" is, for example, a very complex term that is not clearly understood if we think of it as a simple absence of substance. In the *Nan Jing* the triple warmer and master of the heart are said to have a "name but no form" *(NJ 25; NJ 38)*. From this comes a pervasive idea of the triple warmer and master of the heart as "insubstantial organs." This, although "correct" and "properly translated," is far too incomplete to stimulate an appropriately profound understanding of the idea; an idea we must explore in detail if we are to gain a reasonable understanding of how the Chinese saw the processes of change and transmutation.

Zhuang Zhou conceived of no form as absolute jing, the tiniest nondivisible, underlying jing, the underlying substrate of material things.[54] This concept ascribes to the triple warmer some important properties and implications. In addition, the concept of no form has been discussed by a number of classical authors. There have therefore been a number of different ideas about the nature of no form. Although slightly different in their detail, all refer to the same concept: the pure energetic, immaterial precursor of both animate and inanimate matter. Some of these discussions remind the reader so much of the modern relativistic model that it is impossible not to think of no form in those terms.

To reiterate what Zhuang Zhou said:

> Absolute jing has no form. The jing is tinier than [the concept of] smallness. Rough jing has form. No form means that it cannot be divided futher.[55]

Zhuang Zhou, one of the earliest and most famous Daoist masters, seems to be talking about the non-divisible components of matter. The idea of "absolute jing" is almost atomic in nature, perhaps even sub-atomic. Modern physicists tell us that matter and energy are hard to distinguish. We cannot really say that atoms or subatomic particles are material or energetic; they are both and in some sense neither. How they are perceived is dependent on the model, measurements, and techniques used to study them. Yet it is from these basic building blocks that material things are constructed. Thus, in the terminology of Zhuang Zhou, form is composed of something that is insubstantial: no form.

□

There are other ideas about no form. The *Shi Ji,* the book of history, tells us:

> The Daoists cause the person's jing and shen to become one, to move and unite with no form *(Mor).*

Here the term no form is seen in a Daoist context, relative to some Daoist practice. Another Daoist text, the *Huai Nan Zi* from 122 B.C., makes numerous references to the concept of no form. From these we gain greater insight into the nature of no form:

> No form is the great ancestor of matter.
> No sound is the great ancestor of the voice.
> The child [of no form] is light.
> The grandchild [of no form] is water.
> All are created from no form *(HNZ 2:59-60).*

Because of the grammatical structure of these lines we can see this passage as referring to no form, the parent, giving birth to light, the child, and in turn to water, the grandchild.

This passage is describing the materialization of no form, the precursor of material things, from the point at which it cannot be perceived, to a perceived state, light. It then evolves to a materialized state, water. This is remarkably similar to Einstein's idea about the interchange of energy and matter. In this concept, as energy is slowed down it becomes more material. As matter speeds up, it becomes more energetic. Matter and energy are seen as being interchangeable, undergoing changes or transformations back and forth. The same passage from the *Huai Nan Zi* continues:

> Light can be seen; it cannot be grasped. Water can be molded;
> it cannot be destroyed. Therefore, of all things that have
> matter, nothing is more respectable than water *(HNZ 2:59-60).*

Water is again seen as the highest, first, or most respectable material manifestation. This was so clearly understood that it was referred to as obvious: "No form thus creates form, this is obvious" *(HNZ 105).*

Form and no form were found in the Daoist concepts of life, death, and rebirth:

> The form is the abode of life.
> The qi is the fullness [plenitude] of life.
> The shen is the controller of life *(HNZ 77).*

The material manifestation, the form, the body, is the dwelling place of life filled with qi and controlled by shen. No form, on the other hand, was seen in relation to the one, to tai yi.

> It is said, no form is said to be of the one. It is said that the one
> cannot be compared with anything below heaven *(HNZ 61).*

The "one" is the great one, the origin of change and transformation, yin and yang and all things. No form was seen to derive from, or be related to, the great one:

□

All the myriad things, all of them, can be placed in one category. The roots of all material things come out from one gate; its movement is no form; its hua [alchemical transformations] and bian [changes] are like shen *(HNZ 2:62-63).*

No form is the great ancestor of matter, it is that part of the great one which gives rise to matter and all things. The shen is the other part of the great one, which governs and controls the transformations and changes of no form. The interaction of shen with no form, or the derivatives of no form, was seen to be the constant recycling of life and death.

The form, the material things that are derived from no form, also revert to no form:

> Therefore, when the form declines, the shen which [itself] is never alchemically transformed, responds by alchemically transforming [the form]. [Even with] a thousand changes and ten thousand transmissions, it has not yet begun to polarize. [The form that is] alchemically transformed returns again to no form. [The shen that is] never alchemically transformed dwells together with heaven and earth *(HNZ 338).*

Shen as the eternal unchanging principle constantly transforms no form to form at conception and birth and form to no form at death. The passage continues:

> Upon the death of a tree, [the one that made the tree] green leaves the tree. [The one that made] the tree alive is not the tree itself. [The one that makes] the form full is not the form itself. Therefore, [the one that] creates life never dies. [The one that] was created will die. [The one that] alchemically transforms things has [itself] never been alchemically transformed. [The one that] has been alchemically transformed, can be alchemically transformed [is mortal] *(HNZ 338).*

This idea is described again in another passage from the *Huai Nan Zi*:

> [The one that] creates life, never dies, and [the one that] alchemically transforms things, is not [itself] alchemically transformed *(HNZ 120).*

Life and death were seen as transformations back and forth. The shen, which catalyzes or controls the transformations, remains unchanged.

The *Lie Zi* supports the *Huai Nan Zi* interpretation of the cycling of no form between life and death:

> "Having form" [life] is created by no form. [The state of] "having form" returns to no form upon death.[56]

Zhuang Zhou says similar things about life and death. For him, change, bian, rather than alchemical transformation, hua, characterizes the changing or transformative process of life and death:

> If one thinks about the beginnings [of everything], then they basically have no life. Not only no life, but basically no form. Not only no form, but basically no qi. The beginnings are

blending in a dark unclear place. They change and there is qi.
The qi changes and there is form. The form changes and there
is birth. [Then] it changes and passes to [the state of] death.[57]

Understanding the differences between change, bian, and alchemical
transformation, hua, is important for understanding these different but
parallel ideas from Zhuang Zhou and the *Huai Nan Zi*. Bian is more like a
change in nature, almost in the way that one season slips into another, or
how yang at the extreme changes into yin. Hua is a radical change, a
transformation of one thing to another, more in the alchemical sense of
transforming or transmuting one substance to another. The transformations described by Kervran, or the transformation of a seed at germination,
more aptly describe hua.

These differences can be seen in the medical literature and mirror the
polar differences between yin and yang:

> When substance is created it is said to be alchemically
> transformed. When substance reaches its limit it is said to be
> changed. Yin and yang cannot be measured, they are called
> shen *(SW 66:361)*.[58]

This can be seen in relation to the passage from the *Huai Nan Zi*:

> Its hua and bian are like shen *(HNZ 2:62-63)*.

Bian and hua, the yin and yang aspects of change, are like shen.

> Yang alchemically transforms qi; yin becomes form *(SW 5:32)*.

This sentence has been understood in a variety of ways. For instance, the
Lei Jing comments:

> Yang moves and disperses, therefore it alchemically transforms
> qi. Yin rests and contracts, therefore it becomes the form.[59]

Li Zhang Zi comments:

> Yang has no form, therefore it alchemically transforms qi. Yin
> has substance, therefore it becomes the form.[60]

Yin and yang were seen in relation to no form and its transformations.
This returns us to no form in relation to the great one, the center of the
universe, the origin of everything. That no form is related to the tai yi may
be seen again in a passage from *Lie Zi*:

> Form was created from no form. The clear and light [part of
> no form] rose up to become heaven. The unclear and heavy
> [part of no form] went down to become earth *(Mor)*.

The clear, qing, and unclear, zhuo, are themselves dual or polar concepts
closely synonymous with yin and yang. The *Su Wen* tells us: "Therefore
the clear yang becomes heaven, the unclear yin becomes earth" *(SW 5:32)*.
As we have already seen, the tai yi is the north pole star and is synonymous
with tai ji. Both may be seen as the source of all things:

> The myriad things emerge and are created in the great one,
> the alchemical changing of yin and yang.
> Tai ji is the one in which the basic qi is still blending
> together before heaven and earth divide.[61]

□

At the least, we may propose that these creation theories in the medical context describe the interaction of yin and yang, jing, and shen, their changes and transformations, as fundamental to both matter and life.

On a macrocosmic scale shen activates or transforms the jing (no form) to become matter. On a microcosmic scale, the shen activates or transforms the jing (no form) to become a living being. These transformations are mirror images of each other, occurring at the tai yi. Tai yi is on the one hand symbolic of the north pole star and on the other hand is the energetic center of the person below the umbilicus, the moving qi between the kidneys. This makes sense of the comment from the *Shi Ji*:

> The Daoists cause the person's jing and shen to become one, to move and unite with no form (Mor).

In Daoist alchemy one uses breath to bring this about. In Chinese medicine this is one of the functions of the triple warmer. This is why the triple warmer has a name but no form (NJ 38) and is rooted at the moving qi between the kidneys (NJ 8).

What then are we to make of this interwoven, complex and detailed mass of symbols and metaphors? Throughout the whole of Chinese thought, astronomy, meditation, nutrition, and medicine, the idea of a source is pervasive. The thought that the hara, the abdominal center of the processes that create and transform life, is the parallel in the human being of the ultimate universal source is absolutely pervasive. Acupoint names, nutritional theory, meditative practices, the pulse, the most essential and basic theories of qi, jing, and shen, each point to the abdomen as the source. The overall image that is provided by the early Chinese concepts of heaven and earth, form and no form, is that of a complete mirror image in the person of the universe itself. The observations and symbolic functions of the stars, the movements of the heavens, are reflected by name and function in the hara. The transformations that were thought to occur in the universe take place, in human scale, in the vital center of energies, the tai yi of the being. Although the language is far more metaphoric, more replete with symbols and images, than is the language of modern science, there is surprisingly little difference between the ancient Chinese theories and our own.

But, is this fair? Can we, a so-called modern people, possessed of mental habits and attitudes that are distinctly not Chinese, interpret the ideas of Chinese philosophy and medicine through the filters of our own philosophical and theoretical understanding? Some, of course, say no, we cannot. To some extent the Chinese of the last two decades concur by rejecting the "chains of correspondence" in their own philosophical history in favor of the empirical pragmatism of pre-relativistic Western science. The answer must be that the question itself is full of impossible presumption. We have no choice but to interpret through our own understanding. There is no other form of study available to us; we can not become ancient Chinese. No vastness of scholarship can restore the essential suppositions and cultural *sine qua non* of the generative age of Chinese medical theory. The choice is, shall we presume that Chinese thought, being ancient, must be interpreted through our own oldest and most pervasive suppositions, or shall we interpret it through what seems to us to be the most useful ideas

□

of our own time? In short, we can choose, if we wish, to use the layman's understanding of a fixed, material reality to relegate the complex tapestry of Chinese concepts of creation to the pseudosciences. Or, we may apply the philosophical understanding of our own age to what we find. To us, nothing less will do justice to the refinement of these Chinese ideas.

David Bohm, for example, describes a "hidden," "enfolded," or "implicate order" from which the observable world emerges. His descriptions remind us of many of the Chinese ideas. The implicate order is enfolded into what we call "space." The explicate order, the manifest things, are but ripples on the vast sea of energy enfolded into space. As Bohm himself says:

> What we perceive through the senses as empty space is actually the plenum, which is the ground for existence of everything including ourselves. The things that appear to our senses are derivative forms and their true meaning can be seen only when we consider the plenum in which they are generated and sustained, and into which they must ultimately vanish. This plenum is, however, no longer to be conceived through the idea of a simple material medium, such as an ether, which would be regarded as existing and moving only in 3-D space. Rather, one is to begin with the holomovement, in which there is the immense "sea" of energy. . . . This sea is to be understood in terms of a multidimensional implicate order.[62]

This "immense sea of energy" invokes Chinese concepts such as the "sea of qi" and the "yuan qi," the basic or "enfolded qi," an unobservable matrix or order from which all material things manifest, from which all other forms of qi derive. This may even help us understand the concept of no form. Just as no form is like the precursor of the observable world, so too is the implicate order.

The Chinese concepts of the energy centers in the body, the moving qi between the kidneys, the dantian, of internal alchemy, the transformative properties of the triple warmer, are all related. All arise as the essential properties and functions of an "implicate qi." Philosophically and medically, this is why abdominal diagnosis and treatment can be so powerful.

□

Chapter

- 6 -

Source

Theory

Source Theory

Source theory, as we have seen, plays a particularly important role in the theory of Chinese medicine. For Chinese medical theorists beginnings were important. The origin characterized the form and function of everything. The energetics of the human body have a compound beginning: cosmologically in the heaven—person—earth continuum; individually in the embryological development of the fetus and the relationship of the fetus to the mother. The energetics of the hara are intimately related to the source. We find the physiological and energetic function of the hara repeatedly mentioned in the context of origins.

As usual, it is the *Ling Shu* theory that has been the basis of later thought and speculation. These comments may be traced to earlier concepts and theories of embryology from the *Huai Nan Zi*. Ideas expressed in the *Ling Shu* are the foundation of *Nan Jing* source theory and later commentary. Among the authors who have commented upon the idea of source, Sosen Hirooka of Japan, who wrote in approximately 1750, and Xie Lin of China, from the late Qing dynasty, make some of the clearest statements. *Nan Jing* source theory revolves around the functions of the triple warmer and the master of the heart. As expected, it is a more developed theory. It traces energetic connections from before birth and details the function of postpartum nourishment. Comparatively, the *Ling Shu* source theory more directly concerns the energetics of prepartum development and nourishment. It also considers anatomical structures that are not frequently the concern of either Western or Eastern medical thinkers. Among these are peritoneal membranes, the systems of fascia, and the connective tissues. However, much of source theory is not obvious. Many of the ideas must be unearthed from careful consideration of the texts, the etymology of the terms, and the conclusions drawn by the classical authors. The connections between the *Ling Shu* and *Nan Jing* source theories are not often clearly stated; however, there are conclusions that may be derived and implications that are clear only in context. These are often fascinating, particularly since modern anatomical and physiological data tends to elucidate, rather than deny, the relationships of classical energetics.

Ling Shu Source Theory

The *Ling Shu* theory of the triple warmer is the groundwork for part of the *Nan Jing* source theory. Although it is different from the *Nan Jing* theory of the triple warmer and is the theory most often cited as *the* triple warmer theory, the differences are interpretive. The *Ling Shu* triple warmer theory involves food and water metabolism, ying qi and wei qi:

> The Yellow Emperor said, "I would like to know where the ying and wei come from."

Qi Bo answered, "The ying comes out from the middle warmer, the wei comes out from the lower warmer."

The Yellow Emperor said, "I would like to know where the triple warmer comes out."

Qi Bo answered, "The upper warmer comes out from the entrance of the stomach, parallelling the esophagus. It passes through the diaphragm and then disperses inside the chest. It goes to the armpits and passes down [parallel to] the side of the lung meridian; it then passes to the large intestine meridian and returns. It passes up and goes to the tongue, then passes down the stomach meridian. . . . With regularity, the ying passes to the yang [areas] twenty-five times and passes to the yin [areas] twenty-five times; this is one circulation. Therefore, after fifty cycles there is a great meeting at hand tai yin [lung meridian]. . . ."

The Yellow Emperor said, "I would like to know where the middle warmer comes out."

Qi Bo answered, "The middle warmer also parallels the inside of the entrance of the stomach. After [the upper warmer qi comes out], the middle warmer qi comes out. This, which receives the qi, separates the useful from the non-useful parts of food. It steams the jin 津 and ye 液. It alchemically transforms it to the tiny jing. [The tiny jing] rises up and passes to the lung vessel [pulmonary arteries and veins?], and then it is alchemically transformed again becoming blood. With this, the living body is nourished. Nothing is more valuable than this. Only this passes to the meridians, it is called the ying qi."

The Yellow Emperor said, "The blood and qi are the same kind, how does one differentiate them?"

Qi Bo answered, "The ying and wei are the jing qi, the blood is the shen qi; therefore, the blood and qi have different names, but are the same kind. . . ."

The Yellow Emperor said, "I would like to know where the lower warmer comes out."

Qi Bo answered, "The lower warmer divides the intestines, goes to the bladder and is absorbed into the bladder. Therefore, water and grains always reside together in the stomach and compose the non-useful parts. The non-useful parts go down to the large intestine. [These functions] compose the lower warmer. [The lower warmer] thus [functions] to absorb and to send the non-useful parts downward. It purifies and sifts the juices, separating them and passing them to the lower warmer and absorbing them into the bladder. . . . The upper warmer is like a mist, the middle warmer is like froth, the lower warmer is like the drain pipes" *(LS 18:197-200).*

In regard to the phrase, "the ying comes out from the middle warmer, the wei comes out from the lower warmer," there is some controversy. Several commentators feel that this is a textual mistake, that the wei qi comes out from the upper warmer and not the lower. The *Ling Shu* itself does say "the lower warmer;" however, Sun Si-Mo and the writer of the *Tai*

Su disagree with this. They feel that the "upper" character was replaced by the "lower" character by mistake at some point as the book was being transcribed.[1] The essential information to remember is that the entire meridian system is an extension of the upper warmer, or part of the upper warmer. Thus, the meridian system was seen in relation to the triple warmer. This connection becomes increasingly obvious as we consider further aspects of source theory. In both the *Ling Shu* and *Nan Jing*, the triple warmer is described as a source of the meridian system. This is particularly obvious in the *Nan Jing*.

The *Ling Shu* theory that describes the relationships of certain tissues and organs to a series of source points further develops this connection. The *Ling Shu* tells us:

> The five yin organs have six [corresponding] yang organs. The six yang organs have twelve sources [points]. The twelve source [points] come out at the four joints [wrists and ankles]. The four joints control and treat the five yin organs.
>
> If the five yin organs have disease, treat the twelve source [points]. The twelve sources can give qi and taste [nourishment] to the three hundred and sixty five nodes [acupoints], because of the five yin organs. When the five yin organs are sick, they respond and come out [reflect] to the twelve source [points]. The twelve sources each have places where they come out. [If one] clearly understands the sources and observes their responses, one is able to know the extent of the damage to the five yin organs.
>
> The shao yin of the yang is the lungs, the source comes out at tai yuan [LU-9] at both the left and right sides. The tai yang of the yang is the heart, the source comes out at da ling [PC-7] at both the left and right sides. The tai yin of the yin is the kidneys, the source comes out at tai xi [KI-3] at both the left and right sides. The shao yang of the yin is the liver, the source comes out at tai chong [LV-3] at both the left and right sides. The jue yin of the yin is the spleen, the source comes out at tai bai [SP-3] at both the left and right sides. The source of *gao* 膏 comes out at jiu wei [CV-15], only one point. The source of huang 肓 comes out at po ang 脖胦, only one point.
>
> These twelve source [points] control and treat diseases of the five yin and six yang organs (LS 1:13).

The ideas relative to gao, huang, and po ang provide the most important information, though many interesting concepts in this passage deserve discussion. First, the source points are reflex points for internal problems. These points are easily diagnosed by palpation and are featured in the treatment protocols of a variety of styles. Further, the idea that the twelve sources nourish, "give qi and taste to the three hundred and sixty-five nodes [acupoints]," is important. This implies that the qi of the acupoints is ultimately derived from the correct function of the five yin organs which have twelve corresponding sources. This relationship is more clearly stated in the *Nan Jing* where the twelve sources emanate from one single source in the hara, the moving qi between the kidneys, which is considered to be the ultimate source of living energies in the body. However, the source points described by the *Ling Shu* and the *Nan Jing* differ slightly. Another noteworthy idea is that the four "joints" (ankles and wrists) treat the five yin organs. This has many implications for exercise and movement therapies.

The most intriguing part of this passage lies in the question, what do the gao, huang, and po ang reference? Gao and huang are usually seen to refer to fatty tissues. Huang has another common meaning, the "space below the heart and above the diaphragm."[2] Huang connotes a "missing" or "hidden" organ. One modern Chinese commentator sees gao as referring to the extensions of the peritoneal membranes that encapsulate each of the yin and yang organs. Huang would thus be perceived as the fascia, mesenterium, and omenta that connect the various organs to one another.[3] Gao also refers to the melted form of animal fat *(Kad)*. These definitions seem strange in relation to source theory in Chinese medicine. If we investigate po ang, relevance begins to unfold.

Both the characters *po* 脖 and *ang* 胅 refer to the umbilicus. This was true in classical times as well.[4] Thus, the source of huang can be considered as the umbilicus. This is not a universal interpretation. Many scholars have interpreted po ang in the *Ling Shu* as CV-6, qi hai.[5] Determining an overall sense of the idea is difficult when we take po ang as CV-6. Except that it implies some important energetic connections, we are left with little further relationship.

Nonetheless, there are good reasons for interpreting the source of huang as CV-6, or at least as a point below the umbilicus. The *Su Wen* talks briefly about the source of huang as being below the umbilicus.

> [If the] qi is full in the large intestine, it thus manifests at the huang. The source of huang is below the umbilicus; therefore, if it encircles the umbilicus, there will be pain *(SW 47:260)*.

It is possibly this passage on which later texts base the interpretation of the source of huang as CV-6, though no compelling identity of CV-6 and the source of huang is to be found here.

On the other hand, there are basic physiological and anatomical structures that support the interpretation of po ang as the umbilicus. Etymologically, the character *po* 脖 is derived from the pictogram of a baby in the womb *(Fuj)*. The character refers to fetal growth in a sense parallel to the sprouting of seeds into young shoots. This embryological implication may also be seen in other aspects of the *Ling Shu* source theory. For example, gao also relates to fetal development. In the *Huai Nan Zi*, gao is that which exists or comes into being during the first stage of fetal development:

> Jing and shen are received from heaven, subsequently, the form and the body are received from earth. Therefore it is said, one creates two, two creates three, three creates the myriad things. The myriad things carry yin on their backs and embrace yang in their arms. Using harmonious qi it creates harmony.

Therefore it is said: In the first month, there is gao 膏. In the second month, there is a fleshy swelling 胅. In the third month, there is a pregnant uterus 胎. In the fourth month, the skin can be recognized. In the fifth month, the muscles. In the sixth month, the bones. In the seventh, there is completion. In the eighth, there is movement. In the ninth, there is rowdy movement. In the tenth, there is birth.

The form and the body are complete, then the five yin organs take form.

Therefore, the lungs control the eyes. The kidneys control the nose. The gallbladder controls the mouth. The liver controls the ears. The spleen controls the tongue. The outside becomes superficial. The inside becomes the lining 裏. Opening and closing, expanding and contracting, each of these have rules (*HNZ 7:322-323*).[6]

The relation of gao to the first month of fetal development is most relevant to the interpretation of the meaning of huang, po ang, and gao in source theory. During the first stages of fetal development not much is obvious without the use of a microscope, except that there is a cluster or lump growing in the uterus. Visually, this lump is an apparently undifferentiated mass of tissue. Perhaps, it is this basic tissue to which gao refers. Through the later stages of development this tissue becomes the fetus. It is the origin or source of what becomes human life. This seemingly homogenous tissue gives rise to the differentiated tissues of the muscles, bones, and organs, an important part of which is the connective tissues. Since gao and huang both commonly refer to fatty, greasy membranes or tissues, and gao is particularly related to fetal tissue, we feel that in the context of source theory these characters refer to the membranes and peritoneal tissues (mostly composed of connective tissues), the physical substrate of the hara. This interpretation is not so mundane as it first appears.

A very large part of the body consists of connective tissues and membranes functioning in such a way as to hold the body, as a whole, together. These structures connect every part of the body to every other part, at a gross anatomical level through the fascial planes, and microscopically through their component tissues, the connective tissues, enabling the communication of every single cell to all other cells. These tissues are a vast reservoir for the body and meet the requirements of any structure or energetic entity that would be capable of the mediation and transference of energy required of a "source." The parallels of Chinese medicine with embryological development and the nature of the fundamental tissues of the body, the connective tissues, of which the gao and huang are composed, are discussed in greater detail in later sections of the text. For now it is sufficient to note that the context in which these three characters, huang, gao, and po ang, are used relates to tissues and to embryological development. There are both prior and later texts that describe the relationships of these concepts and the area around the umbilicus, the womb, and the hara.

There is another level at which we can understand all this. As we have shown, gao is related to the early stages of fetal development. Huang, through its relationship to po ang (the umbilicus), may also be seen to relate to the fetus. Fetal nourishment is derived through the umbilicus. In this context, it is not unreasonable to think of the alternate meaning of huang, the missing organ, as a reference to the placenta or the whole uterus-placenta complex. As such, it represents both the source of nourishment of the fetus and its protection. After birth this organ disappears, as the infant no longer requires it. The "hidden organ" has similar connotations; it implies some deep part of the body that is not obvious or visible. There is an interesting quote from the *Zuo Zhuan* commentary on the *Chun Qiu (The Spring and Autumn Annals),* which could well be older than any of the references from the *Su Wen* and *Ling Shu:*

> Above the huang and below the gao [is a place that] cannot be
> attacked. It is not possible to reach to and touch this. Even
> herbs cannot reach to it *(S&C 2:606).*

Usually this passage is thought to imply that a problem of this place, which lies above the huang and below the gao, is very hard, if not impossible to treat, since "even herbs cannot reach to it." At the very least it refers to a deep part of the body that is not obviously visible or accessible.

While etymologically there is reasonable sense to the idea that these characters reference a deep, embryologically significant structure, this idea is further developed when we ask, why are CV-15 and the umbilicus (or po ang) seen as the source points of gao and huang? It is possible to answer this question anatomically. There are frequently ignored anatomical structures that directly link these two points to each other through the liver. The ligamentum teres (or round ligament), the falciform ligament, and the coronary ligament demonstrate a firm anatomical basis for the *Ling Shu* source theory. Before birth the fetus derives its nourishment from the placenta. This nourishment passes through the umbilical cord to enter the umbilicus where it passes through the umbilical vein to the liver. At the liver it is processed and absorbed into the blood and thus the body. After birth, the infant loses this connection when the umbilical cord is severed. Yet, the umbilical vein remains, eventually becoming the ligamentum teres that runs from the umbilicus along the interior surface of the abdominal wall to the liver. This remnant of the umbilical vein ascends from the umbilicus upward through the free margin of the falciform ligament to the liver. The falciform ligament continues to ascend through the right and left lobes of the liver to meet the coronary ligament, both of which then attach to the underside of the diaphragm. Where the coronary and falciform ligaments attach to the diaphragm, they pass beneath CV-15. Thus, the anatomical structure of these ligaments provides a physical relationship between CV-15, the umbilicus, po ang, and the liver.

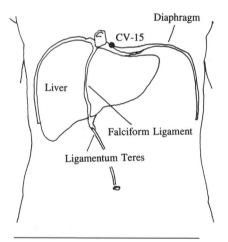

Figure 6.1 Anatomic relationship of the navel (po ang), the liver, and jiu wei, CV-15.

The liver is an interesting organ in Chinese medicine. Corresponding to the wood phase, the spring season, it is said to be the origin of processes in the body because of its correspondence to spring, the season of growth and development in the yearly cycle. Physiologically, the liver has a very similar "origin" function. In the fetus, it is the organ to which nourishment comes; it then processes these nutrients and nourishes the other organs and parts of the body. In the developing embryo and in the newborn, the liver

□

is very large relative to the other organs. The weight of the liver in relation to the total body weight is about double that of an adult. We know that some anatomical studies were performed during or before the Han dynasty; it is not unlikely that these qualities were known. It would be natural to ascribe special qualities or functions to the liver.

This can be seen in some of the ideas of the Han dynasty and earlier. The character for the liver, *gan,* 肝 is of etymological interest. The left part of the character 月 is a common character used to refer to organs, or flesh. 干 is the "stem" of the "ten stems" of Chinese astronomy, astrology, and medicine. Etymologically, 干 is the origin of 幹 which means "stem" *(Fuj).* We can also note that 肝 is the liver and 肢 the limbs. If we remove the flesh radical 月 we are left with 支, the "branch" of the "twelve branches." If we see 月, the radical of both, as a general term for a part of the body, we can see the other characters as the "stems" and "branches" respectively. Symbolically, this suggests that the liver has a stem function relative to the four limbs, the branches. It is very probable, based on these observations, that the liver represents the stem of the body. It is the first organ to receive nourishment from the mother, it is the wood — spring — developmental organ and therefore the stem organ of the body.

This is also explained in other classical texts. The *Shuo Wen Jie Zi* defines the liver as "the wood organ" *(Mor).* The *Shi Ming* says of the liver, "[It] is a stem; in the five phases it belongs to wood" *(Mor).* Clearly, the liver holds a particularly important place and function in the body relative to the other organs. this is referenced by the *Ling Shu* source theory, specifically in regard to the sources of gao and huang as CV-15 and the umbilicus.

This emphasis on the importance of the liver can be found quite often in the medical texts; for instance, when stating important correspondent and generative principles of organ—phase complexes the *Su Wen* tells us:

> East is in the heavens, this is the dark green heaven,
> from the dark green heaven shen is created.
> Shen in the heavens then creates wind.
> Shen in the earth creates wood.
> Shen in the body creates the muscles.
> Shen in the organs creates the liver.
> Shen in the colors creates the cyan color *(SW 5:36-37).*

This passage continues, listing similar principles for each of the other organ—phase complexes. However, its emphasis is different for the liver—wood complex, since it stresses shen as the generative and underlying principle.

Shen is generally seen as one of the original substances or energies from which life springs. It is not incorrect to think of shen as coming into the body from the mother through the umbilical cord to the liver. This is probably why the acupoint in the center of the umbilicus was named *shen jue* 神闕. Jue commonly refers to a special gate that only one as exalted as the emperor may pass. This point is thus the "shen gate." However, this name was not used for the point in the umbilicus, until at least as late as the Tang dynasty.[7] It is possible that the oldest name for this point is po ang. The name shen jue is closely related to po ang. Inside the character

□

jue 闕 is *jue* 欮 which means upside-down, and refers to the body upside-down in a fetal shape *(Fuj)*. This interestingly reflects the meaning of the character po, the fetus upside down, in the womb.

There are other interesting ways of looking at the *Ling Shu* source theory. The text itself actually says:

> The five yin organs have six [corresponding] yang organs.
> The six yang organs have twelve sources [points]. . . .
> If the five yin organs have disease, treat the twelve source [points].

In effect we are told that the twelve sources are of the six yang organs, yet the source points themselves are bilateral points on five of the yin meridians (excluding the heart), CV-15, and po ang. This seems to indicate that the yin organs have corresponding yang organs, which in turn have corresponding source points on the yin meridians that treat the yin organs. Schematically, this can be seen as follows:

Right	Yin Organ	Yang Organ	Left
PC-7	pericardium	triple warmer	PC-7
LU-9	lung	large intestine	LU-9
SP-3	spleen	stomach	SP-3
LV-3	liver	gallbladder	LV-3
KI-3	kidney	bladder	KI-3
CV-15	?	small intestine	
Umbilicus	?	small intestine	

The sixth yang organ would be the small intestine, suggesting that po ang and perhaps CV-15 correspond to the small intestine. The heart may not have been included in this schema because the heart has a different function:

> The Yellow Emperor asked, "The hand shao yin vessel alone has no shu [transformation], what does this mean?"
>
> Qi Bo answered, "The shao yin is the vessel of the heart; the heart is the great controller of the five yin and six yang organs. This is the place where jing and shen stay. This yin organ is tight and hard. Evil can not be accepted here. When evil is accepted, this means the heart will be injured, the shen will leave and this means death. Therefore, every evil [that would come to the heart] will stay at the wrapping luo of the heart [the pericardium]. The wrapping luo is the vessel of the master of the heart; therefore, this is the reason why [the heart has] no shu [transformation] points *(LS 71:494)*.

The heart is of a different energetic order. This is also indicated by the internal trajectory of the heart meridian. The heart may correspond to CV-15 and the small intestine to po ang; however, because the heart is of a different energetic order, considering the small intestine as the yang organ corresponding to CV-15 and po ang is reasonable. In the medical literature, the small intestine also is described differently than the other organs. In the *Zhen Jiu Jia Yi Jing* of 282 A.D., it states:

The small intestine is related to the supporter of the testicles, it belongs to the spine, it passes through the liver and lungs, spirally wraps the supporter of the heart, rises up and harmonizes the intestines and stomach. It smokes [fumes] the liver and lungs and then disperses at huang. It knots itself at the umbilicus. Therefore, using the huang source 肓原, disperse it.[8]

The huang source is usually thought of as CV-6, but as we have discussed, this is not obviously the case. The passage does not explicitly state that it is the small intestine meridian described; it is reasonable to see it as such. Thus, the small intestine may be related to huang or the source of huang. This is somewhat nebulous and not at all clearly defined. Some passages do make clear statements. In two similar passages in the same chapter of the *Su Wen* we are informed:

> If cold qi visits between the stomach and intestines, below the membrane's source 膜原, the blood is not able to be dispersed. The small luo 絡 becomes tense and pulls, therefore there is pain. Press it, then the blood and qi can be dispersed. Therefore, pressing it can stop the pain. If cold qi visits between the small intestine and the source of the membrane 膜原 into the blood luo, the blood becomes stagnant and is not able to pass through to the big meridian. The blood and qi are stagnant and not able to move. Therefore, it becomes chronically stuck and consequently becomes a lump [yin lump] 積 *(SW 39:219-220)*.

In his Tang dynasty commentary on the *Su Wen,* Wang Bing describes "below the membrane's source" as "the membranes separating the organs" *(SW 39:220)*. Although the character translated as membrane 膜 is different from huang and gao, it has a similar meaning. Thus, the small intestine is here related to the place from which blood is dispersed to the body, from between the small intestine and the "source of the membrane."

This membrane may be the omentum or the mesenterium, both of which cover or connect the intestines and stomach. Embedded within the mesenterium are the mesenteric arteries that supply the intestines with blood. Returning from the small intestines is the hepatic portal vein, carrying food-enriched blood from the intestines to the liver. The hepatic portal vein has a parallel function (for the child and adult) to the umbilical vein in the fetus, implying a similar function for the liver after birth. Perhaps the *Su Wen* was stating that the small intestine is related to this process. It is the small intestine where most food is absorbed. The mesenteric artery and hepatic portal vein are further indicated in this context by the idea that when cold qi invades there is a resultant stagnation of blood and ultimately a lump. Both are easily related to impaired circulation.

That the small intestine may be related to CV-15 and po ang, the source of gao and huang, is possibly what the writers of the *Zhen Jiu Juying* and *Zhen Jiu Da Cheng* had in mind when they said,

> Fire yang goes back to wangu [SI-4]. This is the center of the source.[9]

The small intestine — fire yang — is seen in relationship to the source. What this source may be remains to be fully clarified. One modern researcher suggests that the small intestine is the source of the normal, non-stressful production of red blood cells. He states that under stress the body produces red blood cells in the marrow of the bones, but that normally they are formed from protocellular cells in the small intestine.[10] This theory has not gained much recognition in the West, but is worthy of further research, as it has the potential of relating processes described in Western physiological terms to the processes described by Oriental medicine.

What may we take from all this discursive material that furthers our understanding? Clearly, the classical medical theorists believed that there was a source, a significant center which played an important, if not uniquely central, role in the energetics of the human body. Certainly, each of these central energetic functions occur within the hara. This source is related, if not explicitly or exactly, by an overwhelming preponderance of etymological, energetic, and functional concepts to both prepartum and postpartum processes. At least the liver, the heart, the source points, and the placenta—womb complex are attached to the source. The source is associated with shen, the particular generative energy central to Chinese cosmology, the elemental starting point of wood—spring and the nutritive energies of food. Given only the vagaries of translation and the relative scarcity of English-language efforts to which we may compare, one could not fairly propose that the idea of a specific, uniquely central source is textually proven beyond question. However, the questions that remain are those that concern specific functions. The idea of a source is sufficiently established to serve as an organizational concept by which we may understand and utilize the thoughts of the classical medical authors.

Anatomical Relationships

One association we may take from *Ling Shu* source theory is the admittedly random, yet frequent relationship of organs, energies, and pathways to membranes, a pervasive infrastructure that was certainly familiar to the authors of these texts. Gao and huang may reasonably refer to the membranes that line the peritoneal cavity and the organs. However, it is sufficiently unusual to relate internal anatomical structures and processes, other than the organs themselves, to Chinese medical theories, that the idea itself seems oddly foreign. There is a considerable tendency to think of even the organs themselves only in their energetic aspect. This is a trend in Western thought that some translators of Oriental medical literature attribute to an unjustified overstatement of the functional aspects of organ theory encouraged by mistranslation and zealous typographical concentration.[11] Of course, we are all quite accommodated to point and meridian descriptions that depend on superficial anatomy. Ligament, vein, and membrane relationships are certainly not the commonplace conversation of most modern acupuncturists. Yet, on close inspection, the classical medical texts are frequently aware of the body's inner structure. The passages describing the gao and huang and embryonic development demonstrate this awareness, as do the specific and detailed concepts of internal meridian pathways.

□

The early Chinese medical theorists did not think of the body as an empty energetic sphere. The idea of a "lining" of the body and of the organs, the *li* 裏, is quite prevalent in early Chinese medical literature. Today, this character is commonly translated as "inside" or "internal," as in the "internal — external" duality of the eight principles. In the Han dynasty, li definitely meant a lining *(Fuj; Mor)*. This case clearly demonstrates one pitfall of translating a character language. The meaning of a character depends on use. Was li originally used in the inner — outer pair because it meant "lining," and was handy, or seemed appropriate to the unnamed author who first wrote of the system? Or was it used because the dichotomy was indeed intended to mean between the superficial lining, the skin, and the interior lining, the superficial and deep fascia? From our viewpoint, this second choice would indeed make a perfect logical parallel. Did it simply change meaning over time? Did the scholars or typesetters of some great dictionary make a mistake? In short, there are only context, scholarship, and an individual sense of the text itself on which to rely. Absolute meanings are not to be considered reliable. The distinctions are important. Translating li as the "lining" and not as the "interior" provides a markedly different connotation. Perhaps lining refers to the membranes that cover the body, the superficial fascia. In this context, we can persuasively associate energetic concepts with interior membranes such as the gao and huang, which are part of the body's fascial system.

Such an association is not without textual justification. A quote from the *Huai Nan Zi* discussing embryological development includes this passage:

> The outside becomes the superficial; the inside becomes the lining *(HNZ 7:323)*.

In numerous places, the *Su Wen* distinguishes the lining from the outside. The *Nan Jing,* for example, discusses the "tension of the lining" *(NJ 29:17).* as one of the symptoms that would suggest treatment of the chong mai. This passage is usually interpreted to reference the tension of the abdomen, a phenomena created by the condition of the abdominal fascia. As we will see in succeeding chapters such references are by no means rare.

Perhaps the fascia, the tissues that cover and line the body and organs, have some special qualities, properties, or functions that were recognized by the medical authors of the Han dynasty. As we have argued, it is reasonable to see these tissues in relation to the *Ling Shu* source theory, gao and huang. From the sense of the texts, the classical physicians were familiar with the body's interior and the interior structures, particularly the fascia, which were considered important to the concept of source. The evidence is sufficient to indicate that the body's fascial system was considered central. At the very least, it is clear that *Ling Shu* source theory pertains to some fundamental underlying tissues and energies in the body that are critically important during embryological development and throughout life.

In following discussions, we will describe the hara in relation to these tissues in a variety of ways. For now, there is one practical evidence of such a relationship. Let us align the points that have names involving gao or huang:

Point	Name
BL-38	gao huang
KI-16	huang shu
BL-46	huang men
BL-48	bao huang

There are energetic and therapeutic connections of these points with CV-15 and po ang. Bunshi Shiroda, a modern practitioner and scholar of acupuncture and moxibustion, quotes his teacher, Takeshi Sawada, as saying that by treating CV-6 we can treat problems reflected at CV-15 and BL-38 and vice versa.[12] There are also connections between KI-16 and BL-46. KI-16, huang shu, is on the front of the body, where shu points are generally on the back. BL-46, huang men, is on the back of the body where the men points are generally on the front. In discussing these points in relation to each other, Shiroda and Sawada recommend the treatment of these points to eliminate pressure pain at the associated points.

Since we cannot possibly make a final judgment that po ang is CV-8 or CV-6, we must propose that based on the *Ling Shu* theory, CV-15, CV-8, CV-6, BL-38, BL-46, KI-16, and possibly BL-48 and LV-3, KI-3, SP-3, LU-9, and PC-7, all have some relationship to each other. Further, there is possibly some underlying energetic or physical substratum. When we find reaction on any of these points, we should check the others. Regardless of what organ or meridian problems there may be, we may treat these points. The results of experienced practitioners such as Shiroda and Sawada indicate that stimulating these points may have profound effects. Their advice is particularly effective regarding the treatment of reactions found on KI-16, the umbilicus (CV-8), CV-6, and CV-15. When standard treatments of the extraordinary vessels, meridians, or five phases have not produced adequate results, attending to these points expands our therapeutic repertoire.

Shiroda and Sawada's discussions of the huang and gao and their related treatment points are based on extensive studies, practice, and research. They quote Ippo Okamoto, a Japanese acupuncturist who wrote a commentary on the *Su Wen* in 1703, the *Shinkyu Aze Yoketsu*,[13] as positing a relationship between the extra point, *bi gen* 痞根, and huang men, BL-46. Bi gen lies half a division lateral to BL-46. Okamoto points out the relationship of the huang to the triple warmer and the triple warmer to the kidneys and the source. This discussion is pivotal to understanding the *Ling Shu* and *Nan Jing* source theories and forms a bridge between the two. Before examining this more complex relationship, we should first describe the *Nan Jing* source theory and its descriptions of the triple warmer.

Nan Jing Source Theory

The *Nan Jing* source theory is among the most important theories in Oriental medicine. It describes the root or core of the body, the root of all the organs and meridians, as being located in the abdomen below the umbilicus at the gravitational center of the body. The hara is considered the root of life processes. The *Nan Jing* states the basic principles but is lacking in detail. Many commentators have explained the theory in greater detail than has the *Nan Jing;* we have included several lengthy comments that expand and clarify the basic ideas.

Essentially, the theory revolves around the functions of the triple warmer and the master of the heart. These have been considered difficult subjects for a long time. As with the various commentaries describing the internal pathways of the meridians, there is not a simple consensus of a few unquestioned facts. Again, it is important to remember that the existence of contradictions in the discussions of the triple warmer and master of the heart represent differences of emphasis and are the result of the complexity of these functions themselves. Often, one author will present a specific facet of their function while another will concentrate on a different phenomenon. What is important in this context is a thorough knowledge of the *Nan Jing* source theory, the fundamental nature and importance of the hara diagnostically and therapeutically.

Although these discussions are theoretical, there is a considerable practical dimension to the *Nan Jing* theory. Waichi Sugiyama has said, for example, that we cannot understand this theory if we don't palpate the abdomen. It is only in touching that we can grasp it.[14] This is one of the reasons hara palpation and treatment is so important to the practice of Oriental medicine in Japan and why it was of concern to the classical authors.

The theory states that there is an energetic center to the body. This center has a physically central location and more importantly is the root of the body energetically. It is an underlying energetic substratum called the source 原. Around this substrate revolve all the other strata of energetic manifestation and function. The meridians, the five yin and six yang organs, stems, branches, phases, all are the concentric ripples of this energetic vortex. The source has certain qualities. It is the source of all movement in the body and is itself described as a moving qi. Most frequently, it is known as the "moving qi between the kidneys." Many propose that this moving qi is felt as a very slight pulsing on palpation of the abdomen below the umbilicus. Often, it is perceived as a sensation of movement rather than movement itself.

This moving qi between the kidneys is thought to be a manifestation of an even more profound energy in the universe. It is constant; when it ends the person dies. It regulates and is interdependent with other energetic properties, the jing, shen and qi. When it is healthy and strong, it is easier for the person who has a disease of any other energetic strata, the meridians and organs for instance, to recover from the disease. If it is weak and poorly nourished, or itself is diseased, no matter how strong the energetics in the other strata, it will be difficult for the person to fully recover. Thus, the moving qi between the kidneys, the source, is extremely important and one of the first things that we must diagnose. It is most easily diagnosed by palpating the abdomen. All problems that can cause disease can be seen to react through or manifest in the hara; thus, they may be diagnosed and treated there. The source is the "gate of breathing." Poor breathing habits can weaken the source. Since the source is at the physical center of the body, physical imbalances can also affect its energetics. Emotions affect energetics and can affect the correct functioning of the source. Problems of diet manifest in the hara, partly because of the proximity of the digestive organs and partly because of the close energetic link between the source and the energies derived from food.

The energetic continua that link the source to the other energetic strata are the triple warmer and the master of the heart. These links receive nourishment from eating, drinking, and breathing, and nourish the moving qi that generates other energies, for example, the source qi 原氣. These energies then nourish the meridians and the yin and yang organs. The moving qi between the kidneys is a manifestation of the source itself. It is like the body's generator. When it is cared for, it has a healthy, generative function that supports all other life processes. Not only is this important to diagnose, but it is very important to be able to treat what one finds. Treatment of the source is root treatment. Over time a variety of techniques that focus on the hara have been developed.

The centrality of the source is very clearly stated in the *Nan Jing*:

> The Yellow Emperor asked, "The pulse is normal and yet sometimes people die, why is this?"
>
> Qi Bo answered, "Each of the twelve meridians has a relationship to the source of the vital qi [living qi]. The source of the vital qi is the root-origin of the twelve meridians, it is the moving qi between the kidneys. This means that the source of the vital qi is fundamental to the five yin organs and six yang organs; it is the root of the twelve meridians, the gate of breathing. It is the source [origin] of the triple warmer. Another name for it is the shen [that] protects against evil; therefore, qi is the root of the person. This is why if the root is dying, the stems and branches [organs and meridians] will be drying [out], yet appear normal. The vital qi is dying inside, but it is still there on the outside [the pulse is still normal]" *(NJ 8:11).*

We can see here an immediate and simple diagnosis, the examination of breathing ability. If the breathing is shallow and does not reach into the abdomen, the nourishment that the moving qi needs is not adequate. Practice of deep breathing is therapeutically useful, providing immediate relief and a source of energy for the moving qi. The "gate of breathing" is an important Daoist concept. In the first chapter of the *Lie Zi* the "gate" and "root" are described in relation to heaven and earth's energies, life and death:

> Jing and shen are of the category of heaven.
>
> The skeleton and bones [the physical body] are of the category of earth.
>
> [The nature of] the category of heaven is clear and dispersive.
>
> [The nature of] the category of earth is unclear and contractive [convergent].
>
> The Yellow Emperor said, "Jing and shen return to the gate.
>
> The skeleton and bones return to the root."[15]

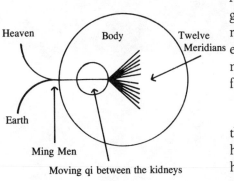

Figure 6.2 Diagrammatic representation of the continuum of cosmological and human energetic interactions.

These gate and root characters are the same as used by the *Nan Jing.* After death, jing and shen which are originally from heaven return to the gate. The skeleton and bones which are originally from earth, return to the root. The moving qi between the kidneys is the place where heaven's energy enters or attaches to the body. This parallels the discussion of how ming attaches to the body at ming men, connecting to earth's energy, that is found in chapter 25 of the *Su Wen.*

We can understand ming men as a concept intimately involved with the *Nan Jing* idea of a gate of breathing. This also parallels the idea of the hun from heaven and po from earth entering at birth and returning to heaven and earth at death. Similarly, the source, the root of the twelve meridians, is the place where earth's energy reacts with heaven's energy. This may be why the meridians were named the twelve branches in relation to the cosmological concept of terrestrial branches. In effect, the source is the point of interaction for the cosmological energies that comprise man. Diagrammatically we can see this in Figure 6.2.

The moving qi between the kidneys is the "shen that protects against evil." This establishes for us the relationship between the moving qi and the shen that the classical texts tell us is stored in the heart. However, this idea is more intricate. In his commentary on this idea, Sosen Hirooka says:

> The moving qi is called the shen of protecting evil. This means heaven's qi is in the person. Inside the qi, shen is created. This shen protects. It means that all kinds of evil cannot invade the person's body.[16]

This attraction of "heaven qi" into the person and the resultant creation of shen which protects the body is part of breathing. When breathing is correct, this process functions well. Like most concepts that relate to the source, this idea has multiple applications. Correct breathing may be utilized for good health and it is the root of Daoist contemplative practices. Henri Maspero's excellent text, *Taoism and Chinese Religion,* is a source of many specific discussions of Daoist breathing techniques.[17]

The moving qi is also the origin of the triple warmer. According to the *Nan Jing,* this relationship is quite complex. The triple warmer transports source qi from its origin to the source points of each of the twelve meridians. Chapter 66 of the *Nan Jing* states:

> The triple warmer is the alternative messenger of the source qi.

Thus, it maintains the basic energetic connection of twelve meridians to the source. The idea of an alternative messenger of the source qi may be understood if we examine a quote from Wang Shu He:

> The triple warmer unites qi at the kidneys. The kidneys are the regular [messenger] of the source qi. The triple warmer is the alternative [messenger] of the source qi.[18]

This knowledge allows us to treat problems of the organs themselves (*NJ 66*) and to diagnose the condition of the organs by palpating the source points.

□

Again, the character used is significant. *Yuan* 原, the source, has connotations that relate it to the five phases, expanding the concept relative to five-phase treatments. Yuan refers to a spring, as a spring of water that flows from behind the rocks of a ravine (Kad). The *Shuo Wen Jie Zi* states, "Yuan is the root origin of water" (Mor). It is the place where an underground source of·water reaches to the surface. The analogy is too clear to ignore. Source qi is the spring of qi which rises from a deeper level. The yuan, basic qi, the original or fundamental qi, prenatal qi, is the surfacing underground river. As the *Shuo Wen Jie Zi* says, "Yuan 元 is the beginning 始" (Mor). Yuan is the precursor of all else. If we recall the ideas of origin discussed in chapter 5, we find that the basic qi, the energetic substrate that underlies all other qi and precedes the separation of heaven and earth, is strongly reflected. No form, the pre-energetic state that precedes the development of form, material things, and the living body is just as strongly recalled. There is a clear relationship between the basic, fundamental qi and the source qi. Basic qi is the "enfolded or implicate" order; the source qi is the first unfolding of the basic qi. The Chinese metaphors of origin and beginning that are implicit in both concepts support this interpretation, as do the notions that the basic qi precedes and underlies all else, while the source qi is one of the first manifestations of this original qi. In the largest philosophical sense, what is seen on the macrocosmic scale is found microcosmically in the body. The basic qi is the prenatal qi, while the source qi is the root of postnatal qi.

According to *Nan Jing* theory, source qi is formed when the breath comes to the moving qi between the kidneys, the gate of breathing. It is derived from both prenatal and postnatal sources of energy. The triple warmer, which is also rooted in the hara, carries the source qi to the source points of the twelve meridians. The *Nan Jing* presents no discussion of any pathways by which this occurs. The source qi manifests at the source points synchronistically. Remembering that many Chinese authors allude to qi as water, or like water, and that water is the first of the five phases and the root of the following four, the water that metaphorically "wells" at the jing points may be the completion of an extended metaphor which begins with yuan, the origin of water. The source qi may be seen to supply the qi that manifests at the jing points of the twelve meridians.

This relationship is not clearly stated in the *Nan Jing*, nor is it found in commentaries. It does, however, explain one major paradox of five-phase theory, the idea of jing, yong, shu, jing, and he points. The jing points are seen as the places where the qi wells out. The yong points are where the qi streams, the shu points where the qi gushes. The jing points as where the qi moves and the he points are where the qi enters or unites.[19] This flow of qi thus described is always from the fingers and toes back towards the body. This contradicts the usual description of the circulation of the twelve meridians where six of the meridians pass towards the fingers and toes away from the body. The contradiction may be resolved by assuming that the source qi that moves through the five-phase points is not simply the meridian qi. If this assumption is correct, it gives great significance to the five-phase points in treatment. Treatment of these points would directly affect the flow of the source qi. Since the triple warmer is the medium through which this process occurs, it is even more significant.

□

Wang Shu He's commentary on the passage from the *Nan Jing* concerning the pulse and the abdomen discusses the triple warmer in relation to the water — fire duality.[20] The triple warmer is a product of the kidney — ming men interaction.

> The kidney belongs to water, ming men belongs to fire. The qi comes out from inside of the water — fire. The qi of the triple warmer starts [occurs] there. Therefore, the source of the triple warmer is the shen that protects against evil. Breath reaches to the inside; the qi grows and then becomes solid. This protects the body against injury by evil. Protecting on the inside and defending on the outside, this is the qi.[21]

Ming men is the fire aspect of water; it is the deeper energetic aspect of the body from which the moving qi between the kidneys manifests. The *Nan Jing* states that ming men is the right kidney and that it is the place where jing and shen reside (*NJ 36*). In his commentary on the *Nan Jing*, Sosen Hirooka distinguishes ming men and the moving qi:

> How does one differentiate between the moving qi between the kidneys and ming men? When thinking of material things, we may say ming men has form. When thinking of qi, we may say the moving qi between the kidneys has no form.[22]

Ming men is the place or terrain of the moving qi. Both the *Nan Jing* concept of ming men and Sosen Hirooka's concept relate to the *Su Wen* idea of ming men. The *Su Wen* has a cursory discussion of ming men, the "small heart":

> [At the] side of the seventh vertebra [the seventh counting upwards from the coccyx, at the second lumbar vertebra] on the inside, is the small heart (*SW 52:275*).

This has been expanded by Yang Chang Shan, the author of the *Tai Su*, who states that ming men is "the palace of the true heart's shen and ling" (*TS 331*) and that:

> The small heart makes the will of the heart.
> The kidneys stay below the seventh vertebra.
> Jing and shen are the will.
> All the ling of the five yin organs are called shen.
> The place of shen is conception.
> The name that becomes the will is the shen of the heart.
> The will of the heart is the shen of the kidneys (*TS 331*).

This passage demonstrates a close connection between the small heart, ming men, the true heart, and the kidneys.

In an interesting and surprisingly clear statement, Zhang Jie Bin says of ming men:

> Ming men totally controls the kidneys and both kidneys belong to ming men. Therefore ming men is the *fu* 府 of water and fire. It is the home of yin and yang. It is the ocean of the jing qi. It is the passageway of life and death. If ming men is depleted, then the five yin and six yang organs all lose some of their function; yin and yang are diseased and changed. [Therefore] there is no place unaffected [by this depletion].[23]

□

Ming men is the active aspect of water. Water was seen as the creative principle from which life comes into being. In the earliest ages, water was seen as primary in the creation process. In the *Shu Jing (Classic of Documents)*, water was number one, the first created of the five phases (*Mor*). In the *Lun Heng*, circa 82 A.D., the human form was seen to derive from a condensation of qi, much as water becomes ice:

> Qi creates the person.
> Water makes ice.
> Water becomes solid, making ice.
> Qi becomes solid making the person [body].[24]

The qi—water parallel may be seen in the names of many acupoints, particularly the five transporting points, the jing, yong, shu, jing, and he points. The names of these points, as we have previously detailed, describe the movement of qi in a manner that is analogous to a spring becoming a stream and finally a river. A famous Japanese practitioner, Waichi Sugiyama, also stressed the water—fire duality.[25] Water is the first created phase from which all else is created. Fire is like the yang line in kan, the water trigram ☵, without which the water (yin lines) would be inactive.

The interaction of the active and creative principles, ming men and the kidneys, produces the triple warmer. Li Shi Zhen, agreeing with Wang Shu He's comment, defines the triple warmer as "the function of ming men."[26] Given this view, we could consider that the various functions of the triple warmer are extensions of ming men. The triple warmer has digestive functions, as emphasized by the *Ling Shu (LS 18)*, but its theories are somewhat different than the *Nan Jing* theory. The *Nan Jing* says:

> We have the triple warmer, but where does the triple warmer accept qi, where is the beginning and end of the triple warmer? The triple warmer is the pathway of water and grain, the place where qi begins and ends. The upper warmer is below the heart [sternum], below the diaphragm at the entrance of the stomach. The upper warmer can accept things, but cannot get rid of them. The treatment point is CV-17 [1.6 divisions below CV-18]. The middle warmer is at the inside of the stomach [CV-12], neither above nor below, between the sternum and the umbilicus. It controls the transformation of food into energy, the treatment place is at the side of the umbilicus [possibly KI-16 or ST-25]. The location of the lower warmer is around the entrance of the bladder. Its function is to divide the clear and unclear; there is an exit but no entrance. The treatment place is one division below the umbilicus [CV-7]. This is why it is called the triple warmer. The storage place of the triple warmer is qi jie [ST-30] *(NJ 31:19-20)*.[27]

This passage is useful in a practical sense, as it informs us that CV-17, CV-12 (and possibly KI-16 or ST-25, CV-7, and ST-30), are each potential reflex points for the triple warmer or treatment points for problems in each of the warmers.

□

The triple warmer also functions in relation to the master of the heart—pericardium and thus to the heart and to the kidney. This relationship establishes a link to the energies of shen and jing. Perhaps this is why the *Nan Jing* states that ming men is the place where jing and shen reside. Shen is said to be stored in the heart and jing in the kidney *(SW 23; LS 8)*. The triple warmer function relative to the heart and kidneys is the transportation of the jing and shen through the body. This was described by Sun Si-Mo, a famous seventh-century herbalist, acupuncturist, alchemist, and Daoist sage. He wrote:

> The triple warmer's other name is the three gates 三關.
> It has a name but no form.
> It controls the five yin and six yang organs,
> the circling of the way of shen.
> It helps the jing qi pass and the water way pass.[28]

As these classical quotations demonstrate, the source — moving qi — ming men — triple warmer relationships are matters of essential energies. The theories relating to these functions are theories of life itself. The triple warmer is identified as the basic energies, not just their pathways. There is a Western mathematical set that parallels the manner in which the triple warmer is described. By analogy, the triple warmer is the sum of the energies of which it is comprised. Each function may be identified singly, yet it is the sum of those energies acting synchronistically that is the triple warmer. Unfortunately, the functional aspects are not clear. Most of the medical theorists who have attempted to explain the energetic phenomenon on which the principles of acupuncture are based have found it necessary to grapple with the classical concept of the triple warmer. Many commentaries help to detail these energetic relationships more clearly.

One commentary by Sawada extends these ideas and includes the relationship to Western anatomical and physiological structures:

> The triple warmer is where the mysterious qi 妙氣 of the living spirit 生靈 resides.
>
> The person who accepts life as a gift is between heaven and earth. Therefore, the principle of life and existence also exists.
>
> The triple warmer is the dividing messenger of the source qi and becomes the basic [part of] respiration. In what way can we describe the triple warmer? The nature of the warmer is as heat. Heat is the fire; fire is the body temperature. Therefore, this also is the regulator of the body temperature [like a thermostat].
>
> There are three kinds of fire: yang fire, yin fire, and ministerial fire. Yang fire is of two organs, the heart and lungs. When one breathes, one accepts yang qi and makes the blood warm; this is the heat of the upper warmer. Yin fire belongs to the kidney. The kidney controls water. The *Su Wen* says the fire in the water is called "dragon fire." When the dragon moves it makes fire come out; therefore, yin fire is the heater of the lower warmer.

The ministerial fire is controlled by the middle warmer. The middle warmer is the spleen—stomach—pancreas. These are three that become one. [This] one becomes three. These control the heat of the middle warmer; therefore, this becomes the ministerial fire.

The triple warmers are the upper, middle, and lower warmers; these three become one, this one becomes three. The three warmers have three qi: the zong qi, the ying qi, and the wei qi.

The zong qi is the qi of the upper warmer, it accepts yang qi from heaven at the heart and lungs. Zong qi and blood circulate throughout the whole body, they are steamed, it is like cloudy fog. Ying qi is the qi of the middle warmer, it accepts nourishment at the stomach; the spleen absorbs the five tastes; subsequently [these five tastes] are alchemically transformed to blood. [The ying qi] provides nourishment for each organ; therefore, the spleen—stomach is the official of storing grain—food.

The five tastes by themselves come out at it [the middle warmer]. Will, intelligence, and the flesh belong to the spleen; therefore, it is also the postnatal source qi. The wei qi is the qi of the lower warmer. The milky nourishing liquid [chyle] is absorbed into the lacteal ducts from the small intestine and then to the superficial [layers of the] skin of the whole body.[29]

Sawada's descriptions integrate some of the *Ling Shu* and *Nan Jing* theories of triple warmer function. The role of chyle and the lacteals will be discussed in the next two chapters. Again, we are shown processes that are essential to life. The triple warmer is the process by which the functional energies of the digestive and transformative organs are distributed. However, it is an essential process itself. In particular, the idea that the person who has accepted the gift of life "stands between heaven and earth" intimates that these energies reach beyond the body. The set of energies that we call the triple warmer is itself a member of a larger set, the energies of heaven and earth.

In Chinese mythology the dragon is an important and interesting figure. Etymologically it is associated with the origins of the shen and tai ji characters. The *Kadokawa Etymological Dictionary* describes how the ℓ line in the shen character ⅞ represents a dragon. It also suggests that it is related to 震 from the *Yi Jing*, based on considerations of pronunciation and because 申 represents lightning and 震 represents thunder *(Kad)*. In her book, *Chugoku no Yokai (Mythical Creatures of Chinese History)*, Miyoko Nakano discusses how the earliest form of the dragon derived from the image of a snake devouring itself. This is related to the origin of the tai ji symbol where each half represents a snake/dragon devouring the other. *Fujido's Etymological Dictionary* states:

The dragon is a mythical animal that looks like a giant snake. It has four legs, horns, and long whiskers/antennae. The dragon creates the clouds and causes rain to fall to the earth. In the spring it rises up to heaven, but at the autumn time it is hidden in yuan.

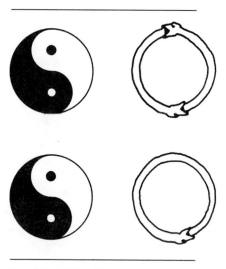

Figure 6.3 Origin of the tai ji emblem.

The symbolism of the dragon is clearly that of deep, generative, cosmic forces. This dragon "makes the fire come out." The generative energies are activated and the nutritive "yin fire" comes into play. The association of the water symbol furthers the description of the kidney energy as primary and creative.

The *Tong Su Shang Han Lun,* a *Shang Han Lun* commentary from 1916, provides another dimension of this picture:

> Yin fire is the basic yang of ming men.
> Its other names are the basic qi and the true fire.
> If one tries to see it, one cannot.
> If one tries to search for it, one cannot find it.
>
> Ming men attaches internally to the qi and blood
> and controls the precursor of the qi and blood.
> Therefore, the root exists.
> The existence of the root [is described as] dantian in Daoism,
> and as ming men in the *Nan Jing,*
> and as "at the side of the seventh vertebra" in the *Nei Jing.*
>
> Yin and yang unite, separate, and exist here.
> Exhalations and inhalations, entering and exiting, are connected here.
> This is not the fire that is able to warm the body.
> This is not the water that is able to moisten the body.
> There is one line on the inside that has not yet peaked.
> This is the living qi, the single line, that has not yet been lost.
> Even with anatomy one can't find it.
> Even with a microscope one can't see it.
> This is ming men.[30]

Here, the author relates the function of ming men to blood production, dantian, breath, and the basic qi. Yin fire is synonymous with all these and is the "living qi." Unlike Sawada, this commentator does not relate the triple warmer to the body temperature. Sawada does explain the "non-temperature" function of the triple warmer as a relationship to the source, the shen, and jing. The following passage from his work states the principle succinctly:

> Shen is the heart, it is the yang-fire; it is the emperor-fire.
>
> The heart organ is the official of royalty; it is the true shen which has form.
>
> The supporting fire is the triple warmer, which accepts the emperor-fire and stores it at dantian; this is the shen of no form. This is the principle of the descending yang.
>
> Jing is the kidneys; it is the yin-fire. The kidney organ becomes the prenatal source qi and stores the jing; this is the place where the true jing has form. When the form is full the function is strong, therefore, it is called the official of physical strength.
>
> Water can alchemically transform everything. Jing is mysterious; it cannot be measured. The power of techniques and abilities comes out [from the jing]. Subsequently, this is the jing that has form.

□

The moving qi between the kidneys starts at qi hai; the triple warmer meridian receives it and sends it up to the head and into the brain. This is the jing that has no form. This is the principle of the ascending yin.

Jing and shen are stored at dantian, the two dantian, the upper and lower dantian. The brain is the upper dantian. CV-4 is the lower dantian. These two become one. This one becomes two.

The true principle of between heaven and earth returns to one source. There are also twelve sources; [these] twelve sources are one source.[31]

Sawada's description tells us how the triple warmer moves shen from the heart to the lower dantian and moves jing from the kidneys to the upper dantian. The triple warmer is intimately tied to the function of the heart. The heart is the emperor fire; the triple warmer is the supporting fire. The triple warmer sends jing from the source to the upper dantian. These principles of descending yang and ascending yin further support the concept of the triple warmer as a mediating function. It provides feedback and intercommunication between the more localized functions and energies. Sawada's comments also return us to the concept of a central source.

That there are twelve sources and that these twelve sources are one source is another idea from the old texts that Sawada confirms. A passage from the *Yixue Rumen (Introduction to Medicine)* also notes this:

If we scrutinize the unusual functions of the triple warmer, we can understand that the yin and yang organs are different, yet the same.

The same, yet different.

Upon dividing, it becomes twelve. Upon uniting, it becomes the triple warmer. The triple warmer is also one warmer. The warmer is basic. It is the qi of the one basic.[32]

Again, we are presented with another statement that emphasizes the multiplicity of the triple warmer energies. This, the centrality of the source, and the dependency of the other energies upon it, are ubiquitous. However, there are a variety of ideas of the triple warmer relationship to the source, the heart, the master of the heart, the kidney, and ming men. Ryoan Terashima, author of *Wakan Sansai Zue,* an early eighteenth century treatise, draws an interesting parallel between the creation and development of the human and a plant. In doing so, he makes important statements about ming men and the heart — kidney relationship.

When the mother and father's jing are united, there is not yet any form. This is primarily a symbol of the connection between the fetus and placenta. This just-manifesting connection, the one stalk, is like the lotus flower's stigma [female part of the plant]. First there is creation and then the umbilical cord. The one point inside the stigma is truly the source of the created body and established life, it is ming men. Both kidneys are then the fruit of created life, the place of extreme yin. Even if it is the water organ, it lets the helping fire reside; it symbolizes the dragon fire in the water. With activity it forcefully pushes open to left and right; it is exactly symbolized by the cross bar that locks the gate. With quietude it closes and moistens, nourishing the true water of the one yin. Water is constant, fire is changeable. The kidneys have two leaves; their form is like the kidney bean. They are level with each other and curved. They touch both sides of the spine, one and a half divisions lateral to the spine. Outside of them is a yellow fatty enveloping sac. Each one has two cords and two lines, the upper line is connected to the heart.[33]

This is an interesting embryological metaphor. The "one point" he refers to is an expression of the universal qualities of fertilization. Pollen particles settle on the stigma inside the flower of the plant. Terashima refers to this point as the equivalent of ming men. Ming men is in some way the place where the male and female jing unite at conception. It is the result of prenatal energies. This idea is not unique. Waichi Sugiyama, in his work *Sugiyama Ryu Sanbusho,* offers a stimulating discussion of the triple warmer and the moving qi:

> The basic qi of before heaven [prenatal]
> is said to be the moving qi between the kidneys.
> The prenatal basic qi was accepted
> before the body was completed, before
> the five yin and six yang organs were completed.[34]

He continues this discussion with a review of the process of creation of the five phases from the *Yi Jing* where water is the first created.[35] In his work, the moving qi between the kidneys is also described as the "yang qi" of the kidneys. This yang qi is like the light of a lighthouse. If the flame is full and strong, one can see about the lighthouse — the body is well nourished and healthy. Sugiyama presents an interesting and more detailed discussion of the moving qi between the kidneys, explaining what he considers to be an important distinction:

> The moving qi between the kidneys is the yang qi in the kidney organ. It means that yang is in the yin [part]. This understanding is like ☵ of the *Yi Jing.* The upper and lower lines are yin; separating these is a yang line. The yang is connected to and dependent on the two yin. This is not the yang of yin. The nature of the kidney organ is of water and yin. The moving qi between the kidneys is the yang qi of the kidneys. We should not confuse this idea ☵ with the general idea of yin and yang ☯. The *Nan Jing* writer says that the moving qi between the kidneys is two divisions below the umbilicus, it is the vitality of the person, the root of the twelve meridians. This refers to the principle of heaven, the first principle, creating water.[36]

In talking about the moving qi between the kidneys we are not talking about ultimate concepts of yin and yang, rather dependent concepts of yin and yang. This is not the ultimate source of life, it is rather a manifestation of it. The "yang of yin" is like ☯. The yang is not dependent on the yin, it is contained within the yin. The moving qi between the kidneys is dependent on the yin, the kidneys. Sugiyama also draws an interesting parallel between the triple warmer and the moving qi. He states:

□

The triple warmer and moving qi between the kidneys are basically the same, but later they divide. The *Nan Jing* says that the triple warmer has a name but no form, it is like bubbles in water or droplets in fog. The triple warmer is the primary verbal knowledge of the medical Dao. Reading chapter 18 of the *Ling Shu* and chapter 31 of the *Nan Jing*, one can understand. The lower warmer of the triple warmer is the root, the lower warmer is the same place as between the kidneys.[37]

Two lengthy quotes from Sosen Hirooka demonstrate exactly what Sugiyama named the "primary verbal knowledge of the medical Dao." The first passage is part of his commentary on *Nan Jing* chapter 8 which refers to taking the pulse and examining the root:

Below the umbilicus is the dividing earth of dantian, qi hai [CV-6] and yin crossing [CV-7]. These are the places at which we can feel this tiny movement of the moving qi. Below the umbilicus is the ocean of yang qi and the crossing [place] of yin—blood, the root of yin—yang, the person and the body. [Here] is the prosperous field 福田 of the stirring dan 錬丹 which makes life long.

[Using] Daoist inhalation and exhalation makes the jing harmonized and stirs the internal dan 內丹; it can be the most essential part of heaven and earth. Gathering this [by Daoist breathing practices] in the world, one can later become a sage.

Dantian is the earth of fertility. This can create the person's body. The father — jing — is like the seed. The mother — blood — is like the fertile earth. The embryo is like the fruit. That which wraps the embryo is like the flowers and leaves. The lining is like the fruit. The umbilicus is the place of the stem.

When fruit and cucumber grow, all have stems. The person also has the umbilicus-stem, which becomes the root. Therefore, the umbilicus exists to the center of the right and left, upper and lower parts of the body. The umbilicus becomes the shu no 樞紐 "pivot rope," it symbolizes the north star of the person. It becomes the source of the living qi, the shen that protects against evil, the most noble. Because of its respectability, it is called shen jue [CV-8], zhongji [CV-3], qi hai [CV-6], and yin jiao [CV-7], shimen [CV-5], dantian. All these are based on the pulse of shen.[38]

Many concepts referenced in this passage have been elucidated by other authors. Some points mentioned, especially CV-3, relate to the north pole star. The "prosperous field" characters refer to greasy fatty tissues and together commonly mean fertility. This is likely a metaphor for fat people, who were considered wealthy, living off a fertile land.

The following quote requires little explanation. It is one of the most insightful passages in Chinese medical literature:

□

Nan Jing 25 says, "There are twelve meridians, five yin and six yang organs." These are eleven. What is this one meridian? The meridians are the branches and leaves; the yin and yang organs are the basic root. If there are roots, there must be branches. If there are branches, there must be roots.

Now [in this case] there is a branch but no root, what is this? Surely, this meridian is the divided vessel of the master of the heart which belongs to hand shao yin [heart meridian]. The heart and master of the heart are one. Thinking about the yin organ's symbol, it is called the heart. Thinking about the function of shen, it is called the master of the heart. Thinking about the meridian, it is called hand shao yin. Shao yin divides; from this comes a meridian. This is called hand jue yin. Hand shao yin permeates [belongs to] the heart, subsequently jue yin has no place to which it belongs; therefore the master of the heart controls this. The master of the heart is the master of the twelve meridians. If there is an empty space, then everything is permeated by the master of the heart.

The five yin and six yang organs total eleven. Each controls one of the twelve meridians. Upon dividing, one meridian comes out permeating the master of the heart; consequently, the total becomes twelve.

How does one differentiate between the master of the heart and the moving qi between the kidneys? With the master there is subsequently a place in the upper [part of the body]; it is called the master of the heart. With the root, there is subsequently protection of the lower [part of the body]; it is called the moving qi between the kidneys. The moving qi becomes the root of the yin and yang organs and the meridians. Therefore, on the larger [macrocosmic] scale, the master of the heart and the triple warmer become the surface and the lining. On the smaller [microcosmic] scale, the master of the heart is respectable; thus, it is the master of the moving qi. Therefore, on the larger scale, this is the master.

The source is created from the moving qi. It is like this: the emperor is the most respectable; consequently he controls the great land. This respectability also issues forth from the earth. This is how one differentiates between the master of the heart and the moving qi. The master of the heart and the triple warmer become the surface and the lining, both of these have names but no form. The master of the heart is the master of the five yin organs. The triple warmer is the most superior of the six yang organs.

The divided vessel [hand jue yin] and the triple warmer together become the surface and the lining. The master of the heart controls the lining. The triple warmer controls the surface. The triple warmer manages the qi alchemical transformations. The qi roots between the kidneys, subsequently, it becomes function and movement. The master of the heart substitutes for the shen functions. The shen stays between the

kidneys and comes out at the heart. This becomes consciousness. Shen and qi both have names but no form. Therefore,
no form responds to matter. Its function is to work without
limit.

As a rule, between heaven and earth, having both form and
no form is like spring and autumn, wind and heat, the stems
and branches, the voice and the tones. Form is already derived
from no form and then it can function. Therefore, the function
of the yin and yang organs and the meridians is also truly
brought about by the functions of the master of the heart and
the triple warmer.[39]

There is an empty space, because there is nothing for the master of the
heart to belong to, no organ for it to permeate. This empty space is said to
relate to the twelve meridians and since the master of the heart controls this
space, it also controls the twelve meridians. The author references
emperorship to emphasize the relationship; without rule of a great land one
cannot become truly respectable. The great land is the moving qi between
the kidneys; the emperor is the master of the heart.

Again, the idea of no form directs our attention to the distinction
between potential energies, which work without limit, and kinetic energies,
which work on matter. The dualities mentioned are each phenomena we
experience and describe yet are without form. Pure energy is the precursor
of matter or form.

Both Sawada's and Hirooka's commentaries offer some of the clearest
explanations we have found. They have historical context; they are not
fanciful speculations by latter-day scholars and practitioners. Their studies
and commentaries were based in part on other commentaries on the *Nan
Jing* written in the third, fourth, and seventh centuries and compiled by
Wang Jiu Si in his *Nan Jing Ji Zhu (Collected commentaries on the Nan Jing)*.
In a number of other texts different aspects of the *Nan Jing* theory were
discussed by both herbalists and acupuncturists. Several passages selected
from these commentaries demonstrate the historical background from
which Sawada and Hirooka absorbed ideas. The commentary of a Mr.
Yang, who lived from 618 to 670 A.D., made some points that parallel those
of Hirooka about the master of the heart and the moving qi between the
kidneys. He described the area between both kidneys as "the great
ocean."[40] The moving qi between the kidneys resides between the kidneys;
it is metaphorically both the great ocean and the great land; it represents a
vast reservoir. Yang also identified the moving qi with dantian:

Below the umbilicus is the moving qi between the kidneys.
It is dantian.
Dantian is the root of the person,
the place where jing and shen are stored.[41]

The principles of ascending yin, or jing, and descending yang, or shen,
arise from dantian. This is also seen in a another comment ascribed to a
Mr. Wang, quoted by Hua Shou in his commentary on the *Nan Jing*, the
Nan Jing Benyi:
□

The triple warmer has a name but no form.
The upper [warmer] unites with the master of the heart.
The lower [warmer] unites with the right kidney.[42]

In the *Nan Jing,* the right kidney is ming men, where the jing and shen reside *(NJ 36).*

The scholar, Ding, from 338-379 A.D., defines the moving qi:

> The moving qi between the kidneys is the basic qi that occurs
> in the infant. The *Huang Ting Jing* says, "This is the jing of
> water, the qi of kan ☵." Now, it is said to be between the kid-
> neys; it is the source qi of the person. The Daoists say between
> the kidneys is called dantian; it is also called the hidden ocean
> in which is the shen-turtle, inhaled, exhaled, and source qi.
> Therefore it is said to be the gate of breathing.[43]

These concepts are strictly consistent through each of the various aspects of Chinese philosophy, cosmology, and medicine. The energetic center of the body, below the umbilicus, is related to the north pole, the "great one," the "great ultimate." It is correlated to the lower dantian, qi hai dantian, at which the shen and jing are stored and interact. Each of the ideas is also the moving qi between the kidneys in a different aspect. We can see each as equivalent concepts, each discussed and commented on in a variety of texts and styles. This provides the energetic source for the meridians, the organ functions, and the triple warmer. The triple warmer is comprised of all these and all these comprise the triple warmer. Also, as Yang states, it is different from the five phases; it does not belong to the normal cycling of the phases:

> Only the source is not according to the five phases. The source
> is the basic. The basic qi is the qi of the triple warmer. This qi
> is highly respectable; therefore, it does not belong to the
> category of the five phases.[44]

The triple warmer and master of the heart are different from the organs of the five phases. They have a more central role and greater significance because they are the precursors of all the phase, organ, and meridian relationships. We can see this clearly in the theoretical descriptions of the cycles of open points that are found in Ming dynasty texts. Unfortunately, space does not allow us to detail these cycles; we will do this in a later work.

The distinctions between the triple warmer and pericardium and the organs and phases could not have been more succinctly stated than in the Jin dynasty (1115-1234) text, the *Zi Wu Liu Zhu Zhen Jing,* believed to have been compiled by He Ruo Yu:

> The ten meridians, the blood and qi all come out at the jing
> [points] and enter at the he [points]. Everything flows through
> the jing, yong, shu, jing, he [points] without depending on
> them.
>
> It is also said that the vessels have twelve meridians. Why
> are there said to be only ten meridians? What are the other two
> meridians said to be?

□

It is said that the two meridians are the triple warmer, this is the yang qi of the father; the heart-wrapping luo [pericardium], this is the yin-blood of the mother. These two meridians are respectable, they are not connected to the five phases. Mainly they accept the ten meridians. The blood and qi and nourish and feed them.[45]

This short text also describes the uses of the stems and branches in acupuncture theory. It was probably quite influential for Xu Feng who wrote the *Zhen Jiu Da Quan* nearly three centuries later. In that text, full descriptions of the open point cycles are found. The references to father and mother in the preceding quote are derived from Wang Shu He:

The triple warmer is the father of the qi, the pericardium is the mother of the blood.[46]

There are a great many concepts that are essentially the same concept. There are a great many phenomena that have a common origin. All these functions, actions, and energies center in the umbilicus and the abdomen. As Yang says:

One name for the umbilicus is the "life of the person," another name for it is tai zhong ji, the great middle pole [CV-3]; another name for it is tai yuan [LU-9]; another name for it is kun lun [BL-60]; another name for it is wu cheng, the five mansions. The five mansions have [house] the true people [realized sages]. It means the five emperors. Outside the wu cheng are the eight messengers, these are the eight trigram-shen. The eight trigram-shen are united with the tai yi, the great one, these become the nine noble ones. Outside the eight trigrams, there are the twelve towers; the towers have twelve children. These unite with the triple warmer. The shen becomes the twenty-seven physicians and also unites with the four supporters. The shen becomes the eighty-one officers [gentlemen]. The center of the umbilicus is called the tai yi, the great one.[47]

This passage is explicit. All of the facets of the medical model are centered in the umbilicus, the great one, the tai yi.

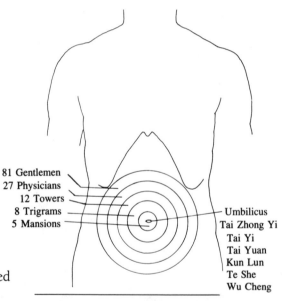

Figure 6.4 Energetic rippling from the center, the umbilicus.

The numerological sequencing is important and requires some examination. It is tempting, though not necessarily justified, to see the five mansions as related to the five phases. The eight trigrams, however, are related to the eight extraordinary vessels. This is supported by the fact that they unite with the center, the tai yi, to become the nine nobles. In the Ming dynasty the eight extraordinary vessels were equated with the eight trigrams of the *Yi Jing* temporal sequence, which is based upon the magic square of nine.[48] The twelve towers and their children are the twelve branches and their meridians. These unite with the triple warmer; all have a common origin at the moving qi. The twenty-seven physicians are most likely the twenty-seven jing-luo. In the *Nan Jing*, there were said to be twenty-seven jing-luo, twelve meridians, and fifteen luo vessels. The reference to the eighty-one gentlemen is not clear, perhaps it is another symbol for the myriad things. We can see this diagrammatically.

□

Yang continues his explanation with a reference to meditative practice:

> Jing is the basic part of the living being, therefore, we know
> dantian is the basic part of life. The Daoists, Buddhists, Zen
> monks, all move their mind qi [heart qi?] to below the umbil-
> icus. Therefore, the source is the respectable title of the triple
> warmer. The triple warmer unites with the qi at the kidneys.[49]

The practices of the Daoist, Buddhist, and Zen monks were well
known at this time; it is clear from this passage that many of the concepts
we have been discussing — the jing, the dantian, the mind-heart, the
source, the triple warmer, the kidneys, the shen and the moving qi — were
important in both meditation and medicine. This is not just true of the
Nan Jing, but of the medical corpus as a whole. The medical practices are a
natural extension of the contemplative practices. This is evident in much
of the medical literature.

In the *Huang Di Nei Jing Tai Su,* Yang discusses the moving qi in relation to the chong mai, notably integrating the systems of Chinese medicine:

> Below the umbilicus is the moving qi between the kidneys, the
> living energy of the person. This is the root of the twelve meri-
> dians. This "blood ocean" is chong mai, the ocean of the five
> yin and six yang organs and the twelve meridians *(TS10:153).*[50]

In a previous work we have shown through an examination of the origins and natures of the ren mai and du mai that they too are related to the
chong mai and thus the moving qi between the kidneys.[51] This can be
clearly seen in a quotation from Wang Bing:

> This is why we can say that the du mai, ren mai and chong mai
> have different names but are all the same.[52]

Similarly, from Li Shi Zhen:

> The triple warmer is the function of ming men. The ren mai
> and du mai make contact together at the chong mai.[53]

The extraordinary vessels, at least the chong mai, du mai, and ren mai,
have their origin at the moving qi. Thus, the meridian, organ, extraordinary
vessel, and triple warmer systems have a common origin. However, it is
more effective, and truer to the sources, to think of these different systems
as different energetic levels or strata in the body. The source is much more
than a junction box in a wiring diagram.

In his 1895 commentary on the *Nan Jing,* the *Nan Jing Zheng Yi,* Xie Lin
details the same connections and adds several other concepts:

> Both kidneys belong to water. Between them the kidney sup-
> porter belongs to fire; this is ming men. *Su Wen* chapter 52
> said, "At the side of the seventh vertebra in the middle, there is
> the small heart." This is ming men. The person, heaven, earth
> are three. Ming men and tai ji are similar. Tai ji creates the two
> poles; the poles create the four phenomena; the four
> phenomena create the eight trigrams; the eight trigrams create
> the sixty-four hexagrams. Ming men creates the two kidneys;
> the two kidneys create the six yin and six yang organs; the six
> yin and six yang organs create the four limbs and all the bones.

Before the person's conception, before the jing gathers, there is first a meeting of fire. This fire becomes the root [beginning] of the prenatal. Water becomes the true yuan [basic] of heaven. The fire between the kidneys is called the "helping fire." Ming men is the root of the triple warmer; it becomes the home of the helping fire; this disseminates to the triple warmer. Therefore, ming men is the beginning.[54]

The inseparability of ming men and the moving qi between the kidneys and the unstated equation of these concepts cannot be ignored. They are the yin and yang poles of the same concept; ming men is on the back [yang] and the moving qi is at the front [yin]. Xie Lin makes some immensely interesting statements in his *Nan Jing Zheng Yi.* He first quotes from the *Su Wen:*

The sage standing, faces the south direction.
His front is called the guang ming [extensive, broad brightness].
His back is called the dai chong [the great chong of chong mai].
It is called the shao yin (SW 6:49).

He then comments on this passage:

Dai chong is the unity of the kidney meridian and chong mai; when it expands and becomes large, it is called the dai chong. Between the kidneys is the terrain [place] from which the chong mai emerges. On the surface its [reflex] area is around guan yuan [CV-4, the qi hai dantian area]. This is the source of the triple warmer's qi transformations, the qi of the twelve meridians. All these are connected here. Therefore, it is called the root. It rises up parallel to the ren mai to the throat, with inhale and exhale; therefore, it is called the gate of breathing. Those in the upper parts connect to the arm three yin and three yang; these become the branches. Those in the lower parts connect to the leg three yin and three yang; these become the root. This is qi; it becomes the source of the twelve meridians, the fu of the triple warmer. It controls the movements of the ying and wei. It also becomes the secure place of the jing and shen, the connection, supporter of the basic qi. One more name for it is the shen which protects against evil. With the shen of ming men, we can protect with strength.

The moving qi between the kidneys is the source of the vital qi of the twelve meridians; it oversees the ying and wei. It gives exhaustively to the upward and downward motions of the qi and blood. This is primarily caused by breathing and therefore makes a circuit. During inhalation, the yang of heaven is drawn in. During exhalation, the yin of earth comes out. The master of the heart and the emperor fire and the qi of inhalation are the heaven yang and also belong to fire. The qi comes in through the nose into the lungs and then timelessly passes to the heart. It attracts the heart fire. Then from the supporter of the heart, it passes down the du mai and comes into the kidneys. Also from the supporter of the kidneys [already said to be ming men], it extends to the lower warmer and the uterus.[55]

From the kidney supporter it [passes to] and reaches the lower warmer qi hai. What is qi hai? It is the root of the triple warmer. It is located below the umbilicus. The text says that this is the chamber of the uterus. The heaven yang of the person's inhalation unites with the heart and passes down to attach to the chamber of the uterus. It goes around the bladder and goes to the lower orifice [of the bladder]. This [moving qi between the kidneys] lets the yang qi of heaven come in through inhalation. It unites with the heart fire and steams the water of the bladder. It alchemically transforms and becomes qi; it passes around the chong and ren mai and rises up, passing through the diaphragm to enter the lungs. It then returns and comes out from the mouth and nose. The qi that rises up and comes out is in the mouth and tongue. In the yin and yang organs it becomes the jin and ye. The qi from each of the qi jie comes out externally to the skin and hair. The fire comes into the water and transforms it. It is the principle of qi. The ☰ and ☷ mutually interact. It is the principle of the three su [roots]. Therefore, this is heaven, person, and earth.[56]

This passage is rich in information; it clearly describes the relationship of the kidneys and chong mai and their relationship to the source. Again, the triple warmer and the twelve meridians connect to the source; the ren mai and du mai relate to breathing. The circuit it describes is intriguing. Upon inhalation, qi passes through the nose to the lungs, to the heart, and down the du mai to emerge between the kidneys and enter into the lower warmer, the uterus, and bladder. During this process a variety of transformations occur. Upon exhalation it passes to the chong mai and ren mai, moving upward through the diaphragm to the lungs, and finally out the mouth and nose. In another description of this circulation the author notes that the qi, once at the diaphragm, passes to the spleen before moving to the lungs. Quite clearly the ability to attain proper breathing has a strong bearing on this process and the condition of the moving qi.

The latter part of his commentary describes how breathing causes heaven and earth to mutually interact resulting in water and fire. This describes the shift from the early heaven sequence of the trigrams to the later or temporal sequence of the trigrams (Figure 6.5).

In another interesting passage, Xie Lin describes the relationship of the ren mai and du mai to water and fire, the kidneys and the heart.

The prenatal controls the qi.
In the lower parts it crosses in the uterus.
The postnatal controls the blood.
In the lower parts it crosses in the uterus.
All things are of these two vessels.
With the water and fire theory,
the du mai belongs to the qi and to water,
the ren mai belongs to the blood and to fire.
The ren mai most certainly also belongs to the heart.
The heart and kidneys are associated with each other.

Water and fire are ☲☵
Everything results from this.
Therefore, the ren mai is the ocean of the yin vessels.[57]

These interactions are fundamentally important: "everything results."

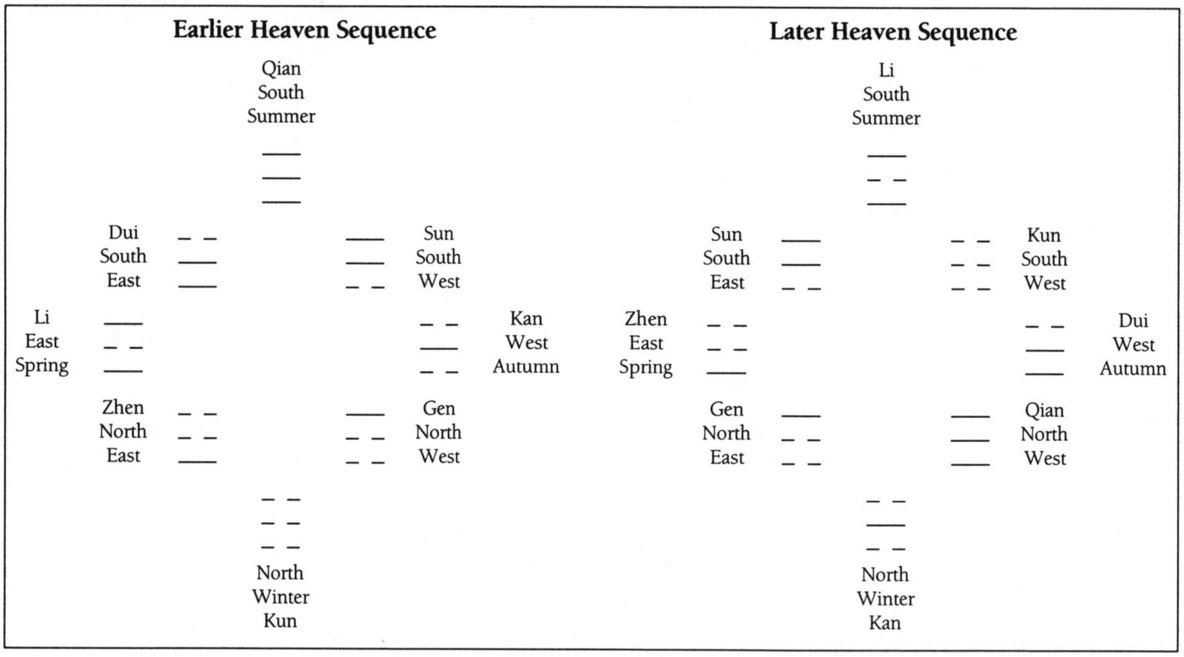

Figure 6.5 The Early Heaven sequence of the trigrams is transformed by correct breathing to the Later Heaven or Temporal sequence.

All important energetic concepts in Chinese medicine are linked to the source, the abdominal area. From a diagnostic perspective palpation of the abdomen is critical. It enables us to diagnose all that reflects there, the moving qi between the kidneys, the source. Since everything springs from the tai ji, which is equivalent to ming men and the moving qi, the extraordinary vessels, the organs and their meridians are all reflected in the abdomen. Treating the indications found on the abdomen is equivalent to treating the problem that created the indication. Eliminating pressure pain on a point will treat the problem that caused the pressure pain. For example, treating points known to alleviate pressure pain on KI-16, in a case of kidney vacancy, will treat the kidneys. Treating points that alleviate pressure pain on KI-16, in a chong mai problem, will treat the chong mai. The cases differ in regard to the energetic levels reflected and affected.

This therapeutic principle is stated succinctly by Liu Wan Su in his *Su Wen* commentary:

> When you treat disease, you have to focus on and differentiate the symptoms [local problems] and the basic [root] problems. The symptoms [express themselves] above the neck; The basic problems [express themselves] at the origin or basic [level].[58]

Since not all symptoms of disease occur above the neck, the reference here is to symptoms that manifest as changes in facial color or tongue body, etc. According to the *Su Wen,* when treating disease, "One should first treat the root, then later treat the symptoms" (*SW 65:357*). The source,

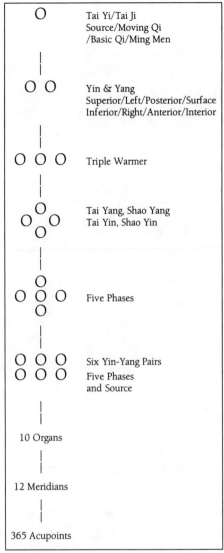

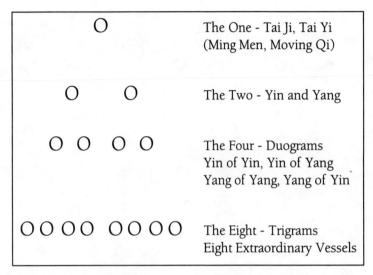

Figure 6.7 Symbolic derivations — the one gives rise to the eight.

the moving qi, ming men, represents the root, the deepest level of the body's energetic strata: the one, the unity, which manifests in the center. Treating the abdomen, the root, should be the main focus of treatment.

Essentially, those things that arise directly out of the ocean of qi lie closer to the moving qi than those phenomena that are branches or extensions. This is an important diagnostic and therapeutic distinction. The one gives rise to two, to four, to eight and on:

Figure 6.6 Symbolic derivations - the one gives rise to the many.

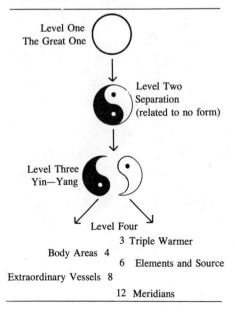

Figure 6.8 Common origin of energetic sequences.

The first sequence shows the relationships of the extraordinary vessels to the source. There is a parallel sequence in which we may see other facets of the medical theories. It is wise to keep the extraordinary vessel sequence and the phase — meridian — organ sequence separate, even though both have a common origin at the moving qi. This is derived from the *Nan Jing:*

> If the [twelve] meridians are full [overflowing], this fullness goes into [spills over] the eight extraordinary vessels never to return *(NJ 28:16).*

These are distinct energetic strata and functions. Each is connected but not sequentially or mutually. Thus, we can see these as distinct sequences with a common origin, as shown in Figure 6.8.

Beginning with the *Ling Shu* and the *Nan Jing,* there have been attempts to identify elements of these sequences, such as the triple warmer and ming men, with anatomical structures and regions. In effect, these attempts would turn the preceding symbolic charts into true anatomical representations. These correspondences do exist and represent a further means of understanding the energetic principles of Chinese medicine and predicting the results of therapy. We will describe these correspondences and demonstrate how the physiological properties of these anatomical structures relate to entities such as the triple warmer.

Chapter

- 7 -

Classical Energetic Anatomy & Physiology

Classical Energetic Anatomy and Physiology

A great advantage of the Oriental medical model is what is currently called a "top-down" approach. Each increasingly specialized and detailed element of the study of human health fits within and reflects the preceding more generalized ideas. Thus it is possible to add new data to our understanding of Oriental medicine as it becomes available. The same concepts of energy that explain the macrocosmic ideas of source and unity may be applied to the microcosmic explanations of man's functions.

Though some disagreement regarding the details of the interior energetics of the human body exists among different authors, there is general consensus that the relationships are substantive and important. Less consonance is evident relative to the importance of "anatomy and physiology" in Chinese medicine. Some authors have been conscientious in noting the parallels between the functional observations of Oriental medicine and the anatomophysiological observations of Western science.[1] Other authors significantly understate this aspect of Chinese medical history. Certainly, some have observed a general trend toward ignoring the finer observations found in the classics.[2] Nonetheless, these observations exist, and are important. These classical references lead us to look more carefully at the fascial system, the "fat, greasy tissues" of the human body. These anatomical structures were known, were understood, and were seen to play an important role in the function of the human body.[3]

Sources and Myths

Despite the pervasive misconception that the ancient Chinese had no anatomical knowledge, a study of the classical texts makes it clear that the medical authors were aware of internal anatomy. Even when the earliest Chinese medical texts were written, there was sufficient anatomical knowledge to conduct discussions of tissues, membranes, and fasciae. In fact, there are several medical and non-medical sources from the Han dynasty that specifically discuss surgical anatomy or, by virtue of the content of the discussion, imply that some surgical anatomy was done. For example, in the "Wang Mang" chapter of the *Han Shu*, there is a brief discussion of Prince Mang's order to skilled physicians and butchers regarding the performance of surgical anatomy on political prisoners.[4] From this account, the physicians and butchers were ordered to perform surgery, that is, vivisection, on live prisoners. They cut open the prisoners, removed and measured their organs and probed the various blood vessels to establish the source, course, and outlet of each. They claimed that with this knowledge they might be able to treat disease. In commentary on this passage, Akira Ishihara dates it to around 16 A.D., the end of the Former Han dynasty.[5]

□

Anatomical measurements of the organs were described in some chapters of the *Ling Shu*. Chapter 31 contains discussions of the lengths of the various organs, and chapter 32 contains discussions of the capacities of the organs. Most commentators and scholars agree that portions of the *Ling Shu* were written during the late Zhou dynasty, other portions by the early to middle Han dynasty with some portions added later. Most of the *Ling Shu* was probably written by the time of the above passage from the *Han Shu*. Thus it is quite likely that these discussions from the *Ling Shu* were written by or before the end of the Former Han dynasty. One *Ling Shu* passage clearly references anatomical dissection:

> The Yellow Emperor asked, "On the inside the twelve meridians belong to the five yin and six yang organs. On the outside twelve meridians meet with the twelve water meridians. The twelve water meridians are not alike, there are large, small, deep, shallow, wide, narrow, distant, and near ones. The five yin and six yang organs are higher, lower, larger, and smaller [in different people]. The capacity for receiving the grains is different. How do we understand this?
>
> The water meridians accept water and subsequently move. The five yin organs unite the shen, qi, hun, po, and store them. The six yang organs receive food and then move. They accept qi and distribute it. The meridians receive the blood and nourish [the body].
>
> By combining [all this knowledge] we then treat. So how can we decide the depth of needle insertion and the number of moxa when we treat?"
>
> Qi Bo answered, "Heaven is too high and is unmeasurable. Earth is too wide and is unmeasurable. The person is between Heaven and Earth and is influenced by the six unitings.[6]
>
> [For example] there is a man eight forearm divisions tall. His flesh and skin are obvious. We can measure the external surface of his body by palpation. Also, if he dies, we can observe his internal anatomy.
>
> [We can see] the hardness, weakness of the yin organs, the largeness, smallness of the yang organs, the capacity of the digestive system, the length and shortness of the vessels, the clarity and unclarity of the blood, the fullness and insufficiency of the qi, whether there is too much blood and not enough qi of the twelve meridians, or too much qi and not enough blood of the twelve meridians, or too much blood and qi or not enough blood and qi of the twelve meridians.
>
> [By observing the anatomy of many corpses] we can assess and standardize the correct needle depth and number of moxa [for each meridian and point]" *(LS 12:154-155)*.

While there are many interpretive questions raised by this passage, not the least of which is how "fullness and insufficiency of the qi" was measured, the ancient Chinese clearly did not limit their curiosity and research to non-anatomical pursuits. The scope of their research was less limited than we might presume. The description of "water meridians" on the outside surface of the body is congruent with the lymphatic system and the interstitial fluids; the relationship of the points and meridians to specific anatomical positions is clear.

These passages are not isolated examples. The *Nan Jing* was written at least by 100 A.D., during the time of the Han Dynasty. Chapter 42 of the *Nan Jing* contains similar discussions that describe the relative lengths, weights, and capacities of the organs. Further anatomical discussions and drawings are available in Wang Shu He's commentary on chapters 42 and 43 of the *Nan Jing*, from his text that was written at the end of the third century.

Although earlier discussions of anatomy were rather terse and crude, the *Nan Jing* and *Ling Shu* discussions of source in relation to fascial membranes were backed up by written documentation of first-hand anatomical knowledge as early as the Han dynasty. It is also true that the *Su Wen* discussions of the meridians, the jing, the luo, and the penetration of evil qi into the body, could have been understood in the context of sufficient knowledge of membranes and fascia. Various discussions and commentaries from both older and more recent times make clear statements about the interconnection of these anatomical structures. By studying these we can understand the classical texts in more detail, remembering that these texts used the language of energetics to describe ideas with very old roots that were based on the traditional macrocosmic world view.

In essence, we must bridge the distance between two prejudices. We must avoid misinterpretations that derive from the idea that the ancient Chinese were necessarily so primitive as to have ignored the basic structure of the body and its mechanisms. At the same time, we must avoid the concept that an energetic medicine must not be "scientific" or structural in any regard. While it is true that the tools of microbiology and biochemistry were not available to the ancient Chinese, and that their descriptions of the human body are predominantly functional, it does not follow that their ideas of human function were totally divorced from the observable structures of the human body. It is our opinion that regardless of any of the limitations of science or culture that may have hindered the Han Chinese, they shared the essential curiosity of scientists in any age and the working physician's will to use all the knowledge available for the benefit of the patient.

The Huang, Gao, and Triple Warmer

In the first chapter of the *Ling Shu* is a discussion of specific source theory that describes various "fat," "greasy" tissues, fasciae, and systems of connecting membranes. In particular the *huang* 肓 and the *gao* 膏 were important elements of this source conception. Each of these was associated with specific treatment or reflex source points. The gao was shown to have bearing on early stages of embryological development. Both the gao and the huang were linked to the *Nan Jing* theories of the source and triple warmer.

Further commentary discussing huang in relation to the triple warmer and movement of yang qi in the body occurs in Ippo Okamoto's *Shinkyu Azeyoketsu*, an acupoint book dating from 1703. This discussion comes within a general discussion of the nature of the extra point pi gen 痞根 and why it is able to treat lumps within the body:

Some say that pi gen is huang men [BL-46]. Why does huang men treat problems of pi gen?

To the right and left sides of the thirteenth vertebra [L1] on the shu line is the triple warmer shu point [BL-22] above the kidney shu point [BL-23].

The *Nan Jing* says, "The triple warmer is the alternative messenger of the source qi." The source qi is the basic yang between the kidneys. Therefore, the location of the shu point of the triple warmer is above the kidney shu point.

At the same level [on the outer bladder line] is huang men [BL-46]. Huang 肓 is the space between the organs, bones and flesh. It is that through which the yang qi streams. Therefore, above is the diaphragm, huang, below is the source of huang. All the basic yang gathers and meets here, it is called the huang.

Huang men is to the right and left of the triple warmer shu, because the qi of the triple warmer basic yang comes out from there and goes to the whole body. When the triple warmer moves smoothly, the five yin and six yang organs, the ying and wei move smoothly, therefore one cannot get any lumps. Therefore, if people develop lumps, this is the original place of the lump, treat it. This point also treats pressure pain and tension below the sternum.[7]

In this passage, the key phrase is, "huang is the space between the organs, bones, and flesh. It is that through which the yang qi streams." The characters translated as "space between" are *jian kong* 間空. In this context, where huang is already understood to mean "fat, greasy tissues or membranes," it is most reasonable to consider this a reference to the insubstantial membranes or fasciae that line and lie between the organs, bones, and muscles. Interpreting this statement as saying that the yang qi streams through the fascia of the body fairly resolves the problem of textual definition. In classical source theory the triple warmer is intimately related to the moving qi between the kidneys, and thus it is implicated here. However, this passage does not explicitly state whether the triple warmer is the membranes themselves or is simply functionally related.

In another early eighteenth century Japanese text, the *Wakan Sansai Zue,* written by Ryoan Terashima in 1712 A.D., only nine years after Ippo Okamoto's statement, the triple warmer was not only seen to be related to the functional aspects of the membranes or fascia, it was clearly stated to be those fascia. Though it is difficult to say if the earlier text influenced the later, it is nonetheless important that such an unequivocal statement was made. Terashima begins his discussion by quoting Chen Yan's *San Yin Ji Yi Bing Zheng Fang Lun,* an herbal text from 1174 A.D.. Chen Yan felt that for the triple warmer to be able to carry out its various functions, it must have a form. He identified this form with a certain area of fascia:

Chen Yan said, "The triple warmer has fatty membranes. It is the same size as the palm of the hand. It lies in front of the bladder. It has two white vessels. The membranes [or vessels] come out from inside this to rise up parallel to the spine and pass through the brain."[8]

□

The two "white vessels" in front of the bladder must be the medial umbilical folds (umbilical arteries). The area between these is roughly the size of the palm of the hand. Thus, we can see the triple warmer as being the fascia that lies between these folds. Terashima felt that Chen Yan's comment was only part of the story:

> I feel that this is not the whole story. Because if this is right, why are there the "upper, middle, and lower" warmers? I think the "three," when taken to the extreme, are the upper, middle, and lower [conceptual parts]. The warmer is a symbol of fire. The color red belongs to [the category of] yang. It [the triple warmer] passes around the trunk, abdomen, lower, and upper parts — the whole body; it is like a large envelope. This is the triple warmer.[9]

Aside from the skin itself, the only other "large envelope" is the superficial fascia. Thus, in Terashima's view, the superficial fascia is the triple warmer. He goes on:

> The triple warmer is the external defense of the yin and yang organs. The luo that wraps the heart [the pericardium] is the external defense of the Emperor [heart-shen]. These are the city's inner and outer defense [walls] of the Emperor's gate. Therefore, the triple warmer belongs to [the category of] yang. It is at the same level as the helping fire. Subsequently, the vessels 脈, the luo 絡, and the source 原, are all connected to each other.[10]

For Ryoan Terashima, the "helping fire" is the "luo that wraps the heart," the pericardium.[11] In his description, the triple warmer and pericardium both have the function of protecting the Emperor, the heart-shen function. He analogically compares the triple warmer to the outer defensive walls of the city. The pericardium is like the citadel walls around the Emperor's abode. Just as the pericardium, the "luo that wraps the heart" is a fatty, greasy membrane, a luo that wraps around the heart, so too is the triple warmer a fatty, greasy membrane, the superficial fascia around the body. That the "vessels, luo, and source are all connected to each other," is as clear as possible a statement of the interconnectedness of the various systems of fasciae and membranes in the body.

There are other discussions of the membranes in relationship to the triple warmer. In China, two and a half centuries before Okamoto and Terashima, Hua Shou, in his commentary on the *Nan Jing,* the *Nan Jing Ben Yi,* wrote,

> Gu Yi Yuan Shi said, "That which is called the triple warmer is located inside the diaphragm's membrane, the greasy membrane 脂膏."[12]

Again, the triple warmer is seen in relation to various membranes or abdominal fascia, in particular the *gao* 膏 which plays such a large part in the *Ling Shu* source theory. Gu Yi Yuan Shi continues:

□

[The triple warmer] is the space between
the five yin and six yang organs,
the gate of water and grains, the stream of transformation.
[Its] qi blends in this space.
It heavily steams the diaphragm membrane.
It helps the skin and flesh develop.
It transports to the four parts.
It is called the upper, middle, and lower.
Each of these according to area has its own name.
This is the alternative messenger of the true basic qi 眞元氣.[13]

Thus, all the classical functions and properties of the triple warmer were seen in reference to the "diaphragm's membrane, the greasy membrane."

There are similar passages in other earlier ages. For instance, Yu Bo, who lived from 1436 to 1515 A.D., wrote in his *Dan Xi Yi Xue Zheng Bo*:

It is said that the triple warmer refers to the trunk and the body, and that it is also said to be the wrapping envelope, that it is the total controller of the intestines and the stomach. Inside the chest and above the huang mo 肓膜, the fatty membrane [pleura], is the upper warmer. Below the huang mo and above the umbilicus is the middle warmer. Below the umbilicus is the lower warmer. Therefore, it is called the triple warmer. This has the capacity to receive [things] yet has no place [location]. The body has fatty membranes that exist inside the trunk and the body. They completely wrap the exterior of the six yin and five yang organs. The heart-wrapping luo truly is the membrane that wraps the heart, wrapping the exterior of the heart. Therefore, it is said that the heart wrapping luo and the supporter 系 are connected to the supporter of the triple warmer.[14]

Once more the triple warmer is seen as the fascial systems of the body, in particular the more interior fascial systems and especially the mesenterium by which it is the "total controller of the intestines and the stomach."

Xie Lin, in his Qing dynasty commentary on the *Nan Jing*, titled the *Nan Jing Zheng Yi*, also commented on the triple warmer:

The triple warmer, then, is the abdominal wrapping membrane 腹包膜 [probably the peritoneal membranes]. This is connected to the net-like greasy membrane. All parts of the triple warmer unite and protect the yin and yang organs.[15]

Again, the triple warmer was seen as part of the body's fascia. Wu Kao Pan in his 1980 commentary on the *Nan Jing Zhen Yi*, wrote:

Ming men is the connection 系 of the kidneys, therefore the kidney connection passes down and creates a greasy membrane 脂膜. This is the root of the triple warmer. In Western medicine this is the mesenterium, this is the membrane that interconnects [or controls] the organs in the abdomen.[16]

□

He continues this discussion by explaining in greater detail the various mesenteric folds within the abdomen, the greater and lesser omenta. Xie Lin makes many other interesting comments in relation to the various membranes or fascia. For instance, in discussing the anatomy and connections of the kidneys to the triple warmer and the lower dantian, he says:

> The position of the kidneys is at the same level as the twelfth vertebra. Around them is the triple warmer's greasy membrane [that] wraps [and] lines [them]. Between the kidneys is a single strand of fatty membrane, passing through the spinal bones. It is called the kidney connector 腎系. It passes down to the net-like membrane. There is also [a membrane of] the bronchii of the lungs, which passes downward, attaches to, and surrounds the spine. It goes down to and enters the kidney connector. It passes through and comes into the net-like membrane. It extends to dantian, the source of the lower warmer.[17]

This passage neatly ties together several key concepts in Chinese medicine. The energetic relationships of the triple warmer, kidneys, and the lungs are given a biophysical rationale. This would help explain the idea from the *Nan Jing* that the "moving qi between the kidneys" is the "gate of breathing." The energy drawn down into the abdomen on inhalation may function through these connections. The membranes Xie Lin describes provide the physical pathway by which these energetic exchanges may occur.

What these membranes are remains to be seen. They may be related to the anterior longitudinal ligaments that line the anterior portions of the spine. The "kidney connector" may well be related to the perirenal fascia and the root of the mesentery. Nonetheless, in examining the more classical concepts of human energetic anatomy and the possible relationship to modern anatomical concepts and entities, these connections are a key to our understanding. Other authors in more modern times tend to agree with this identification of the triple warmer with the fascia. The authors of the *Nei Jing Jie Po Sheng Li Xue* paraphrase the theory. They assert that the triple warmer "has form, it is like the greasy membranes."[18]

It is also interesting to note in this context how the assumptions we make about Oriental medicine begin to compound. As we have remarked, most modern Chinese herbal texts, on which a large part of current Oriental medical theory is now based, ignore the finer anatomical descriptions in the older texts. In addition, the functional aspects of the organs and other medical entities are strongly emphasized. These texts usually translate and consider the idea of no form as conceptually equivalent to "of no physical substance." These presumptions combine to permit an idea of the triple warmer as a totally functional entity. This has grievous implications. What, for example, can be the importance of an "energetic medicine" if there is no ground substance for its energetic connections? Why should anyone accept a non-substantive organ, with functions that are only sets of observed events, as anything more than a biological misgrouping that would best be reassigned to metabolism or hormonal stimulants? How would needling triple warmer points effect anything?

□

Clearly, considering the profound interrelationship of source theory, the energetic anatomy of the vessels and points, the transmutation of food and breath, and the various qi, a reassessment of any superficial concept of the triple warmer is required.

One other modern text must be discussed. This is the *Xue Zheng Lun,* a treatise on blood disorders, by Tang Zong Hai, from 1885 A.D..[19] This major herbal text is enlightening not only for its numerous discussions of pathology with reference to the five phases, but also for its discussion of the nature of the triple warmer. Tang Zong Hai points out that the triple warmer's "warmer" character, *jiao* 焦, is related to another character, *jiao* 膲. This relationship is also recognized by authors of the *Guang Ya* from 230 A.D. and the *Ji Yun* from the eleventh century.[20] The *Guang Ya* defines jiao as the san jiao, triple warmer of the person. The *Ji Yun* describes the jiao thus: "The san jiao [triple warmer] is the fu of no form, it is related to jiao - the warmer." In this passage, 膲 refers to the membranes of the body — the parts of the body that have insufficient flesh, the various fasciae. The concept of the "warmer" is here viewed in relationship to the fasciae of the body. The etymology of the "warmer" character, 焦, also has pertinence. The upper part of the character, 隹, refers to a short-tailed bird, specifically the phoenix.[21] The lower part, 灬, refers to the flames of a fire. Thus, the character is a pictogram of a phoenix rising from the flames of a fire. One of the oldest forms of the character shows three phoenixes rising from the flames *(Mor).* Is it a coincidence that there are three warmers?

The image of the phoenix arising from the flames of a fire is a common image in many cultures, usually representing death and rebirth, or transformation. In Chinese culture, the phoenix was important as one of four shen 四神, an animal symbol that related to the southern direction, the color red, and the fire phase. In the character of "warmer" itself there are many meanings beyond "scorching," "burning," or "warming." The best possible translation would refer to the body's essential capability of transformation, for the triple warmer is the medium through which the process of transformation occurs within the human body. It has been noted that this is also an important concept in Daoist practice. The idea of transformation is key for Daoist adepts, as impure energies are transmuted and purified.[22]

The triple warmer was seen as a continuous network of oily membranes connecting the upper, lower, internal, and external portions of the body. As early as the twelfth century in China, and somewhat later in Japan, the triple warmer was identified as an area of fascia, or the network of membranes or fasciae in the body. Both Japanese and Chinese authors derived the justification for their theories from classical texts and classical ideas. According to the later commentaries and texts, the triple warmer is the system of fasciae and connective tissue membranes throughout the body, in particular the superficial fascia that surrounds the body. Ippo Okamoto specifically determined that the triple warmer qi exited at huang men (BL-46); from there it passed through the huang, the fascia, to the whole body. Recall that the huang and gao are the various systems of fascia in the abdomen, and in particular the fasciae that connect the organs and encapsulate them.[23]

☐

The Mo and Luo

Other concepts referred to in the classical literature are worthy of note and further investigation: the *mo* 膜, the *mu* 募, of the mu points, the diaphragm 膈, the concept of the lining of the body, the *li* 裏 and the *luo* 絡 of the luo vessels and points. Careful and detailed examinations of each of these important concepts further reveals the importance of the abdominal and bodily fasciae.

Descriptions in classical texts of the internal trajectories of the twelve meridians note how a meridian "belongs to" or "permeates" its own organ and "spirally wraps" its coupled organ. The character translated as "spirally wrap" is luo *(Fuj)*.

Luo is a difficult character to translate, having a number of different meanings in different contexts. There are the *luo mai* 絡脈, or luo vessels, often translated as the *luo* meridians or as blood vessels. There are the *jing luo* 經絡, or system of vertical 經 and horizontal 絡 meridians that traverse the body. There are the *luo xue* 絡穴, or luo points, one of which lies on each meridian. There is the luo wrapping of coupled organs by the meridians. In several contexts the luo is seen to be an energetic pathway or trajectory, and as such it refers to fascial or connective tissue membranes.

The luo is a branch from the main or vertical meridian. The *Ling Shu* tells us:

> The jing mai 經脈 [meridian] is li 裏 [the lining]. The horizontal branch of the meridian is the luo. The divergent branches are the grandchild luo 孫絡 *(LS 17:190)*.

Here, the luo are described as the horizontal branches of the meridians. From the luo spring other smaller branches, the "grandchild luo." This image is similar to vascular system branches. The blood passes through the arteries to the arterioles and thence to the capillaries. The branching trajectories can be seen in a similar manner. The pivotal concept in the description of the the luo and grandchild luo is that of li, the lining.

In modern times, the character of li has been simplified to 里, meaning inside or interior. In the Han dynasty, *li* 裏 referred to the lining of the body. It was generally seen in opposition to *biao* 表, surface. Since biao, the surface, is usually understood to refer to the skin and body hair, the lining is thus something that covers and lines the body, yet is not the skin itself. We suggest that this distinction is perfectly reasonable and evidences the Chinese understanding of the superficial fascia of the body. In this, we are not alone. In a brief discussion of the yin and yang wei mai, Xie Lin of the Qing dynasty stated:

> The yin wei controls the qi of the greasy membranes 脂膜, it goes to the lining of the body.[24]

Here "lining" refers to the superficial fascia and probably the more internal systems of fasciae as well. This has fundamental implications. Since the "meridian is li, the lining," the meridians themselves are seen as flowing through the superficial fascia of the body. The luo vessels, as the horizontal branches, would also flow through the superficial fascia.

☐

Diagrammatically we can see it thus:

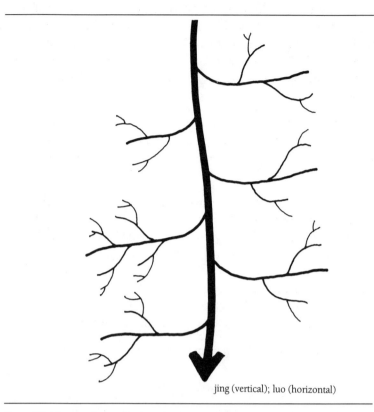

jing (vertical); luo (horizontal)

Figure 7.1 The meridian and its branches.

This system of branches from the meridian is usually understood as traversing the whole body just as the superficial fascia does. When these branches "spirally wrap" the coupled organs they are traversing the fascial envelopes that encapsulate the organs. Anatomically this makes good sense. The various fascial systems of the body are functionally one large interconnected system. Fascial connections from inside the body surround and connect the organs to the surface of the body through the superficial fascia where the meridians and luo meridians lie.

This concept has many practical implications when one needles the acupoints. The acupoints and meridians lie only a few millimeters below the surface of the skin, an important consideration when treating with needles and moxa. Further, it is not a speculative concept. It is described in the *Su Wen* in the context of the origins and transformations of disease:

> The Yellow Emperor said, "This is the origin of disease. It is the tiny, absolute jing. It always comes first into and knots at the skin" *(SW 14:87).*

The concept of "tiny, absolute jing" 微極精 is slightly different from Zhuang Zi's idea of "no form" 無形, as "tiny, absolute jing" 微至精, or that which cannot be further divided. However, the concepts are closely parallel. As we have seen, the "triple warmer has a name but no form." This implies some relationship of the triple warmer to the tiny absolute jing. In this context, the tiny absolute jing of the *Su Wen* discussion might well follow the same idea. Diseases have tiny origins, like the tiny, absolute jing. In coming first to the skin, disease is the smallest perturbation of qi flow in the meridians. This disturbance may be seen to come from within the person and not just from the outside. The *Su Wen* says further:

> This is the origin of all diseases. Evil always attacks first at the skin and hair and then comes into the area between the skin and the flesh. It comes in and stays at the luo vessels. If it does not leave, it transmits to and enters the meridians. If it does not leave, it transmits to and enters the fu 府 and then gathers at the intestines and stomach (*SW 56:290*).

This passage describes disease as originating very superficially, coming in a little deeper to the area between the skin and the flesh, where lies the superficial fascia of the body. From here it is transmitted to the luo, thence to the meridians, thence to the fu and then to the intestines and stomach. In this context, it is very unlikely, as several commentators have said, that "fu" refers to the yang organs 腑.

The term "fu" has been used in a variety of ways over the years. It is generally seen to mean a place of gathering or storing. Fu also refers to the chest, the area around CV-17.[25] This last reference to the area around CV-17 may be construed to great significance. The etymological roots of tanzhong (CV-17) refer to a cooking pot with a lid on it *(Kad)* and also to fat, greasy, smelly tissues *(Fuj)*. Since CV-17 is said to be the "palace of the master of the heart" *(LS 35:288)* and the master of the heart seems to refer anatomically, at least in part, to the major blood vessels exiting and entering the heart, then it may refer to the thymus gland which lies underneath the sternum, roughly level with CV-17. This gland lies over the pericardium and aortic arch. "Fu" further refers to the tendons and the sites at which they attach muscles to bones:

> Yanglingquan [GB-34] is the shu point of the knees.
> The knees are the fu of the great muscles.
> Therefore, this allows stretching and bending [to occur].[26]

Again:

> Many old people wear waist bands [hara warmers]. This is because the lumbar vertebrae are the fu of the kidneys.[27]

The *Nan Jing* distinguishes the triple warmer as the sixth fu *(NJ 38:3)*. This has been interpreted as referring to *fu* 腑, a yang organ. According to some commentaries, the use of the term *fu* 府 in this passage refers to something other than the character used to reference a yang organ. In his commentary on this passage, Wang Shu He actually refers to the "fu of the yang organs," clearly distinguishing fu from the yang organs. Further, he describes each pair of yin and yang organs as having a fu, the triple warmer having or being an "external fu."

In the *Nan Jing Du Ben Mu Lu,* Wang Yi Ren felt that this use of fu referred to the systems of lymph nodes in the body.

□

There are five yin organs and six fu. What is the single fu? It is the triple warmer. The triple warmer is arm shao yang. Shao yang belongs to the kidneys. The upper parts of the kidneys are connected to the lungs. The triple warmer is in between these.

There are lymph nodes in the neck and thoracic regions, the thoracic duct. In the middle warmer there are lymph nodes around the hepatic portal vein. In the lower warmer there are intestinal and abdominal lymph nodes.[28]

Again we find a relation to the source qi and the triple warmer. Also, if fu is related to the area around CV-17, and CV-17 is related to the thymus gland, then the possible relationship of fu to the systems of lymph nodes in the body takes on great import, as both have major immunological functions.

These ideas were clearly stated in 1813 by K. Mitsutane in *Kaitai Hatsumou*. He stated that the triple warmer is related to the lymphatic system in the body, specifically the upper warmer to the thymus gland, the middle warmer to the pancreas and the lower warmer to the systems of the lacteal ducts, especially the cysterna chyli.[29] To be internally consistent it would make more sense to see the middle warmer in relation to the spleen, which has immunological functions after birth. What is important in these correlations, however, is the congruity of the relationships. The involvement of the thymus gland further supports the CV-17 to thymus correlation. The cysterna chyli, lying in the folds of the mesenterium at the level of lumbar one and lumbar two, is in the region of the root of the mesentery and the area of the moving qi between the kidneys. The cysterna chyli is the collecting sac of the lacteal ducts that lie throughout the mesenterium and carry chyle from the small intestines.

Extending the correlations to include the various extensions of the lymph system, the superficial lymph vessels lie in the superficial fascia. We saw above how the flow of qi in the meridians was seen in relation to the flow of fluid at the surface in the water meridians *(LS 12:154-155)*. We now have a possible explanation of this fluid flow, and its relations to the triple warmer and to the meridian systems that are an extension of the upper warmer *(LS 18)*.

This interpretation fits neatly with another usage of the term fu in the *Nan Jing*:

> Therefore when one speaks of the triple warmer fu, it exists at
> qi jie 氣街 *(NJ 31:20)*.

There are said to be four qi jie in the body, in the head, chest, abdomen, and legs. Qi jie is also an alternate name for ST-30, qi chong, which has close proximity to the inguinal lymph nodes.[30]

One last and totally different usage of the term fu comes from the *Huai Nan Zi*. The six fu were seen as the six pairs of opposite earthly branches (e.g., B1-B7, B2-B8). Each pair was described as a "fu" *(HNZ 3:142)*.

Given the considerable use and reinterpretation of the character "fu," it is not impossible and is in fact quite likely that the fu referenced in this context is the lymph nodes. Since fu is generally used to mean a place of gathering or storing, this interpretation is justified. In reference to the movement of the evil from the meridians in the superficial fascia to the fu, it also makes sense to see fu as the lymph nodes. These are places where fluids gather as they stream back towards the interior body. The lymph nodes are also related to the superficial fascia, since the surface lymph vessels that drain into the nodes lie in the superficial fascia. In his 1888 Qing dynasty commentary on the *Su Wen*, the *Huang Di Nei Jing Su Wen Ji Gua*, Zhang Yin An said:

> It [pathogenic qi] does not gather at the intestines and stomach,
> it gathers between the intestines and stomach.[31]

He proposed that the mesenteric membranes between the intestines and stomach were the site of the third stage of disease transmission. In context, this passage can be seen to describe the penetration and transmission of pathogenic qi from the skin to the superficial fascia and through the fascial system to the mesenterium.

In a similar passage, the *Su Wen* describes the penetration of pathogenic qi into the yin organs:

> Therefore evil qi comes slightly to the inside of the five yin
> organs, horizontally connecting to the mu yuan 募原 *(SW 35:402)*.

This brief and seemingly innocuous passage from the *Su Wen* has been richly commented upon. Essentially, it describes the penetration of pathogenic qi to the fascia that encapsulates the yin organs. This is only obvious by examining the meanings of the terms, *mu* and *mu yuan*. In his Tang dynasty commentary Wang Bing says that the mu yuan is "the source connection 原系 of the diaphragm mu." This refers to the mesenteric membranes of the abdomen. It references the ideas of the *Ling Shu* source theory that describe the falciform ligament, at the upper end of which is the *gao* source 膏原. It is attached to the lower edge of the diaphragm, at the lower end of which is the *huang* source 肓原.

Yao Zhi An, in his Qing dynasty commentary on the *Su Wen*, titled the *Su Wen Jing Zhu Jie Jie,* explains that mu yuan is "the source of the *mo* 膜 [diaphragm membranes]."[32] Quoting the *Quan Yuan Qi Ben*, he also explains the *mu* 募: "mu creates the membranes." This passage is cited by the modern commentators of the *Tai Su* as part of their commentary on the explanation of mu yuan *(TS p.448)*. In describing *mo yuan* 膜原, which is seen as the same as mu yuan, since the mu creates the mo or membranes, the *Tai Su* says:

> Each of the five yin organs has a membrane source 膜原. If evil
> qi comes into the five yin organs, it will be horizontally con-
> nected to the transporter 輸 of the five yin organs' membrane
> source.

In other words, each yin organ has a membrane related to it. This membrane has a source, a place of attachment in the body. If pathogenic qi comes into a yin organ, it will be transmitted through the transporter to this source. This is a difficult passage to interpret, but in this context the implication that energy, in this case pathogenic qi, transmits through the membranes, is inescapable.

The commentaries of both Wang Bing and Yao Zhi An present the mu yuan in relation to the diaphragm. In the late Han dynasty, the *Shi Ming* described the diaphragm 膈 as a block 塞 that separated the upper and lower parts *(Mor)*. In the eleventh century Song dynasty, the *Ji Yun,* a massive encyclopedic dictionary, described the diaphragm as "huang 肓 " or "being like leather" *(Mor)*.

As previously postulated, huang refers to certain of the fascia and mesenteric membranes in the abdomen. The diaphragm was also seen to relate to certain fascial tissues. The comment from the *Quan Yuan Qi Ben,* "mu creates the membranes," indicates that the mu is related to the various membranes of the body. Although it is not stated as clearly in the earliest Classical texts, this understanding of the mu existed much earlier, probably as early as the Han dynasty.

A more recent etymological study, the *Shuo Wen Tong Xun Ding Sheng (Explanation Book of the Shuo Wen),* written circa 1848 in the Qing dynasty, attempted to explain the mu character: "Mu was used to substitute for mo 膜" *(Mor)*. The author felt that the term mu, in its earlier uses, was synonymous with mo, the membranes, and was at times used in place of the term mo. The *Shi Ming* of the late Han dynasty saw mo as "like a curtain, spirally wrapping 絡 (luo) the body" *(Mor)*. The mo thus described the superficial fascia of the body. Modern scholars generally agree with this definition of the mo as the superficial fascia, the thin membrane between the skin and the flesh *(Mor)*.

This understanding of mo in relation to the mu and especially the mu yuan can also be found in other texts. For instance Zhang Yin An's Qing dynasty commentary on the *Su Wen,* the *Huang Di Nei Jing Su Wen Ji Gua,* comments on the use of the term mu yuan in chapter 35 of the *Su Wen:*

> The mu yuan is the horizontal connection [that is part of] the gao mo [greasy membrane] 膏膜 of the yin and yang organs.[33]

Mu yuan here is seen as part of the mesenterium or abdominal fascia with a horizontal feature connecting the yin and yang organs to each other and to the abdominal walls, the peritoneal fascia. In another passage Zhang Yin An makes further comment:

> The mu yuan is a greasy membrane. It also has the nature of connecting [things]. Therefore, it is the nature of the skin and the yin and yang organs.[34]

The mu yuan has the nature of connecting things in the body, specifically the yin and yang organs and the skin. This states the same relationship of the superficial fascia and the internal fascia, the meridians and their organs, that the classical authors proposed.

Another possible interpretation of mu yuan is to see it as the "root of the mesentery," which extends from the left side of the second lumbar vertebra to the right sacroiliac symphysis.[35] This is the site of attachment of the mesentery to the dorsal abdominal wall, and holds possible significance since this would place the "root" at the crossing of the lumbar vertebrae at the inferior level of the kidneys, and thus in the region between the kidneys, related to the moving qi between the kidneys. We recall Xie Lin's Qing commentary on the *Nan Jing*:

> The strand of fatty membrane, passing through the spinal bones . . . [is] called the kidney connector. It passes down to the net-like membrane . . . [and] extends to dantian, the source of the lower warmer.[36]

The "net-like membrane" is reasonably seen as the mesenterium and its root as being related to the mu yuan.

Another modern Chinese commentary on the *Su Wen* by Guo Ai Chun defines mu yuan as "the source of the transporting membrane, below the umbilicus."[37] Again, the membranes are seen as having the capacity or function of transportation; they are said to lie below the umbilicus, fitting reasonably with the *Ling Shu* discussions of the source of huang, Chen Yan's statement about the triple warmer, and Xie Lin's discussion of how the membranes extend down to dantian in the lower warmer. Zhang Yin An makes a further relevant comment about huang 肓.

> Huang is the greasy membrane that spirally wraps (luo) 絡 the small intestine.[38]

This is a direct reminder of the relationship of huang to *Ling Shu* source theory. This passage also makes a relatively clear statement about the possible relationship of the small intestine to this theory.

The relationship of the mu points to the fascia is something that can be seen practically in the work of Yoshio Manaka.[39] He has found that often in the prone position the mu points are not reactive when a patient has a problem of the organs and meridians that the mu points are said to reflect. However, by stretching the meridian through rotating, flexing, or extending the foot or hand, the points immediately become reactive. For instance, a patient with a problem of the small intestine as diagnosed by symptoms and point palpation evidenced no soreness at CV-4. After stretching the small intestine meridian, CV-4 became very reactive. Manaka reminds us of the importance of the wrists and ankles in tai ji movements. Given this context, it is quite likely that the mu points are points of specific attachment of the fasciae through which the meridians run. By specific movements of the wrists and ankles, the stretched fasciae acquire a certain tension and changed conductivity. The energy thus freed and the fascial tension induced by stretching establishes a tension at the mu point making it more reactive on palpation. Detailed anatomical studies will help to demonstrate this hypothesis, yet it certainly fits the overall picture.

In his text, *Qian Jin Yao Fang*, Sun Si-Mo provides an idea relating to this picture. Discussing the location of the extra point *huang mu* 肓募, or "fascial mu," he describes its location as follows:

> The huang mu [is found by measuring the distance from] the top of the nipple to the center of the umbilicus [with a piece of thread]. Fold the thread in half. The point is half the distance directly below the nipple.[40]

Sun Si-Mo took as the basis of his idea the *Ling Shu* references to the "source of gao" and "source of huang" and the acupoint huang shu (KI-16); the *Nan Jing* reference to the twelve "source points" on the twelve meridians; and the *Zhen Jiu Jia Yi Jing* references to the mu points. His description of these points, the gao huang shu and huang mu, offers both the concept of a diagnostic point for the fascia and a geometric relationship to determine point location. The umbilicus and the nipples are reference points on the fascial plane. They are areas of attachment and thus points of tension, like a drumskin stretched from three points. The lines of tension within the smooth-surfaced fascia will be determined by the geometric relationship of these attachments. What we propose Sun Si-Mo was describing is the mathematical relationship of the points and angles of the lines of tension created by the stretching of the fascia between the nipples and umbilicus.

The mechanism resembles what occurs with the rotation, flexion, or extension of the fascial attachments at specific joints, as occurs in tai ji or Manaka's meridian stretching. The tensile properties of the fascia change, the geometric relationships to other points of attachment and tension change, and the three-dimensional shape of the interconnected fascial field is itself modified. Since each change relates to the bioelectrical properties of the fascia, specifically its conductivity, there will be both diagnostic and treatment effects.

Muscles and Membranes

Various chapters in the *Su Wen* and *Ling Shu* discuss the different tissues of the body and how they are controlled by the five yin organs. Some of these refer to membranes. For instance, both the *Su Wen* and the *Ling Shu* say:

> The lung controls the skin;
> The heart controls the vessels;
> The liver controls the muscles;
> The spleen controls the flesh;
> The kidney controls the bones *(SW 23:154; LS 78:586).*

A parallel and expanded passage in the *Su Wen* notes:

> The lung controls the skin and body hair of the body.
> The heart controls the blood vessels of the body.
> The liver controls the muscular membranes 筋膜 of the body.
> The spleen controls the flesh of the body.
> The kidney controls the bone marrows of the body *(SW 44:246).*

Again the *Su Wen* says:

> The liver stores the qi of the muscular membranes *(SW 18:110).*

The liver was described as the controller of the muscular membranes. We now call the muscular membranes the deep fascia. For the liver to be seen in relation to the deep fascia, the classical authors must have considered the fascia to be fundamentally important. Some modern commentaries of *Su Wen* chapter 44 also give this passage from the *Quan Yuan Qi Ben:*

> Mo 膜, the muscular membranes 筋膜, are in the person, below the skin and above the flesh (SW 44:246).

Kazunori Shibata, a specialist in Japanese foot reflexology, has made a detailed study of the correspondence of the muscular membranes to the liver.[41] In his description, he differentiates between the muscles and the membranes. To his mind, the term "muscle membrane" does not refer to just the muscles and myofascia, but to both. Based on his research and clinical experience, he distinguishes between the muscles, the longitudinal and vertical fibers in the body, and the membranes, the horizontal fibers. In the context of Chinese medicine he identifies the term "muscle" with the nerves, tendons, and blood vessels as well as the muscle tissues. The term "membrane" he considers to refer to the pleura, peritoneum, mesenterium, myofascia, and superficial fascia. Thus, the term "muscle membrane" refers to all the fibers and membranes in the body. Since these are controlled by the liver, if the liver becomes vacant, all the fibers and membranes can be affected. The liver functions to keep all the fibers and membranes loose and flexible. Using massage of the hands and feet, particularly certain toes, Shibata treats problems that lie in these fibers and membranes.

Another instructive passage from the *Ling Shu* discusses the relationship of gao to digestion and the triple warmer:

> All water and grains enter through the mouth. There are the five tastes; each of them streams to the ocean. The jin 津 and ye 液 run their own individual way. Therefore, the qi comes out from the triple warmer. It keeps the skin and flesh warm. The jin nourishes the skin. The stream that does not move is the ye. The jin and ye of the five grains harmoniously unite and become gao [the membranes.] It is absorbed inside into the holes in the bones, it supplies and nourishes the brain and marrow. Subsequently, it streams downward to the groin (LS 36:295-296).

The jin and ye are the two vital fluids. They flow throughout the body and nourish the tissues. As these two move, the triple warmer qi moves. The jin and ye also create the gao. Aside from the connection of the fluids to the triple warmer and the mesenteric membranes, the gao, this passage has important implications for an examination of the modern anatomical and physiological structures and functions of the various membranes, fasciae, and connective tissues. These water relationships and functions of the connective tissues are an interesting key to modern scientific work, particularly that of Albert Szent Gyorgyi. Modern data also may help us understand the passage from the *Ling Shu* describing the movement of the twelve meridians of the surface in relation to the movement of fluid through the "water meridians" (see page 2 of this chapter). Both the movement of qi, which the ancient anatomists measured for "fullness and insufficiency" and the triple warmer qi which moves with the jin and ye, become less inexplicable as we study the movement and filtration of the interstitial fluids. These fluids play an important role is Szent Gyorgyi's model of bioenergy.

This puzzle has already attracted the attention of scholars and stimulated several hypotheses. Sosen Hirooka, in his wonderful eighteenth century commentary on the *Nan Jing*, makes an interesting comment on *Nan Jing* chapter 42. Referring to the passage from the *Ling Shu*, he says:

> Gao is the product of the water and grains, causing [or stimulating] their transformation to qi. Its color is white. Therefore, it is able to moisten the skin and its interior portions, making it light and moist. Blood is the product of the water and grains causing [or stimulating] their transformation to blood. Its color is red. Therefore, it is able to make the muscles and vessels have a full condition, nourishing and helping them grow. These warm the five yin organs and moisten the whole body.[42]

The water and grain transform into either gao or blood. The gao moistens and nourishes the area of the skin in which the superficial fascia is found. This same area of the body, just below the surface of the skin, seems to be referenced in other passages of the *Ling Shu*. For instance, in chapter 47 there is reference to the *cou li* 腠理. This too refers to an area between the skin and the flesh. One modern Chinese commentary refers to cou li as

> . . . the part of the body between the skin and the inside. The jin and ye, qi and blood, pass through here.[43]

This is the area we call the superficial and deep fasciae.

Another section from the same chapter of the *Ling Shu* discusses the relationship of the wei qi or defense qi to the area between the skin and flesh:

> The wei qi therefore keeps warm the segments of the flesh, gives the skin a full condition, nourishes the tissues between the skin and flesh (LS 47:349).

The *Lei Jing* of 1624 A.D. commented on this:

> The unclear part is of the category of yang. Its character is rapid, therefore it doesn't go through the meridian. Thus, it directly reaches the surface of the skin, making the skin, hair, and space between the skin and flesh full. This is the wei qi [defense qi].[44]

Here the wei qi is clearly seen as passing between the skin and flesh in the superficial and deep fasciae. Another passage from the *Su Wen* states these relationships most clearly, and is probably the oldest concise description of the passage of the wei qi through the membranes:

> The wei qi is the rapid qi of the water and grains. This qi is quick-witted, sharp, and slippery and doesn't enter the vessels [meridians]. Therefore, the wei qi goes between the skin tissues and flesh. The wei keeps the huang mo 肓膜 warm. The wei scatters to the chest and abdomen (SW 43:245).

We have already discussed the relationship of the wei qi to the lower warmer, where it is produced, and to the triple warmer. The wei qi passes through the tissues between the skin and flesh, the fasciae, and keeps the huang mo, the peritoneum, warm. Thus, both the idea of the movement of qi through the fasciae and the hypothesis that the the triple warmer structure is these fasciae, are further supported.

While examples of these relationships are abundant, even this collection of information cannot define the gao, huang, and triple warmer definitively. Among the various classical and modern sources, there have been a variety of slightly different interpretations as to what each of these functional entities may be. However, there is no disagreement as to the importance of the membranes and the fasciae. Generally, the *Nan Jing* source and triple warmer theories were seen in relationship to the earlier *Ling Shu* source theory. Writers who comment on these relationships see the triple warmer as either a system of fascial membranes or as a functional relationship to the system of fascial membranes described in the *Ling Shu*. That the fasciae are important as transporters of qi is clear in all the classical references to transference, connection, and source. The relevance of the fasciae to huang, gao, fu, mu, mo, jin and ye, luo, li, and the meridians evidences a centrality to the energetic anatomy of man that cannot be denied.

One remaining facet of what appears to be a triple warmer function has a notable anatomical basis. Essentially, this function relates the passage of the stomach qi to certain brain structures and seasonal varion of temperature, and thus to bodily thermoregulation. The stomach qi is not often mentioned in classical literature, but existing references seem to suggest a coherent theory. Both the *Su Wen* (SW 18) and *Nan Jing* (NJ 15) describe the stomach qi with reference to the quality of the radial pulse. The *Nan Jing* description explains the normal seasonal pulses and their pathological variations with reference to the stomach qi.[45]

The *Ling Shu* also makes reference to the stomach qi and pulse diagnosis at the carotid artery (ST-9). This passage describes the stomach qi pathway as an explanation for carotid pulse diagnosis:

> The Yellow Emperor asked, "What causes the pulsing at leg yang ming [carotid pulse at ST-9]?"
>
> Qi Bo replied, "The stomach qi rises up to the lungs, the rapid qi ascends quickly into the head, encircling the throat and flowing to the orifices. [A branch] encircles the supporter of the eyes, passes into and spirally wraps [luo] the brain. It then passes out to the temples [around TW-23 and ST-7], circles to the teeth wheel [ST-6] where it meets leg yang ming, then passes down [to ST-9]. Thus, the stomach qi divides and runs from leg yang ming" (LS 62:288).

Most authors agree that the "rapid qi" is the wei qi and should be distinguished from the ying qi that flows through the meridian circuit starting at the lung meridian. Thus Qi Bo's reply could read,

> The stomach qi rises to the lungs. Here it divides, one part
> passing down the lung meridian, the other part, the rapid qi,
> ascending quickly into the head. . . .

The orifices are the seven orifices — eyes, ears, etc. The supporter of the
eyes is probably the optic nerve. When it passes into and spirally wraps
the brain, it is possible to translate this as "passes into and spirally wraps
(some part of) the brain," implying a connection to only a particular structure within the brain and not the whole brain.

The same passage discusses the circulation of the ying and wei qi relative to the invasion of cold or wind. Since we know that the ying qi flows
through the twelve meridians and that the wei qi emerges from the eyes to
circulate around the body, we may again interpret the rapid qi as the wei qi.
Also, since the triple warmer begins in the stomach, and the ying qi and
wei qi are seen as the qi of the middle and lower warmers (LS 18) we can see
the references in this passage as describing some aspect of triple warmer
function.

Further, since the stomach qi is seen with reference to seasonal pulse
variations, it is functionally related to temperature control in the body. The
major variant factor during the progression of the seasons is the temperature. This interpretation is further supported by the discussion of ying and
wei qi circulation and their disturbance by cold or wind invasion, where
circulation to the four limbs is impaired (LS 62). This is, of course, typical
of the body's response to cold. The circulation of blood to the surface and
extremities is decreased. This passage describes the thermoregulatory functions of the stomach qi relative to the ying and wei qi, and indirectly the
triple warmer control of body temperature.

There is considerable physiological significance in the rapid qi of the
stomach rising to encircle the throat, and passing from the eyes into the
brain. The thyroid gland, which essentially regulates metabolism
throughout the body, is in the throat. A significant structure, the
hypothalamus, is found where the supporter of the eyes crosses in the
brain, at the optic chiasm. A major function of the hypothalamus is thermoregulation. There would seem to be no coincidence that two of the
body's most important thermoregulatory structures, the hypothalamus and
thyroid gland, lie on the pathway of the stomach qi. The regulation of temperature begins with the control of blood flow to the surface and four
limbs of the body. When the environment is hot this circulation increases,
when it is cold the circulation decreases.[46] According to *Ling Shu* theory,
when cold invades the body, circulation of ying and wei qi is impaired in
the limbs.

Why these functions are described with reference to the stomach and
stomach qi is another question of interest. When food is ingested and
passes into the digestive system, the circulation of blood to the surface of
the body is diverted to the digestive system to help absorb the nutrients
and fluids of digestion. Since normal thermoregulation varies through the
increase or decrease of blood flow to the surface of the body, we can posit
that the circulatory responses of digestion may create a functional tension
between the control of blood flow arising from hypothalamic function and

□

the control arising as a digestive response. If this is correct, stomach qi describes the body's thermoregulatory functions and secondarily helps explain the temperature-regulating properties of the triple warmer.[47]

Embryological Development

The concept of gao from *Ling Shu* source theory relates the gao to the first month of embryological development as described by the *Huai Nan Zi*. From approximately 400 or 300 B.C. to the seventh century A.D., a series of similar embryological theories developed in China. Although their anatomical descriptions are simple, compared to the microanatomical studies of today, their descriptions are neither essentially inaccurate nor without provocative permutations.

That the Chinese were interested in embryology is very natural; they were fascinated with ideas of "beginning," "root," or "origin" and the "basic" or "source" parts. Many characters in Chinese imply root or origin, not the least common of which is the idea of the "source" 原, the basic idea of both the *Ling Shu* and *Nan Jing* theories. With their desire to understand where things came from, the source or origin of life, it is natural that they would see embryology as an essential study. Looking at embryological development, the fascia and connective tissues, it is possible to understand many of the classical medical ideas about life, health, and disease.

As the most complete and accessible theory, the *Huai Nan Zi* description of the stages of embryological development are a reference to which we may compare several other systems. However, the oldest discussions of embryology can be found in the *Guan Zi (The Book of Master Guan)*, from the late fourth century B.C.:

> The person is [composed of] water.
> The jing 精 of the man and woman unite. Subsequently the water streams and then makes the form.
> At three months it is like masticated food [it has an undifferentiated form].
> What are these? What are the five tastes? What are the five yin organs?
> Acidic controls the spleen. Salty controls the lungs. Spicy controls the kidney. Bitter controls the liver. Sweet controls the heart.
> The five yin organs are now formed, then the flesh is created. The spleen creates the diaphragm. The lung creates the bones. The kidney creates the brain. The liver creates the skin. The heart creates the flesh.
> The five flesh are already created, then the nine orifices occur. The spleen occurs at the nose, the liver at the eyes, the kidneys at the ears, the lungs at the [other] orifices.
> At five months it is already completed. At ten months it is already born.[48]

These early five-phase correspondences differ from the correspondences generally associated with the phases. It is curious that such correspondences are discussed in relation to a developing embryo. The *Huai Nan Zi* also has a brief discussion of other, again slightly different, five-phase correspondences. In later passages, from the seventh century, the five phases were considered fundamental to embryological development.

In the *Guan Zi,* no mention is made of mesenteric or fascial membranes. After the *Huai Nan Zi* in 122 B.C., these tissues, specifically the gao, are mentioned in relation to either the first or second month of development. The *Ling Shu,* believed to have been compiled around 300 B.C., has an interesting brief embryological description. Like the *Guan Zi* it makes no reference to mesenteric or fascial membranes and further has no clear reference to the five phases:

> The Yellow Emperor said, "[After] the person's conception, the jing is first composed. Then the jing composes the brain and bone marrow. The bones become the stem [the spinal column forms?]. The vessels become the ying [nourishment]. The muscles become firm. The flesh becomes [like a] wall. The jing is hard, and then the hair and body hair grow.
>
> [After labor when the] gu [grains] come into the stomach, the vessel-meridian pathways are [all] connected, the blood and qi [begin to] move" *(LS 10:104).*

This passage introduces the description of meridian pathways. It seems to imply that the qi and blood, thus the meridians, begin circulating after birth. In a medical context this is extremely important.

The description of the first month of pregnancy given in the "Shi Qin" section of chapter 6 of the *Guang Ya (Mor)* is the same as the *Huai Nan Zi* description, as is the third month, the "pregnant womb." The description of the second month, zhi 脂 and the fourth month, *bao* 胞 are somewhat different in the *Guang Ya.* Zhi refers to fat greasy tissues and bao refers to the uterus. This passage was probably influenced by the earlier *Huai Nan Zi* because the membranes and fat greasy tissues of the first and second months of embryological development were noted. The fifth through the tenth months described in the *Guang Ya* follow the *Huai Nan Zi* description: muscle, bones, completion, movement, rowdy movement, birth. Since we know that the fascia and membranous tissues are vital in embryological development, their inclusion at this time into the corpus of classical medical theory is significant. It is indicative of an ancient anatomical knowledge of some sophistication.

Another important development of embryological theory came some three hundred eighty years after the *Guang Ya.* In 610 A.D., the physician Chao Yuan Fang published the *Zhu Bing Yuan Hou Lun,* which contained a description of embryological development that included a theory of the origins of symptoms in illness. Briefly, in each of the ten months of fetal development there is a relationship between the mother and the developmental state. During each stage one pair of the mother's meridians nourishes the developing fetus. Chao Yuan Fang's descriptions of fetal development are somewhat different from the *Huai Nan Zi* and the *Guang Ya.* One would be pressed to prove the influence of the earlier works on the latter. However, his discussions of the relationships of the mother to the developing fetus are interesting. They describe a possible mechanism by which the fetus comes into life with inherent problems, strengths, and weaknesses. If

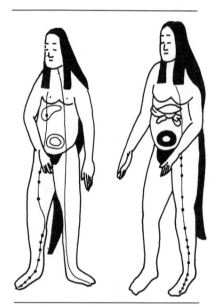

Figure 7.2 - 7.3 The first two months of development (after *Ishin Po*).

the mother has a weakness in a meridian, this would lead to problems during the related stage of development. Although this is not a specific claim made by Chao Yuan Fang, it is a tempting interpretation.

In the following quote, note how Chao Yuan Fang perceived the entry of the five-phase jing into the developing fetus and the development of dantian by the tenth month. The accompanying illustrations are in the style of Tamba no Yasuyori's *Ishin Po,* an important tenth-century Japanese medical treatise.[49]

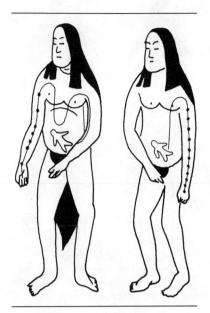

Figure 7.4 - 7.5 The third and fourth months of development (after *Ishin Po*).

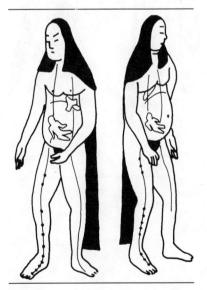

Figure 7.6 - 7.7 The fifth and sixth months of development (after *Ishin Po*).

In the first month it is called the beginning of form 形. Leg jue yin nourishes this. Leg jue yin is the vessel of the liver, the liver controls the blood. At this time the blood flow stops [the menses stop]; therefore, leg jue yin nourishes this.

The second month is called the beginning of gao 膏, the mesenteric membranes. Leg shao yang nourishes this, leg shao yang is the vessel of the gallbladder. The gallbladder controls the jing 精. The jing of the fetus 兒 is composed in the lining of the wrapping [of the fetus, the lining of the uterus, possibly the placenta].

The third month is called the beginning of tai 脂, the pregnant uterus. The arm master of the heart controls this, the arm master of the heart is the jing and shen in the vessels, the inside is connected with the heart, it is able to cleanse the shen.

The fourth month is when the water jing 水精 is beginning to be accepted. With this the blood vessels are composed. Arm shao yang controls this, arm shao yang is the vessel of the triple warmer, inside it is connected with the fu 府 [here, probably the yang organs].

The fifth month is when the fire jing 火精 is beginning to be accepted. With this, the qi is composed, leg tai yin nourishes this, leg tai yin is the vessel of the spleen. Leg tai yin controls the four seasons. In this month the four limbs are completed.

The sixth month is when the metal jing 金精 is beginning to be accepted. With this the muscles are composed, leg yang ming nourishes this. Leg yang ming is the vessel of the stomach. This altogether controls the mouth and eyes.

The seventh month is when the wood jing 木精 is beginning to be accepted. With this, the bones are composed, hand tai yin nourishes this. Hand tai yin is the vessel of the lung and controls the skin and body hair.

The eighth month is when the earth jing 土精 is beginning to be accepted. With this the skin is composed, it harmonizes the heart (or mind) and quiets the breathing, arm yang ming nourishes this. Arm yang ming is the vessel of the large intestine. The large intestine controls the nine orifices.

The ninth month is when the stone jing 右精 is beginning to be accepted. With this, the skin and body hair are composed, leg shao yin nourishes this. Leg shao yin is the vessel of the kidney. The kidney controls the connecting thread [umbilicus].

In the tenth month all the five yin organs are completed, the six yang organs and the umbilicus are connected. Heaven and Earth qi enter at dantian.

The most critical implication in this description is that the nature and origin of disease is prenatal. It does represent one of the clearest attempts by a Chinese physician to demonstrate how prenatal problems can influence our health after we are born. Sun Si-Mo, in his *Qian Jin Yao Fang (Priceless Prescriptions)* from 652 A.D., describes an embryological development essentially identical to Chao Yuan Fang's from forty years earlier. The one simple difference here is that Sun Si-Mo refers to the first month as the "beginning of the embryo," rather than the "beginning of form."[50]

For each month of development, Sun Si-Mo prescribes certain herbs. He also comments that one should not needle or moxa points on the meridian during the month a meridian is in active control of fetal development.[51] This is perhaps medical practice in its most superb and sophisticated aspect. Treating pregnant mothers to ensure healthy children may represent the most advanced form of preventive medical practice possible.

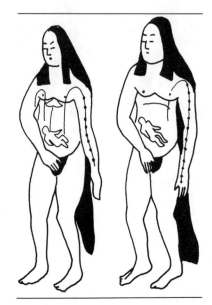

Figure 7.8 - 7.9 The seventh and eighth months of development (after *Ishin Po*).

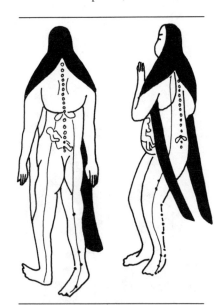

Figure 7.10 - 7.11 The last two months of development (after *Ishin Po*).

Chapter

- 8 -

Modern Anatomy
& Physiology
of the Fasciae &
Connective Tissues

Modern Anatomy and Physiology of the Fasciae and the Connective Tissues

The human body is an intricate set of systems that interact with each other as a functional whole. The nervous, muscular, skeletal, digestive, respiratory, reproductive, excretory, hormonal, and vascular systems each have distinct characteristics and properties. Yet none of these systems are separate entities. When working synchronously they constitute what we call, in a gross sense, "life." Several systems exercise mediation or control of functional interactions. The nervous and vascular systems are, for example, largely concerned with regulation. All parts of the body are to some degree innervated and vascularized. These systems provide a medium that connects the parts through a series of complex interactions and feedback mechanisms. Incorporated within the nervous and vascular systems are various sub-systems such as the hormonal messengers. Each sub-system is itself a categorization that represents another set of specific interactions.

Within the body one system is amazingly pervasive and versatile: the connective tissue. In effect, the connective tissue is a system that totally interconnects all parts of the body at each level from the anatomical to the microscopic. Connective tissues can be found within every single organelle, within every cell, and within every tissue of the body. Most significant for Oriental medical theory and practice are the properties such as energy generation and conduction that these tissues demonstrate.

The various membranes and fasciae discussed in Oriental medical literature are composed of connective tissues. Although modern anatomical, physiological, and embryological knowledge is much more detailed than the discussions in early Chinese medical texts, the essential anatomical details are the same. More noteworthy are the many parallels between Oriental medical concepts, in particular qi movement, and the modern understanding of the properties of the fascia. While there are intimations that the Chinese medical authors were discussing energetic concepts and concurrently utilizing physical knowledge, it is the mass of data compiled by modern physical sciences that compels us to consider these energetic concepts in the light of what we now know of the body's physiological and electrical functions. It is thus possible and intriguing, and in fact necessary, to propose and examine models by which we may explain classical Chinese medical concepts using the data of Western science.

□

Using all the information at hand, what can be demonstrated is the possible means by which at least some organ relationships described by classical medical theory may function. For instance, the five phase, ten stem and yin-yang correspondences and functions can be understood as analogs of biophysical relationships among fascial tissues. The relationship of certain acupoints to certain areas in the body and the probable mechanism by which the lines of energy movement, the meridians, develop and function may also be understood as bioelectrical functions of the fascial planes. The points of connection, the unifying factor of many energetic concepts, may be seen as related to the the systems of membranes and fascia and their connective tissue structure.

The Fascial System

In gross anatomical terms there are two basic systems of fasciae: the subcutaneous and the subserous systems. We can delineate quite clearly whole systems of tissues, accurately defining their anatomy and function.[1] Although these are continuous systems that merge with each other, they are distinct. The subcutaneous system is the system that connects the skin, muscles, and skeletal structures. The subserous system lines the body cavities. Both systems have connected layers.

The subcutaneous system has two distinct layers that form a continuous sheet over the whole area of the body. Properly, we speak of the subcutaneous fascia as having two layers, one more superficial, the other deeper. The superficial fascial layer of the subcutaneous system is itself a double layer that is fused and continuous. Essentially, it is a membrane that varies in depth according to location and individual differences. It also has varying amounts of fatty tissues. The deeper level contains the nerves, the blood, and the lymph vessels that nourish and help maintain the skin. This layer also functions to maintain body temperature and protect the body from trauma.

The superficial fascia tends to be thinner in males than in females. It is quite distinctly deeper over the abdomen and thinnest over the dorsal aspects of the hands and feet, the sides of the neck, the face, around the anus, and over the penis and scrotum.[2] The areas where it is thinner are all areas traditionally classified as yang or relatively yang. The areas where it is deeper, in particular the abdomen, were classified as yin areas. Thus, the yang areas of the body, or the more yang nature of those areas and the meridians located there, have a clear relationship to the depth of the superficial fascia and the amount of fatty tissue.

Since the superficial fascia is continuous with the dermis, it lies just below the epidermal and dermal layers of the skin. Generally this is just over one to just over two millimeters beneath the skin surface.[3]

Beneath this doubled superficial layer is the deep fascia. This includes the fascia that covers all the muscles of the body, excluding the superficial muscles of the head, neck, and palmar brevis, all the large blood vessels, all the large nerves, the deep lymphatic vessels and nodes, as well as certain glands. The deep system of the subcutaneous fascia is the system that passes from the superficial parts of the body to the interior. In the limbs, this layer connects as deep as the periosteum, the connective tissue membranes of the bones. In the trunk, it runs as deep as the interior walls of the thoracic and abdominal cavities. In both these places it envelops the muscles and bones, providing surfaces that form attachments and aid movement. This system is an important part of the musculo-skeletal support structure. By lining the interior walls of the abdominal and thoracic cavities, it becomes continuous with the subserous fascia.

The subserous fascia of the thoracic cavity is called the pleura. In the abdominal cavity, the subserous fascia is the peritoneum. Each of these fascia is layered. One layer lies next to the deep fascia that lines the inside of the cavity, the parietal pleura and parietal peritoneum. The layers that are more related to the different organs in each of the cavities are the visceral pleura and the visceral peritoneum. The visceral layers envelope and connect the various organs. For example, in the abdomen the visceral layer is called the peritoneum proper. Its invaginations and folds form the mesenterium that envelopes, connects, and covers the digestive organs.

The subserous layers of the thorax and abdomen are almost separated by the diaphragm, which stretches between the two. But the parietal layers of each cavity are continuous, since the fascia enveloping the aorta as it passes through the diaphragm merges with the parietal fasciae of the cavities above and below the diaphragm.

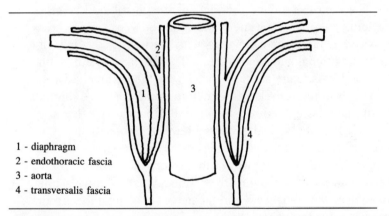

1 - diaphragm
2 - endothoracic fascia
3 - aorta
4 - transversalis fascia

Figure 8.1 The fascial sheath of the aorta is continuous with both the endothoracic fascia and the transversalis fascia on the superior and inferior surface of the diaphragm.

Not only are there fascial continua by which the surface of the body is connected to the interior, but there are also fascial continua that connect all the organs inside the body.

Fascial Connections

By following these various connections or continua of fascia, we can trace pathways from any one part of the body to any other, running up to down, down to up, inside to outside and outside to inside. The examples provided by James Oschman trace these connections quite clearly:

> In principle it would be possible to trace the fascial connections between any point within the body and any other. For our purposes we shall begin by tracing the larger planes of fascia upward from the feet to the top of the head and then back

down through the nervous system. The route followed will be upward through the legs to the pelvis and viscera, diaphragm, mesenteries, sheaths of various organs, the pericardium, the roots of the great vessels emerging from the heart (and thence throughout the branching network of the circulatory system), the trachea, the capsule of the thyroid gland, hyoid bone, temporal bone of the skull, and the fascia ensheathing the brain. From the brain the fascial layers can be traced downward as the sheath of the spinal cord and thence outward along the branching peripheral nerves as the perineural sheaths.

To be more specific, the myofascia and periosteal fascia of the legs are continuous via the acetabuli with the fascia of the general pelvic bowl. This, in turn, is continuous with the mesenteric fascial sheaths that support the abdominal organs. It is through these connections that the walls of the entire digestive tract and its associated organs join the myofascial network. Extending upward, the fascia ensheathing the psoas major and quadratus lumborum muscles blends with the fascia covering the right and left crus of the diaphragm. These crus, in turn, attach to the bodies of the lumbar vertebrae which are sites of attachment of vertebral ligaments, tendons, and myofascia. The central tendon of the diaphragm is contiguous with the pericardium and the roots of the great blood vessels, the aorta, the pulmonary artery and vein, and vena cava. These perivascular fascia are contiguous with the fascial coverings of the entire arterial and venous trees. The fasciae blending with the blood vessels are also associated with the peritracheal fascia, which in turn envelope the thyroid gland, form the carotid sheath, and fasten securely to the hyoid bone. This bone is connected to the styloid process of the temporal bone by a dense fascia, the stylohyoid ligament. The temporal bone, in turn, is the site of attachment of the tentorium cerebelli. These merge with the dura covering the brain and extend down as the covering of the spinal cord and the nerves branching therefrom and extending throughout the body.

At any particular level in the body the connective tissues form a continuous network ensheathing muscles, bones, nerves, blood vessels, and extending down microscopically onto the surfaces of cells and even into the cells themselves. This latter concept is a relatively new way of visualizing connective tissue. It has arisen because of the discovery that every cell has within it types of connective tissue consisting of rigid, flexible, and contractile elements. Moreover, it has been discovered that this cytoplasmic system is linked to the extracellular connective tissue via specific structures that traverse the cell membranes from the inside to the outside.

While the fascial planes are continuous sheets, there are more subtle relationships present. The fibers comprising those sheets are not randomly oriented, but are instead laid down in a precise way. There is a general rule as to how the majority of the fibers orient. This is stated in Wolf's law:

". . .The form of the bone being given, the bone elements [collagen] place or displace themselves in the direction of the functional pressure and increase or decrease their mass to reflect the amount of functional pressure."

Hence, the fibers become laid down along the lines of stress within the organism. This does not mean that all the fibers are oriented along the stress lines, for in much of the fasciae the collagen bundles are woven together to provide a relatively flexible but inelastic material of considerable tensile strength.

There is also a close anatomical relationship between the fascial sheets and the autonomic nervous system, to the extent that the autonomic ganglia are embedded in fascial planes. The precise physiological significance of this has not been given adequate attention. There are many case studies suggesting relief of autonomic dysfunction as a consequence of alterations in the fascia. It is often mentioned that tension in the fascial planes may adversely affect the circulation and hence nourishment of the autonomic ganglia embedded within the fascia. However, we are unaware of any specific research to test this suggestion.[4]

It is quite feasible that the meridians described by Chinese medicine as being in the "lining" (the superficial fasciae) can pass from the surface of the body to the interior, to any organ. There will be numerous variations by which any one pathway may be traced and there will be numerous fascial continua by which the connections may be effected. That these connective lines could be pathways of energy or qi is also quite feasible. The fascial systems are composed of connective tissues that have demonstrated abilities to transmit a variety of biological energies.

Research has shown that the connective tissues are capable of communication, connection, and energy conduction in the form of electron and proton transmission. Thermoelectric properties, pressure-activated responses that result in tissue change and thus functional changes, piezoelectric currents, and a variety of properties have all been discerned. The connective tissues are an amazingly plastic, malleable, changeable, and highly functional group of tissues. That the classical Chinese authors related the triple warmer and the conduction of qi to the fascia and their connective tissues well before scientific measurement was able to demonstrate such activity is a remarkable achievement.

The connective tissues compose much more than just these systems of fasciae. The fasciae are only the visible portion. There is an even more pervasive system of connective-tissue fibers at the microscopic level that extends into every cell in the body. These are the collagen and glycosaminoglycan fibers of the extracellular matrix and the microfilaments, microtubules, and microtrabeculae of the intracellular matrix. Both these connective matrices connect across cell membranes through the action of proteins such as fibronectin.[5] Since each of these microsystems evidences most, if not all, of the communicative properties of the fasciae and is intimately connected to the fascial macrosystem, every cell is explicitly connected to every other cell. This system forms the skeleton of all the cells and

□

ultimately the skeleton of the whole body. Recent electronmicrographical evidence shows that small fibers, the anchoring filaments of the hemidesmosome system, extend through the dermal-epidermal junction, allowing continuity from the collagenous filament system of the dermis through the epidermis to the surface of the body.[6] Thus, we not only have the means of tracing a pathway from the surface of the body to the interior structures and organs, but to virtually any cell in the body. Importantly, the pathway traced is not simply a mechanical connection, but is as well a bioelectrically and biochemically active chain of tissues capable of a variety of communication transfers.

It is because of this biophysical and bioelectrical context, a pervasive strata capable of a variety of informational transfer mechanisms and energy communication mechanisms, that the triple warmer as classically described is a completely justifiable concept. Indeed, it is feasible that all the triple warmer energetic capacities and functions could operate through the fasciae. Clearly, the triple warmer root and origins at the source, the "moving qi between the kidneys," is perfectly rational.

Oschman summarizes the basic physiological model of these structures quite elegantly:

> The connective tissue and fascia form a mechanical continuum, extending throughout the animal body, even into the innermost parts of each cell. All the great systems of the body — the circulation, the nervous system, the musculo-skeletal system, the digestive tract, the various organs — are ensheathed in connective tissue. This matrix determines the overall shape of the organism as well as the detailed architecture of its parts. All movements, of the body as a whole, or of its smallest parts, are created by tensions carried through the connective tissue fabric. Each tension, each compression, each movement causes the crystalline lattices of the connective tissues to generate bioelectric signals that are precisely characteristic of those tensions, compressions, and movements. The fabric is a semiconducting communication network that can convey the bioelectric signals between every part of the body and every other part. This communication network within the fascia is none other than the meridian system of traditional Oriental medicine, with its countless extensions into every part of the body. As these signals flow through the tissues, their biomagnetic counterparts extend the stories they tell into the space around the body. The mechanical, bioelectric, and biomagnetic signals traveling through the connective tissue network, and through the space around the body, tell the various cells how to form and reform the tissue architecture in response to the tensions, compressions, and movements we make.[7]

While there is a considerable and exciting body of detail associated with these ideas, the thrust is clear. The classical descriptions of human energetic functions, both those that are "interior" to the body and those that respond to events in the "exterior" environment, are justified by the properties of the most pervasive of the body's features, the fascia.

☐

The Fasciae in Embryology

To the Chinese authors, the idea of a source suggested prenatal roots. In embryological development we see distinct parallels among the Chinese medical ideas and the data of anatomical research. In particular, the concept of the triple warmer as the system of connective tissues related to the prenatal source of energy becomes clear. As the embryo develops, the connective tissues and planes of fasciae that the triple warmer represents are significant to correct development. There are obvious connections between the yin and yang organs. These can be seen to be the precursors of the various inter-organ relationships. These tissues provide the medium, the lines of communication, the meridian pathways, that Oriental medicine describes.

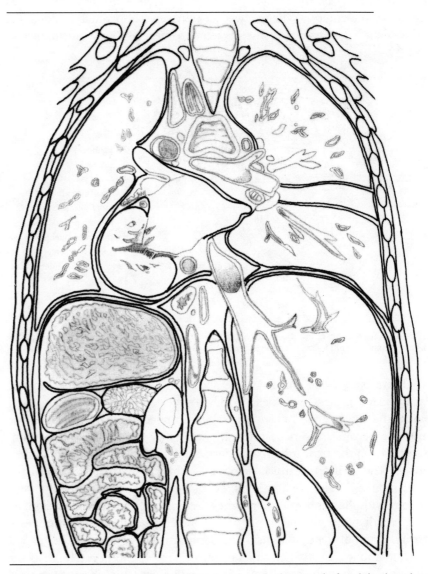

Figure 8.2 In this dorsal view through the thoracic and peritoneal cavities, the fascial sheaths and sacs of the various organs, muscles, bones, etc. are penned in as the darker lines. The interconnectedness of the fasciae from the thoracic to abdominal cavities is clear.

Because our research is still but a fraction of the effort that would be required to justifiably do so, we must refrain from stating definitive, absolute relationships concerning the correlation of the fasciae with classical Chinese theories. However, we can outline some of the most important correspondences and propose models that explain the medical relationships which have been specifically defined through many years of clinical practice.

The following diagram is a sagittal cross-section of an embryo, roughly 7 mm. long and 33 days old. This shows quite plainly the developing liver, gallbladder, stomach, spleen, large intestine, small intestine, and bladder. These early structures are all on the same plane of the body and are interconnected through the single continuum of the mesentery. Toward the front is the falciform ligament; between the liver and stomach is the ventral mesentery; between the stomach and dorsal wall this membrane becomes the dorsal mesentery. When viewed in transverse horizontal sections, the single-plane relationships of the organs and the mesentery are unmistakable.

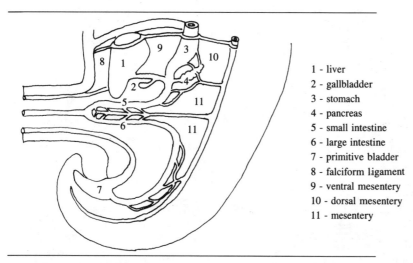

1 - liver
2 - gallbladder
3 - stomach
4 - pancreas
5 - small intestine
6 - large intestine
7 - primitive bladder
8 - falciform ligament
9 - ventral mesentery
10 - dorsal mesentery
11 - mesentery

Figure 8.3 Cross-section of the abdominal region of an approximately five-week old embryo. Note the plane and continuity of fasciae over all organ structures.

There is a continuum from the abdomen to the developing thoracic cavity. This is obscured by later development, as the diaphragm itself blocks the continuum. In early stages, this connection is prominent. This structure becomes the pericardioperitoneal canal which maintains a connection from the pericardium and developing lung buds to the abdominal cavity. The pleuropericardial membrane, which initially lies between the heart and the developing lung buds, extends into this canal and is thus continuous with the peritoneal membranes. As the lungs and heart develop, by the seventh week, the pleuropericardial membrane fuses with the mesoderm in front of the esophagus. The diaphragm as it develops fills the pericardioperitoneal canal. Remnants of the original connection remain as the membrane around the esophagus. The membrane around the esophagus is a clear analog for the *Ling Shu* reference to the origin of the upper warmer "coming out from the entrance of the stomach, parallelling the esophagus, passing through the diaphragm to disperse inside the chest" *(LS 18)*.

☐

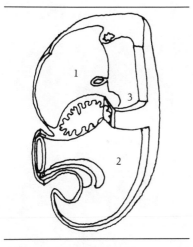

Figure 8.4 The developing thoracic cavity (1) and abdominal cavity (2) are connected via the pericardioperitoneal canals (3)

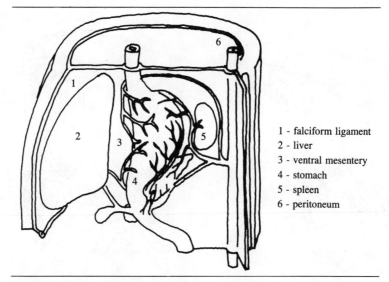

1 - falciform ligament
2 - liver
3 - ventral mesentery
4 - stomach
5 - spleen
6 - peritoneum

Figure 8.5 The plane of fascia is very evident.

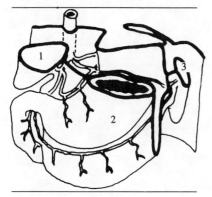

Figure 8.6 The dark line shows the continuity of the planes of fasciae as the organs begin to move.   1 - liver   2 - stomach   3 - spleen

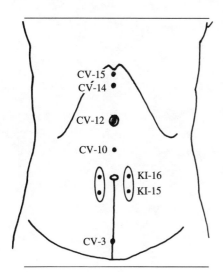

Figure 8.7 Tohaku Ishi's embryologically based abdominal diagnosis.

Thus, we see the connections between the abdominal and thoracic organs and a continuous system of membranes within which all the organs first develop. As the organs develop further, these connections become obscured. For instance, the liver shifts upward to the right and fuses with the lower portion of the septum transversum. On the upper surface of the septum transversum the embryonic heart is developing. The stomach migrates to the left, as does the spleen. As this occurs, the mesenteries begin to fold and invaginate; both the small and large intestines begin to migrate.

The small intestine and large intestine arise from the primitive intestinal loop. This loop communicates with the yolk sac by way of the vitelline duct. Because of this connection, a portion of what later becomes the small intestine can be found within the umbilical cord itself. This portion later retracts as the primitive intestine and the mesentery that suspends it go through an approximately 270-degree rotation.

Tohaku Ishi, a practitioner and scholar of Oriental medicine who was particularly interested in early embryological development, determined that these initial positions and movements reflect in later life. Thus, when we palpate the abdomen we are able to diagnose different organs because of their positions during certain embryological stages. He describes the following diagnostic correspondences:[8]

Area	Point	organ
1	CV-15	heart
2	CV-14	liver
3	Around CV-12	stomach/pancreas
4	CV-10	large intestine
5	KI-16, KI-15	kidneys, ovaries and testicles
6	linea alba below the umbilicus	liver
7	Anterior lines of the iliac crest	sexual organs
8	CV-3	bladder

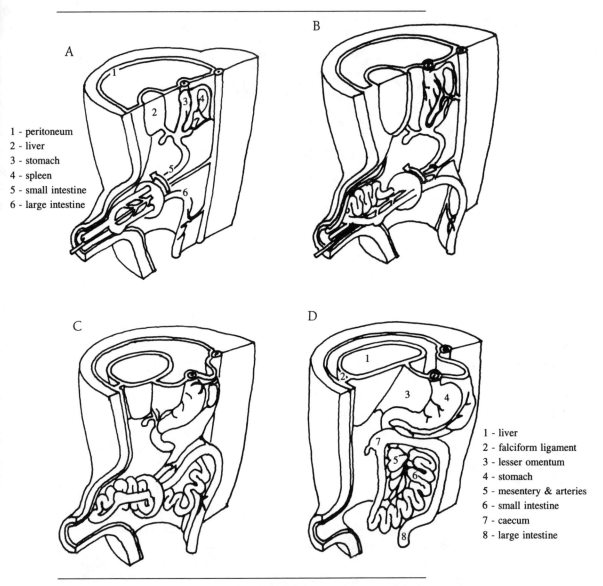

1 - peritoneum
2 - liver
3 - stomach
4 - spleen
5 - small intestine
6 - large intestine

1 - liver
2 - falciform ligament
3 - lesser omentum
4 - stomach
5 - mesentery & arteries
6 - small intestine
7 - caecum
8 - large intestine

Figure 8.8 As the intestinal loops rotate, the other organs begin to swing toward their resting places, and the intestines retreat into the abdominal cavity; the planes of fasciae are still evident here.

Ishi further comments that tension to the right or left of the linea alba can reflect tension along that whole side of the body. He utilized this particular form of abdominal reflection in his clinical practice. Ishi's work also helped Yoshio Manaka develop one of his abdominal patterns for five-phase diagnosis.[9]

The small intestine is for a time connected to the yolk sac and closely related to the umbilicus. This is intimated by the classical medical literature wherein the small intestine was seen by some as related to the source. Also, in migrating to the left, the spleen establishes a clear connection with the left kidney, the lienorenal ligament. This ligament connects to the left kidney from the fusion of the dorsal mesentery with that portion of the peritoneum that lines the dorsal aspect of the abdominal wall over the left kidney.

☐

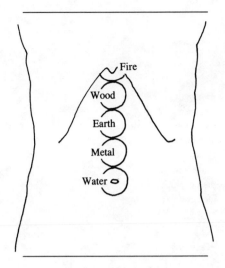

Figure 8.9 One of Dr. Manaka's phasal diagnoses.

In the *Nan Jing*, the left kidney is seen to be the real kidney. The right kidney is ming men *(NJ 36)*. Within a standard five-phase sequence the left kidney is thus more significant. In the developing embryo, the mesentery connecting the liver and gallbladder to the stomach and spleen is also continuous with the left kidney. It is in turn continuous with the membranes of the lungs and heart (pericardium). Embryological development further describes the formation of communicative, biologically active connective tissue membranes that could serve as the physical medium of communication for the cycles and relationships described by Oriental medicine.

Of course, the right kidney is not out of the picture nor out of contact with the system. At this stage of development it lies on a different plane and is open to slightly different channels of communication. Later, after the liver has shifted to a position in front of it, the hepatorenal ligament forms. However, for a number of days during development, before the liver becomes attached to the dorsal wall by the hepatorenal ligament, an open circuit through the five-phase organ cycles exists through the fascial continua.

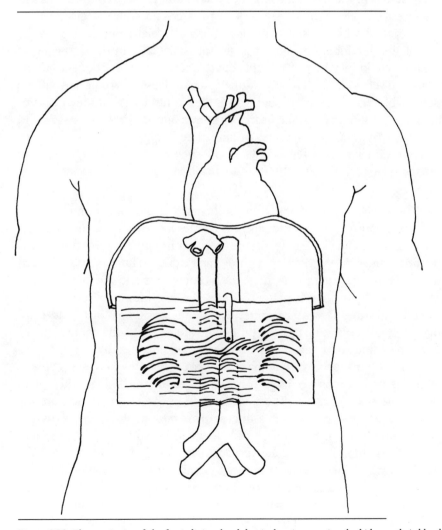

Figure 8.10 The continuity of the fascia lining the abdominal cavity covering the kidneys, their blood vessels and the aorta and vena cava can be seen here.

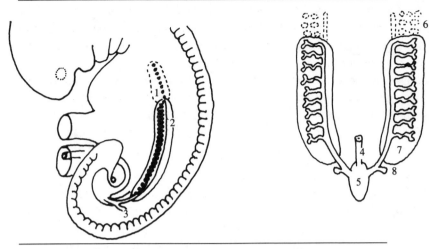

Figure 8.11 The primitive excretory system which later gives rise to the kidneys.

1 - pronephros
2 - mesonephros
3 - metanephric diverticulum
4 - allantois
5 - cloaca
6 - pronephros
7 - mesonephros
8 - metanephros

According to the *Nan Jing*, the right kidney is not a true kidney. It is ming men, "life door," where the jing and shen reside. The shen is normally stored in the heart, the jing in the left kidney. As we have seen, it is possible to see the right kidney, at least for a certain embryological period, as positioned within a somewhat less marked fascial continuum with the rest of the developing organs. It is also possible, later in development, to see the right kidney in a very simple but clear anatomical relationship to the heart and left kidney. The two kidneys themselves are connected via the perirenal fascia.[10] The perirenal fascia is then continuous with the fascia of the aorta stemming from the heart. The aorta and renal blood vessels and their associated fasciae present a striking picture (Figure 8.10). If the heart and left kidney are the repositories of the shen and jing, it is quite easy to see the relationship of the heart and left kidney to the right kidney, ming men.

The development of the kidneys themselves is also worthy of note. The sexual organs, the testicles and the ovaries, develop from the same tissues as the kidneys. These tissues, the nephrotomes, give rise to the nephric tubules in the developing urogenital ridges. These may be divided into three systems: the pronephros, the mesonephros and the metanephros. These three lie in lines on either side of the midline of the embryo and extend upward as far as the somites that are the precursors of the developing cervical vertebrae. They extend downward as far as the somites of the developing lumbar vertebrae. The pronephric system lies in the upper portion. It is a transitory structure that will later degenerate. The mesonephros in the central portion seems to function as an interim kidney, then gives rise to the sexual organs. The metanephros in the lower portion are the precursors of the permanent kidneys. The mesonephric tubule tissues extend up to the sixth cervical and down to the third lumbar somites. Thus, the kidney functions are related to tissues that traverse nearly the whole length of the embryo, from head to tail. Although most of these tissues degenerate and are reabsorbed as the permanent kidneys develop, the communicative pathways of the kidneys are probably established during these stages. The initial internal pathways of the kidneys are described as running up the spine for an indefinite distance, then turning downward to exit at KI-11 *(LS 10)*.[11]

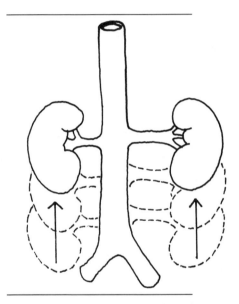

Figure 8.12 The dotted outlines show the previous location of the kidneys and renal blood vessels in the upward migration of the kidneys.

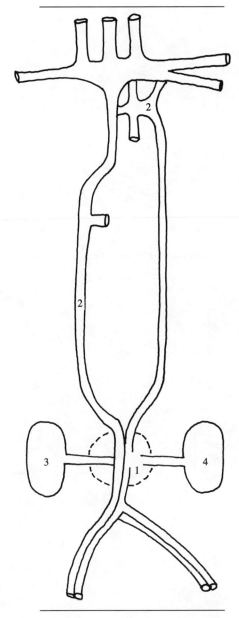

Figure 8.13 The moving qi between the kidneys.

1 - area of moving qi between the kidneys
2 - major blood vessels
3 - right kidney
4 - left kidney

As the kidneys develop from the metanephric tissues, they migrate up the inside of the abdominal cavity on the dorsal wall until they reach their position in the upper part of the abdominal cavity. This movement itself probably creates other lines of communication. As the kidneys rise up the dorsal abdominal wall, numerous renal blood vessels form to maintain the blood supply from the aorta to the kidneys, then degenerate. During this process, in the whole area between the aorta and the line of movement taken by the kidneys, there are probably numerous communicative links established between the aorta and the kidneys.

In Chinese medical terms, this is the area of the moving qi between the kidneys. We know that the abdominal aorta was seen in relation to the master of the heart which communicates with the kidneys and the moving qi between them. The anatomical and physiological connections that establish these links can be most clearly seen during embryological development. Once the tissues and organs are more fully developed, these connections are more obscure in the more complex anatomy of the fully-formed body.

A Japanese herbal text written around 1800, the *Fuku Sho Kiran*, by Inaba Bunrei, gives a very clear reference to the moving qi between the kidneys issuing forth from the region where the renal arteries and veins branch out from the aorta and vena cava. This supports our anatomical interpretation of the moving qi and its relation to the major abdominal blood vessels.[12]

That the organs of generation, the gonads, derive from the same tissues as the kidneys, helps us understand the role of the kidneys in Chinese medical theory where they are main repositories of the generative energies. This area of the developing kidneys also evidences relationships to the extraordinary vessels. Dr. Manaka, citing the work of Tohaku Ishi, describes some of these structures in relationship to both the ren mai and du mai:

> The ren mai is affected by the uracus, the umbilical arteries, and vitelline vessels. The du mai is also affected by the cardinal veins and the nephric tubules. Therefore, both of these are affected by the kidney meridians.[13]

Another organ of particular interest is the heart. The development of the heart conjoins the development of the diaphragm. The heart begins as clusters of mesenchymal cells in the cardiogenic area that lies cranially to the neural plate. These mesenchymal cells originally migrated forward toward the notocord from their position in the primitive streak. When the embryo is still just a layered plate of cells lying mostly in one plane, the heart tissues lie above what later becomes the brain. As the plate of cells folds, the heart tissues retract to below the developing brain. During these stages the tissues that become the septum transversum, which is part of what later becomes the diaphragm and the primitive ventral mesentery, lie still further above or anterior to the heart tissues. As the heart folds underneath the neural plate, the septum transversum and the primitive ventral mesentery tissues follow. The ventral mesentery of the gut is derived from the same cardiogenic tissues as the heart. This parallels the yin-yang, heart-small intestine relationship.

As the mesenchymal cells move forward from the primitive streak, they stimulate and influence structures in their path. They have been found to influence the eyes. For the correct development of the optic vesicles and thus the eyes, it is necessary that heart mesenchymal cells and/or head mesenchymal cells and foregut endodermal cells come to close proximity with the diencephalon where the optic vesicles form.[14] In anatomophysiological science the role that the heart mesenchymal cells play is not clear. However, in Oriental medicine we may propose that this influence is part of the energetic mechanism by which the heart meridian connects to the eyes permitting the shen to be seen in the eyes. Similarly, the foregut endodermal cells, which later participate in the composition of the stomach and parts of the small intestine, influence the development of the eyes. Again, the Oriental medical analog is the beginning of the stomach meridian in close proximity to the eyes.

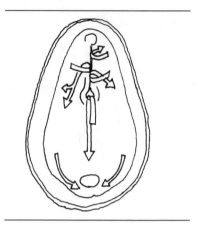

Figure 8.14 The arrows represent the movement of mesodermal cells between the endodermal and ectodermal layers.

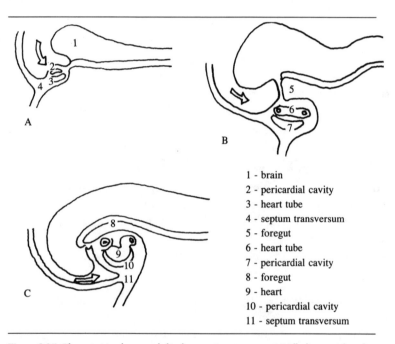

1 - brain
2 - pericardial cavity
3 - heart tube
4 - septum transversum
5 - foregut
6 - heart tube
7 - pericardial cavity
8 - foregut
9 - heart
10 - pericardial cavity
11 - septum transversum

Figure 8.15 The primitive heart and diaphragmatic precursor originally lie cranial to the neural plate - primitive brain - as the head folds, the heart and diaphragmatic structures are retracted into what will become the thoracic and abdominal cavities.

Another developmental parallel of interest is the major part of the diaphragm, the septum transversum. At the upper surface of this structure the pericardium develops. On the lower surface the liver grows. Development of the septum transversum begins at the most distal part of the embryo, the cranial end. It arises from the tissues that develop where the tissues of the embryo and blastocystic wall merge. During this growth and for a short time after, there is a space between the diaphragm (septum transversum) and the developing heart. This may be the area to which the character huang refers. We have already noted its meaning as membranes or greasy tissues. It also refers to the area "below the heart and above the diaphragm." Once the heart membranes, the pericardium, fuse with the septum transversum, there is no longer an obvious space. However, before this stage of development there is a space created by those tissues having branches into the wall of the mother's uterus. The energetic implications of this process are hard to hypothesize. Perhaps the diaphragm, the developing heart, and the space between the two are simply more directly communicative with the mother.

Since the septum transversum provides the medium for the liver and heart to fuse with and grow into, it also provides a direct line of communication between the liver and heart. This is further reinforced by the fact that as the blood supply passes from the mother through the umbilical vein to the liver, a certain amount passes directly from the liver through the ductus venousus to the heart.

In the last chapter we discussed the possible correlations of the triple warmer to the lymph vessels and nodes. We saw how this may be related to the triple warmer's fascial basis, since the deep lymph vessels in the abdominal region lie enfolded within the mesenterium, while the surface vessels of the body lie within the superficial fascia. We further saw the relationship of the triple warmer to the "fu" and "qi jie" and the interpretation of "fu" as referring to the lymph nodes. When we trace the development of the lymph system embryologically we find further interesting correlations. At an early stage of development, there are found to be six "lymph sacs" which precede the development of the lymph vessels. The jugular lymph sacs lie in the neck and head region; the iliac lymph sacs lie in the leg and leg joint regions; the retroperitoneal sac and cysterna chyli lie in the abdominal region. The jugular and cysterna sacs send outgrowths that meet to become the thoracic duct in the chest. The possible correlations arise when we look to the four qi jie described in chapter 52 of the *Ling Shu*. These lie in the head, chest, abdomen, and legs. We feel that there is enough proximity of these qi jie to the major lymphatic sacs or vessels to justify a correspondence.

We also saw, due to location of tissues, a close correlation between the cysterna chyli and the area of the moving qi between the kidneys level with Lumbar 1, Lumbar 2. A further correlation may lie in the triple warmer being "rooted" or having its source here *(NJ 8)* and carrying source qi from here to the source points of the twelve meridians *(NJ 66)*. If as we suggested, this source qi "wells" out at the jing points, to run back towards the body through the yong, shu, jing, he points; then further evidence for the relation of the triple warmer to the lymph system can be seen in the unidirectional flow of lymph from the fingers and toes towards the body. The function of moving qi between the kidneys to protect the shen against evil *(NJ 8)* can be seen in relation to the immunological and protective roles of the lymph system.

Also, we should not ignore the *Ling Shu* statements concerning the flow of qi in the meridians relative to fluid movements *(LS 12)* and the movements of the triple warmer qi with the movements of the jin and ye *(LS 36)*. Since the triple warmer may be related to the lymph vessels and fluids, anatomical and physiological correlations begin to appear.

Finally it is worth noting Takeshi Sawada's correlations of the chyle and lacteals to the wei qi and lower warmer, from whence it springs. To reiterate these correlations:

□

The wei qi is the qi of the lower warmer. The milky nourishing liquid [chyle] is absorbed into the lacteals from the small intestine and to the superficial [layers of the] skin of the whole body.[15]

He goes on to state the role of the chyle:

The wei and ying qi are the lacteal fluids [chyle]; this is why the child's skin is beautiful and moist, because there is much chyle. After labor the woman loses a great amount of 'white blood' [chyle], therefore her skin becomes dry, this is a lack of wei qi and is why we moxa the two yang points. This will prevent this loss. Women with excess hair and dry skin also suffer a lack of wei qi.[16]

Embryological Development of the Meridian System

We can see the potential lines of communication for many of the organ system relationships described by Oriental medical literature. Most, if not all, of these relationships can be seen to occur within the development of the various fascial systems and planes. To understand the connections of these planes to the limbs themselves and thus to the meridian branches, it is necessary to examine the development of the connective tissues of the mesoderm. To further understand the utility of these structural communication links we must examine the various electrical currents and magnetic fields of the embryo and the body.

The limbs first develop as limb buds near the end of the fourth week of embryonic life. These limb buds consist of mesenchymal tissues covered by an ectodermal layer. The mesenchymal tissues are derived from the paraxial or somatic mesoderm. The upper limbs develop about one week before the lower limbs. By the end of the sixth week, the digital rays of the upper limbs are apparent. The digital rays of the lower limbs are not apparent until the end of the seventh week. As the limb buds grow outward, the tip of the limb bud, the apical ectodermal ridge, exerts influences on the mesenchymal tissues which then differentiate, forming the bones, cartilage, and muscles of the limbs. Further differentiation occurs as the nerves from the spine invade the mesenchymal tissues. Thus, the bulk of the limb tissues, the bones and muscles, are derived from this mesenchyme, itself derived from the paraxial mesoderm which has a common origin with all the other forms of mesoderm.

The three major classes of mesoderm are the paraxial, the intermediate, and the lateral plate mesoderm. These have essentially the same origin in the intraembryonic mesoderm, the tissue from which virtually all connective tissues in the body originate. To restate this, the bulk of the limb tissues derive from the same tissues as the rest of the connective tissues of the body. In the early stages of development, up to the end of the third week, the embryo is a plate of cells consisting of three layers — the ectoderm, the endoderm, and the mesoderm. Though there is very little sign of the coming differentiation of tissues into definite structures, these three layers of cells are the origin of all the different systems in the body.

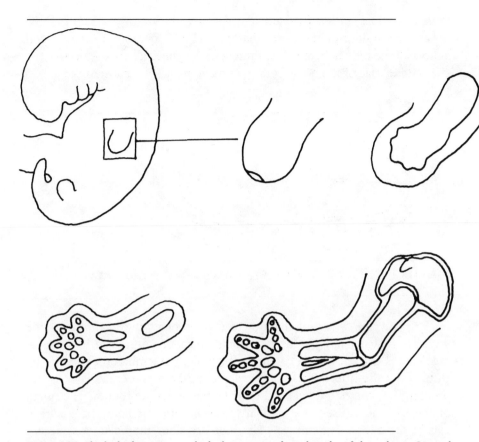

Figure 8.16 The limbs first appear as buds that grow out from the sides of the embryo. Outward growth is accompanied by differentiation of tissues giving rise to the cartilage, mesenchyme, muscles, etc. of the limbs, and finally the bones.

1 - ectoderm
2 - mesoderm
3 - notocord
4 - endoderm
5 - paraxial mesoderm
6 - intermediate mesoderm
7 - neural groove
8 - parietal mesoderm layer
9 - endoderm
10 - visceral mesoderm layer
11 - somite
12 - intermediate mesoderm

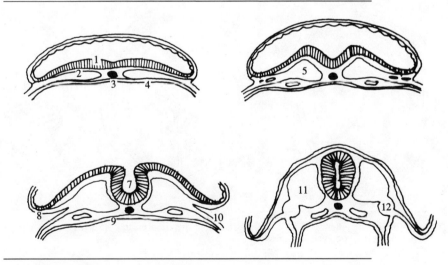

Figure 8.17 Origins of the mesodermal segments.

The ectoderm gives rise to the skin, nervous system, parts of the eyes, the epithelium of the nose, mouth, and anus. The endoderm gives rise to the epithelial lining of most of the alimentary canal, larynx, trachea, bronchi, and parts of the epithelium of the bladder. The intraembryonic mesoderm gives rise to the connective tissues, virtually all of the muscles of the body, the blood, the blood and lymph vessels, the heart, the cartilage and skeletal systems, most of the urogenital system including the kidneys, the mesothelial linings of the pericardial, pleural, and peritoneal cavities, and almost all the mesenchyme. The mesoderm becomes all the connective tissues and fasciae of the body, both the subcutaneous and subserous.

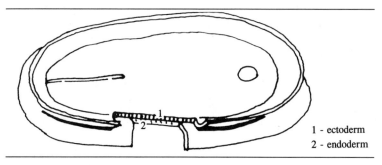

1 - ectoderm
2 - endoderm

Figure 8.18 The bilaminar germ disc. Note the contact between endoderm and ectoderm.

Virtually the whole of the system that becomes the medium for the meridian systems and the energetic communications described by Oriental medicine is derived from a common origin, the intraembryonic mesoderm. Until about the fifteenth day of development the mesodermal layer is not present, only the ectodermal and endodermal layers are found. The origin of the mesoderm itself is particularly relevant, arising along the electrical axis of the developing embryo. This axis lies along the polar axis present in the ovum itself.[17]

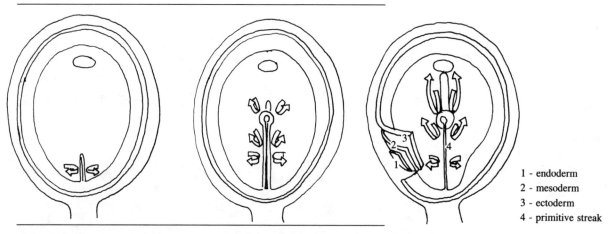

1 - endoderm
2 - mesoderm
3 - ectoderm
4 - primitive streak

Figure 8.19 The primitive streak is an invagination of the ectoderm that spreads cranially from its beginnings at the caudal end of the embryo.

Many eggs and developing embryos, from the least evolved to the most advanced, exhibit electrical polarity.[18] Within the ectodermal layer, a small ridge forms down the center line or polar axis at the tail or caudal end of the embryo. This ridge is the primitive streak. A very rapid proliferation of cells occurs from this primitive streak. As cells pour in from the ectodermal layer, they pass in all directions between the ectodermal and endodermal layers to form the intraembryonic mesoderm. Some of these cells also displace endodermal cells laterally and become endodermal cells themselves. The intraembryonic mesoderm further differentiates into the paraxial, intermediate, and lateral plate mesoderm, which then differentiates into all the structures we have previously described. The primitive streak forms along the polar axis of the developing embryo. Since the primitive streak forms in the ectodermal layer of cells, at the tail end of the embryo, it is forming along that portion of the embryo which later becomes the lower back, or at least the lower portion of the spine. It is possible that this is related to the Chinese concept of ming men. By full term, the primitive streak itself becomes an insignificant structure in the region of the sacrum and coccyx. Before any major differentiation of structures and tissues occurs it extends virtually half the length of the embryo, receding as the embryo grows. For some time during development, it is high enough to correspond to the second lumbar vertebrae where ming men is located.

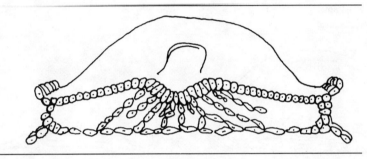

Figure 8.20 Ectodermal cells pour into the primitive streak invagination, splitting off to become the mesoderm.

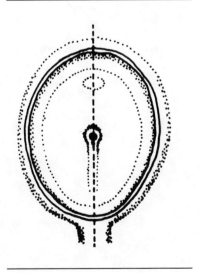

Figure 8.21 The primitive streak lies along the polar axis of the embryo.

At the cranial end of the streak is a small node or knot, the "primitive node" or "knot," which later becomes the neurenteric canal. This node is the point from which the mesodermal tissues proliferate to become the notocord which later helps comprise the vertebral column. Ming men may also be related to this node. From its position along the axis of the embryo, it plays a pivotal role in the communication between the ectodermal and endodermal layers. It also provides a connection between the yolk sac and the amniotic cavity as it becomes canalized.

Both Tohaku Ishi and Yoshio Manaka propose that the neurenteric canal plays an important role in development.[19] By allowing communication between the ectoderm and endoderm, it actually facilitates communication between the neural tube of the ectoderm and the lining of the intestinal tract, the endoderm. Thus, for a time during development, nascent brain tissues have communication via the neurenteric canal with the developing gut tissues. This fact can be seen to have importance in interpreting the research of Taro Kashio M.D., PhD., who has demonstrated that there is a strong relationship between the intestines and the brain; specifically, blockage of the descending colon has been shown to produce cerebral hemorrhages in the left hemisphere.[20] The embryonic communication established by the neurenteric canal may be responsible for this relationship.

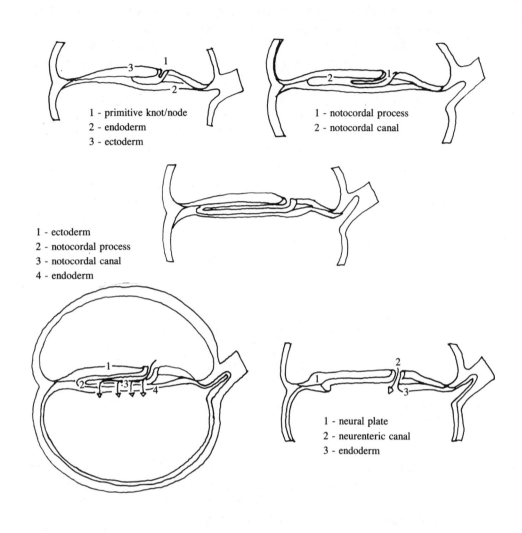

1 - primitive knot/node
2 - endoderm
3 - ectoderm

1 - notocordal process
2 - notocordal canal

1 - ectoderm
2 - notocordal process
3 - notocordal canal
4 - endoderm

1 - neural plate
2 - neurenteric canal
3 - endoderm

Figure 8.22 The primitive node or knot is a small depression at the cranial end of the primitive streak. It continues to grow into the mesodermal layer, finally becoming a hole that shows continuity across the embryo between the endoderm and ectoderm.

A second point of importance is that the areas of ectoderm and endoderm that are in open communication through the canal later become the upper back and lower abdomen. This produces a potential relation to the du mai and ren mai. This is another relationship that Ishi and Manaka feel is important.[21] It is Ishi's thesis that areas where the ectoderm and endoderm interact — for instance, the optic vesicles or the hypophysis — are fundamentally important and express ren mai and du mai relationships and connections. Equally indicative is recent research that has determined that the gastrointestinal mucosa contains certain cells of the A.P.U.D. series which act like endocrine cells, secreting neurohormones and neuro-transmitters.[22] Several of these neurohormones and neurotransmitters are also secreted by the brain. Some of the peptides common to both struc-tures are: somatostatin, bombesin, neurotensin, cholecystokinin and encephalin.[23] It is particularly interesting that encephalin, an opiate neuro-transmitter, is secreted by these A.P.U.D. cells. This neurochemical is thought to play an important role in the control of pain by acupuncture. Encephalin is secreted by the mucosa of the duodenum and upper parts of the small intestine.[24] That parts of the foregut and the brain secrete the same chemicals may also be a phenomenon due in part to the neurenteric canal connections of embryological development.

The primitive streak and node are also places at which considerable growth and differentiation occur. These are highly active centers in the embryo. If for some reason this proliferation fails to slow down, the baby can be born with a tumor in the area of the primitive streak, a sacrococcygeal teratoma. Such tumors are full of a variety of different tissues that have differentiated and developed from the early mesodermal tissues. This attests to the "high potency or energy" state of these tissues and supports the hypothesis that these structures are related to the concept of ming men, a potent source of energy in Oriental theory.

Thus, embryological development shows us possible anatomical analogs, which develop and then recede, having correlation to both the *Nan Jing* ming men, the right kidney, and the alternate theories of ming men which place it below the second lumbar vertebra or just lateral thereto. It is also possible to follow the connections of the source points, on or around the wrists and ankles, to the source and triple warmer.

If the triple warmer is the functional aggregate of the systems of fasciae and, as detailed by the medical classics, it has its root at the source, then it is likely that the source itself and the connection of the source points to the triple warmer will also act through the fasciae. We can see a possible fascial connection in the growth of the limb buds. When the limb buds first form, they are comprised of undifferentiated mesenchyme. The upper limb buds first appear at the end of the fourth week. At this time the mesenteries of the cavities are already present. Perhaps, the connections between source points and the source stem from this early stage. The mesenchymal tissues grow out from the body before they differentiate. The tissues that later become the wrists and ankles have been in contact with the internal fasciae and mesenteries throughout development. There is no clear expression of the limb bud differentiation in the Oriental medical literature. We can only hypothesize that this connection is a reasonable parallel of the others. There is research which supports this idea.

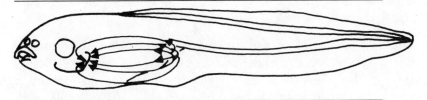

Figure 8.23 Small currents exit the embryo at the site of the lower limb bud to reenter under the gill flaps. The existence of these currents is significant support for our bioelectrical theories.

Research done on chick embryos has shown that relatively strong electrical currents leave the primitive streak to reenter the embryo elsewhere along the ectoderm.[25] These currents are thought to be responsible in part for the proliferation of cells which begins at the streak. Also, these currents may control or even organize the development of the embryo. ☐

Research on Xenopus embryos (African clawed toad) has demonstrated that electrical currents leave the lower limb buds to reenter the embryo under the gill flaps:

> Two preliminary observations suggests that this limb bud current precedes the site of bud formation and that it is closely correlated with bud growth.[26]

Similar work done on other developing embryos, for instance the axolotl, shows that there are ionic currents associated with limb development. These seem to predict the site of limb formation.[27] Although not yet demonstrated in the developing human embryo, it is likely that similar "bud currents" influence the development of the limb buds and their growth. If this is so, it is an immensely important discovery. These currents will not only influence the development and growth of the limb buds, but will also arrange and structure the developing tissues within the limb buds. This may well be the earliest development of the electrical properties in the limbs we call the meridians.

Other research has demonstrated the possibility that the developing spinal nerves, which pass to the mesenchymal tissues in the limb bud, are important in differentiation and are guided by the natural electric field of the embryo.[28] Other research has indicated the possibility that electrical currents and gradients play an even earlier role in development by helping guide the cells migrating from the neural crest.[29] Can we think of the development of the nervous system as an anatomical extension of this natural electric field? This is a hard question to answer, for the situation is not simple or clear. Speculatively, we need to note the Chinese medical de-emphasis of the nervous system. The functional importance of the nervous system is quite markedly lacking in the medical literature. Is it because they conceived of functions we normally ascribe to the nervous system as due to the source?

The natural electrical field is centered on the source, the gravitational center of the body, and pre-exists the formation of the primitive streak, which emanates currents through the embryo as it forms. If these currents are related to the field that guides the nerves, we could then conceive of the nerves as an outgrowth of this field and the source itself. Speculatively, this suggests that the Chinese de-emphasis on the nervous system in classical times was not an anatomical ignorance, but an emphasis on the source's functional, energetic nature.

While the identity of the nervous system with the source is hypothetical, it is no speculation to propose that the bioenergetic, ionic, and electric functions of the human body are centrally important. In this century, a substantial amount of work has been done since the 1920's on developmental electrical currents and fields. It has become quite obvious that these currents and the fields associated with them are vital factors in development. Some researchers and authors posit that these fields are actually the main determinants of pre- and postnatal development.[30]

The natural field is seen to arise from the ovum itself. Various ova have been found to be polarized. Many factors can cause this polarization or influence and change it, including direct electrical current, unilateral light, the presence of neighboring eggs, acidity differences, temperature gradients, calcium ions, gravity, and the entry point of the sperm.[31] The point at which the sperm penetrates the ovum is significant.[32] The original polar axis determines at least the early cell divisions which occur along this axis.[33] In a more complex pattern, division in relation to this polar axis probably continues through development.

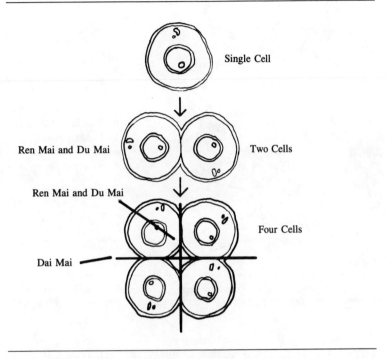

Figure 8.24 The first division gives rise to the ren mai — du mai axis.
Figure 8.25 The second division gives rise to the dai mai axis.

This polar axis is critical in the context of classical Chinese medical theory. It is reasonable that because of the nature of this polar axis and its electrical polarity and electrical field, this axis field is related to the the source or *yuan* 原, which was seen as so important in the medical literature. Yoshio Manaka proposes that the first division of the fertilized ovum along the polar axis gives rise to the ren mai and du mai, the oceans of yin and yang.[34] Further, the second division forming four cells creates the dai mai. In the very early stages of development, after the first divisions, it is possible to see this pattern of differentiation continue. Later, it is only apparent in a more general sense because of the increased complexity that accompanies development.

Manaka cites the work of Tohaku Ishi in discussing the ren mai and du mai polarity.[35] Ishi suggests that if we were to think about the connections of the twelve meridians to the brain, we would see that these exist through the ren mai and du mai. He notes that the ren mai is embryologically connected to the developing optic and nasal vesicles and to a point near GV-28 on the frenulum of the upper lip. From here, it extends to the anterior hypophysis or pituitary gland where it meets the du mai, which has ascended up the developing spine through the posterior pituitary.

□

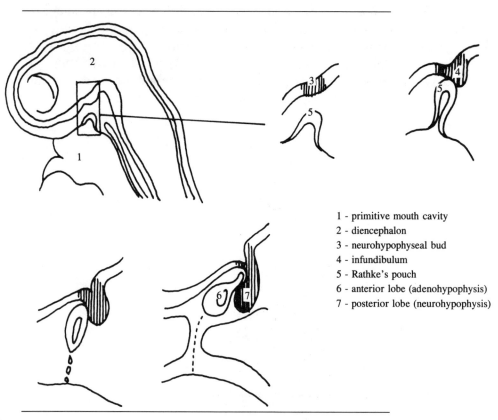

1 - primitive mouth cavity
2 - diencephalon
3 - neurohypophyseal bud
4 - infundibulum
5 - Rathke's pouch
6 - anterior lobe (adenohypophysis)
7 - posterior lobe (neurohypophysis)

Figure 8.26 A downward growth of tissues from the prebrain (neurohypophyseal bud) meets with an upward growth from the stomodeum (Rathke's pouch) to form the anterior and posterior hypophyses.

The anterior pituitary and posterior pituitary have different origins. However, both form from the interaction of the ectoderm and the underlying ectoderm or endoderm. The anterior portion of the pituitary forms from a pocketing of the ectoderm or endoderm of the oral cavity, this is known as Rathke's pouch. Some authors feel that this is only ectoderm, others feel that it occurs at the junction of ectoderm and endoderm. The posterior portion forms from a downward extension of the brain, the diencephalon. This is known as the infundibulum.

Ishi suggests that the neural tube components forming the posterior pituitary are related to the du mai, where the gut components, specifically the ectoderm-endoderm of the mouth, form the anterior pituitary which is related to the ren mai. We can extend this idea further. The posterior hypophysis is of neural ectodermal origin and is structurally of neural tissue. The anterior hypophysis is of epithelial ectodermal and gut endodermal origin and is of a glandular nature; it is the master gland of the endocrine system. A distinction may thus be proposed where the ren mai is relatively more related to metabolic hormonal function and the du mai is more closely associated with neural hormonal function.

This structural genesis shows us why the ren mai and du mai start on either side of the anus and end either side of the mouth. Being related to the ectoderm-endoderm interactions, the mouth and anus are where ectoderm and endoderm overlap. While "overlap" is a rough image of this three-dimensional interaction, the ectoderm does extend down into the throat and up into the rectum. This provides a possible physical connection of the ren mai and du mai in the brain and establishes a connection of the yin and yang qiao mai to the ren and du mai. We should remember that the *Ling Shu* describes the yin and yang qiao mai as branches splitting outward from the brain *(LS 21:215)*. With all four of the extraordinary vessels meeting or branching out of the brain, this embryonic connection and early electrical polarity may be the genesis of their connection and development as coupled pairs.

This basic system of polarity of ren mai and du mai, which is derived from the polar axis of the embryo and the dorsal-ventral axis of the dai mai, remains throughout life. In a sense, these circuits or lines of division are major lines of force or communication which are both produced by the field of the polar axis and modify this field. In Oriental medicine, they are seen as major lines of division of the body into yin and yang, left and right, upper and lower, and are also seen as deriving from the root or source. Derivation from the source is not so clearly stated for the dai mai.[36] However, both the ren and du mai lie on the polar electrical axis along which the spinal cord grows. If, as Ishi and Manaka posit, the ren and du mai have some connections to the brain and nervous system as a whole, then it is also possible to explain how this pair, the oceans of the yin and yang, relate to the source.

Since the ren and du mai have their origin at a source which we propose to be the embryonic bioelectric field influencing the growth of the spine and the nervous system, the course of their growth will be subject to the same influences as the developing nervous system itself. As noted,[37] the nerves that grow outward from the spinal cord follow the natural electrical field of the embryo. These grow into the limb bud mesenchyme causing the limb tissues to differentiate and grow. It is likely that the meridians form in response to these growing nerves or in response to the common electrical field. We can visualize the ren mai and the du mai as initial bioelectric pathways from which the nerves and meridians may develop. In effect, the patterns they establish direct and stimulate the development of the meridians. If we image these patterns as the "oceans of yin and yang," as did the classical Chinese, the meridians and nerves complete the analogy as energetic streams.

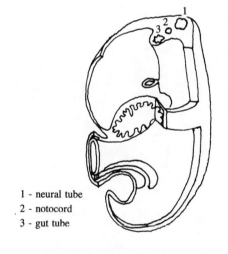

1 - neural tube
2 - notocord
3 - gut tube

Figure 8.27 Sections showing the parallel axes of the neural tube, notocord, and gut tube.

The polar axis of the embryo is also related to the source itself. This axis clearly correlates with electrical gradients through the developing embryo and with the fields associated with these gradients.[38] The idea of the source includes the concept of underlying or prenatal energies. The polar axis is present from the very earliest stages of development, possibly before conception itself. Both the source and the polar axis are prenatal. The early medical authors described both the ren mai and du mai as having their origin at the source, the moving qi between the kidneys. Both these energetic entities were sometimes equated with the uterus, or described as located below the umbilicus. The chong mai also originates in this place. The role of the chong mai in embryological development leads us back to the source.

During the period following the development of the notocord, the embryo contains three parallel central axes. These are the neural tube, the notocord, and the gut tube, which lie on the same plane. The neural tube is

□

of ectodermal origin and is related to the du mai. The gut tube is of endodermal origin and is thus related to the ren mai. The notocord is of mesodermal origin and we propose that it is related to the chong mai since it too parallels the genesis and structure of the other extraordinary vessels.

The ren mai rises up the midline of the front of the body; the du mai up the back on the midline and the chong mai up the inside on the midline in front of the spine. The disposition of all three extraordinary vessels evidences the structure we would expect from their ectoderm, mesoderm, and endoderm origins. The same is true for their relationship to the neural tube, notocord, and gut tube. Further, the ren mai and du mai are known as the oceans of the yin and yang vessels.[39] This is often interpreted as referring to the meridians, just as we proposed in regard to their bioelectrical generation. However, the expression is also given without specifying vessels or meridians, nor is the ascription exclusive. The chong mai is said to be "the ocean of the twelve meridians, the five yin and six yang organs and the ocean of the blood" *(LS 38:308; LS 62:434 LS 65:463; TS 10:153)*. If we follow the derivatives of the ectoderm, endoderm, and mesoderm, we may note some definite relationships that conform to the classical description of chong mai.

The ectoderm gives rise to the epidermis, the surface of the body, and the nervous system. The endoderm creates the endothelium of the stomach, the small intestine and large intestine, the liver and gallbladder, and most of the bladder and the lungs — in effect, most of the interior portions of the body. The mesoderm produces the heart, blood vessels and blood, the kidneys, spleen, connective tissues, fasciae, muscles, cartilage, and bones. The du mai as the ocean of the yang vessels is related to the yang areas, the surface of the body, and the spinal cord and brain. This we would expect from its ectodermal genesis. Ren mai too expresses its prenatal origin in its classical appellation. As the ocean of yin (vessels) it relates to the interior portions of the body, the yin areas. The chong mai as the ocean of the twelve meridians can be understood in context as the mesodermic origin of the connective tissues and fasciae. Here, it shares a prenatal base with the meridians. As the ocean of the blood its mesodermal origin is again predictive. However, it is the chong mai in its aspect as the ocean of the yin and yang organs that merits the closest examination because most organs develop from the endoderm and mesoderm, not exclusively the mesoderm.

The smooth muscles of the gastrointestinal and urogenital tracts arise from the mesoderm, but the endodermal derivatives are not so clearly seen. However, the organs of endodermal origin all arise within the planes of subserous fasciae. This relationship is not mere coincidence. In some cases it has been found that the organs will not develop in the absence of these fasciae. Thus, the organs arise from endodermal interaction with the mesoderm. The mechanism of this interaction remains to be seen.

Quite possibly, the bilateral columns of somites which are of mesodermal origin are involved, in addition to the notocord, in the chong mai relationship to the polar axis. While there are clearly areas where the appropriate research questions have not been posited nor solutions found, it is evident that the embryonic polar axis is an important energetic determinant.

☐

At certain stages, this axis is related to electrical gradients and fields, the neural tube and ectoderm, the notocord and mesoderm, and the gut tube and endoderm. Each of these corresponds to one of the principal extraordinary vessels in terms of function, derivation, and location as we would expect from the classical description of each vessel. These axes change physically as development progresses, but remain as the du mai, chong mai, and ren mai.

The pathway of the du mai across the midline of the skull and down the spine strongly suggests a direct relationship to the central nervous system as a physical correlate, which may explain why it is called the "governing" vessel, possibly referring to the governing functions of the central nervous system. The ren mai pathway does not have such a clear physical correlate except in the abdominal region. Here it follows the linea alba from the pubic symphysis to the sternum. It is possibly called the "conception" or "pregnancy" vessel because in many pregnancies the linea alba becomes pigmented to a reddish brown, in which case it is called the "linea nigra." These color changes can persist for some time after birth.

Manaka feels that the ectoderm, mesoderm, and endoderm axes may be responsible for or give rise to the pattern of meridian relationships described in the classic literature as tai yang—shao yin; shao yang—jue yin; and yang ming—tai yin.[40] The origins of this idea are not entirely clear, but it remains worthy of note.

The electrical axis that coincides with the polar axis is itself a concept important to understanding embryonic development. It has been described in various ways. This axis and its associated electrical gradients form part of a larger scheme which Harold Saxton Burr has called an "electrodynamic field":

> The pattern or organization of any biological system is established by a complex electrodynamic field which is in part determined by its atomic physio-chemical components and which in part determines the behavior and orientation of those components.
>
> This field is electrical in the physical sense and by its properties relates the entities of the biological system in a characteristic pattern and is itself, in part, a result of the existence of those entities. It determines and is determined by the components.
>
> More than just establishing a pattern, it must maintain that pattern in the midst of a physio-chemical flux. Therefore, it must regulate and control living things. It must be the mechanism, the outcome of whose activity is wholeness, organization, and continuity.[41]

Many of these properties and functions have been accurately measured and documented by Burr and his colleagues.

> [This electrical field] can be measured with considerable certainty and accuracy and shown to have correlations with growth and development, degeneration and regeneration, and the orientation of component parts in the whole system.

□

> Perhaps more interestingly than any one thing, this field exhibits remarkable stability through the growth and development of an egg.[42]

This stability and governing control is what sets the climate for many things to come as the egg develops into an embryo, an infant, and an adult. The patterns it describes are strong determining factors in later life.

These fields also have cyclic variations mirroring the cyclic variations described by the Chinese in the cycles of the stems and branches. Burr discusses how in a variety of different living organisms the field has been measured at a distance from the organism, both in embryological and adult stages.[43] For example, in the obelia the voltage gradients of the field were measured through the life cycle of the organism. They were found to increase steadily to a point at which they plateaued and then declined.[44] This is remarkably similar to the cycles of energetic activity described in the branch cycle of the *Shi Ji*. Similar measurements have been made on trees for a number of concurrent years, the relative strengths of the field of the trees varying regularly according to the time of the year.[45] As early as 1959 similar measurements were made on humans showing regular variations of the field strengths according to seasonal changes and progressions.[46]

The Russian scientist, A. S. Presman, feels that the electrical and magnetic fields have three basic communicative functions:

- Through the process of evolution, electrical and magnetic fields were used by living organisms to obtain information about changes in the environment.

- Electrical and magnetic processes are involved in informational interconnections within living organisms.

- Electrical and magnetic fields facilitate informational interchange among living organisms.[47]

Presman discusses a large number of experiments showing how tissues and living organisms respond to electrical and magnetic fields. He discusses how these fields have much broader spheres of action and influence than is often believed.

Robert O. Becker has done some interesting research in the United States on the nature of the body's electric field. Using the adult salamander as his experimental animal, he found evidence strongly suggesting that the field pattern correlates with the nervous system.[48] He distinguished two types of electrical systems in the body. The first is the more specialized and evolutionarily advanced system, the nervous system. The second is a more basic or primitive system able to communicate information in the form of direct electrical current. Information such as the "injury potential" and the ability to detect changes in the environmental electrical and magnetic fields are processed by the more basic system. He concludes that the nervous system at least determines the pattern of the field, but that there are many electrical activities within this field that do not originate with the nervous system and that serve as information channels for the whole body. He posits that these are derived from the most ancient life forms.[49]

☐

The existence of these systems and fields is beyond doubt. They have been measured in the lowest and highest forms of life, in living things with and without a nervous system. From the perspective of Oriental medicine, the most significant property of this field is that in a living being the core or center of this field will lie at the center of gravity, just as in non-living systems. This core will lie somewhere on the polar axis as the polar axis itself will pass through the center of gravity. The center of gravity of a person lies somewhere in the abdomen below the umbilicus. It is sometimes seen as being located roughly two inches in front of the second sacral vertebra. During normal gait, it oscillates up to two inches in a vertical direction.[50] Thus, the center or core of the field and the polar axis will be centered in the abdomen below the umbilicus. This has a remarkable similarity to the Chinese concept of the source.

If the body is imbalanced or distorted for any reason, the center of gravity will shift slightly so as to lie off the center of mass. Thus, someone who has a slightly curved spine, one shoulder higher than the other, or the hips and pelvis slightly tilted in an abnormal gait, will have a center of gravity that is off center. These distortions may lead to disorders and diseases. Those involved in bodywork can describe many such disorders. The Japanese therapeutic exercise system, Sotai, devised by Keizo Hashimoto, is based on this perception.[51]

Distortions also result from functional or structural changes in the internal environment. As the various organs become weakened or hyperactive, different tissues are affected, resulting eventually in structural changes and functional disorders. Each of these circumstances will affect the underlying electrodynamic field and the polar axis. Again, this is similar to the idea of the source underlying the various organ and meridian functions. In five-phase diagnosis and treatment, we are essentially assessing the condition of the source. As we use our skills to identify a weakened or imbalanced organ or meridian, we are identifying what it is that has affected the source. A similar analogy is true for the eight extraordinary vessels.

As Yoshio Manaka explains, the extraordinary vessels affect both deep energetic levels and gross structure.[52] In assessing which of the extraordinary vessels is imbalanced, we are assessing the cause of the physical distortion that has weakened the source and engendered the disease. All disease may be seen as resulting from disorders or imbalances of the source regardless of the origin of the distortion. Both prenatal weaknesses and a wide variety of postnatal causes may have introduced the distortion.

Manaka feels that the relative symmetry of the body is extremely important in determining the relative health of the individual.[53] He traces the development of this symmetry to the earliest stages of development. As the body develops, it progressively loses its symmetry. Manaka describes this progression as an adaptation that allows for an increased ability to act and perform after birth, thus enabling greater survivability of the organism. Initially, there is a direct and simple symmetry in the single cell. However, it is not absolute. For instance, scientists have demonstrated animal and vegetal poles within the egg.[54] Each pole has a different effect on the nature of the cell divisions and cell differentiations. The single cell splits into two cells, almost mirror images of each other, that become the left and right sides of the embryo. Further divisions also produce near mirror images. However, with the development of the internal organs, the rotations, migrations, and the singularity of many of the organs, the initial symmetry becomes less dominant. The original, nearly perfect symmetry is still reflected in the bilateral ears, eyes, legs, arms, and other body parts. Eventually, the body becomes imperfectly symmetrical, retaining its only real symmetry on the surface.

Manaka views these symmetries as important in the nature of the extraordinary vessels. He also feels they are important structurally and energetically. He proposes that topological geometry, the geometry of three-dimensional objects, will provide greater insights into the significance of the body's relative symmetries. Simply stated, his idea is that the body retains a memory of the symmetry lost through embryological development and that its state of imperfect symmetry expresses many of these memories. With any distortion of the body, either physically or energetically induced, the body will respond in some manner that will symmetrically reflect that distortion. For example, problems of the left leg can often reflect on the right arm. Problems of the lower right abdominal quadrant can reflect on the upper left abdominal quadrant; problems of the lower abdomen on the midline may reflect on the midline of the upper back.

Manaka proposes that these symmetries and the body's natural ability to compensate symmetrically for distortion are mathematically precise. If such mathematical relationships exist, it is very likely that there are some components of the body that are able to transmit or communicate the information by which these compensations are directed. The extracellular matrix and intracellular matrices of microtubules and microfilaments that are the whole system of the connective tissues are likely candidates for research into this communication mechanism. These provide a pervasive skeletal structure. Perhaps, as distortions occur in the physical or energetic body at the macrostructural level, these distortions transmit through the connective tissue matrices, producing symmetrically opposed reactions. As Oschman states:

> All movements of the body as a whole, or of its smallest parts, are created by tensions carried through the connective tissue fabric. Each tension, each compression, each movement causes the crystalline lattices of the connective tissues to generate bioelectric signals that are precisely characteristic of these tensions, compressions, and movements. The fabric is a semiconducting communication network that can convey the bioelectric signals between every part of the body and every other part.[55]

This idea is important not only to body workers but also to acupuncturists because of the energetic nature of the connective tissues. Whatever the physical basis of such symmetrical relationships and expressions, they are quite likely part of the mechanism of acupuncture. Indeed, Manaka feels that the ancient Chinese physicians were concerned with reinstating the prenatal symmetry lost through development.

□

An Electrodynamic Model
of the Triple Warmer

The electrodynamic field model describes a field with strong regulating properties. It is simultaneously determined by its components and determines the orientation, pattern, and organization of the components.[56] This mutual interaction of the electrodynamic field with the body is analagous to the mutual interaction of the body's different systems with the source. The source is the root of the twelve meridians, the source of the triple warmer and fundamental to the five yin and six yang organs *(NJ 8)*. There is a constant interaction among all these. In a human electrodynamic model the body's field would thus be central to all biophysical and bioelectrical functions, and any theory of how the human body functions must explain these interactions.

As previously discussed, the triple warmer may be either functionally or actually identical to the fascial system. Remembering that both the polar axis and the electrical axis of the embryo have effects on embryological development, we may associate the known qualities of these fields to the fully-formed energetic system. Thus, the control and regulation functions of the electrodynamic field are reasonably examined through the Chinese theories of triple warmer function.

As we have discussed, the *Ling Shu* described the upper warmer as "coming out from the entrance of the stomach, paralleling the esophagus, passing through the diaphragm to disperse inside the chest" *(LS 18:197)*. As noted, the pleural and peritoneal fasciae are continuous and wrap the esophagus. Thus, the upper warmer is easily identified with the fascia of the upper stomach which lines the esophagus. It becomes continuous with the pleura of the lungs, to "disperse inside the chest." According to the *Ling Shu* theory, the upper warmer then passes "to the armpits and down [parallel to] the side of the lung meridian; it then passes to the large intestine and then down through the stomach meridian" *(LS 18:197-198)*. That is, the chronobiological cycle of meridian energy flow is itself a function or extension of the upper warmer. Thus, the theoretical correspondence of the functions of the upper warmer and the fascial system is justified.

The middle warmer is described by the *Ling Shu* in terms of digestive function. It is difficult to see a relation to the fasciae unless we posit that the bioelectrical regulations and controls that govern the digestive system operate through the electrical and communicative qualities of the fasciae. The fasciae would be thus the interconnecting lines of the communications network.

The lower warmer is easily associated with the peritoneal fascia or mesentery. The *Ling Shu* says, "The lower warmer divides the intestines, goes to the bladder, and is absorbed into the bladder" *(LS 18:200)*. This passage is not traditionally related to the mesentery. It is most often thought to refer to the lower warmer division of the intestines, or a qualitative division of the clear and unclear elements of food and water. The peculiarity of the original text allows all three interpretations to claim textual authority. However, we feel our interpretation, that the division of the intestines refers to the mesentery, is grammatically correct. Clearly, the relationship to the

□

mesentery neither limits nor contradicts the other interpretations. It provides a method of interpreting and studying the means by which these processes may function.

The mesentery both supports and separates the intestines. It also provides the physical analog of going "to the bladder" and being "absorbed into the bladder." Connective tissues have important water components. The more hydrated they are, the more energetically conductive they will become. The drier they become, the less conductive they will be. Due to the connection of the mesentery to the other fasciae, it is also continuous with the fascia surrounding the bladder. As with the development of organs in the presence of fascial tissue, this connection is not merely coincidental. Experiments where toad ureters were clipped so that no urine could pass into the bladder demonstrated that fluid is nonetheless absorbed from the surrounding tissues, which include the fasciae.[57] Water is also absorbed in the peritoneal cavity through the peritoneum.[58] This fits the *Ling Shu* concept of triple warmer water metabolism.

It has also been noted that "respiratory movements" expedite the absorption of water in the upper part of the peritoneum.[59] This underlines the classical importance of breathing with regard to triple warmer function. Deep abdominal breathing would stimulate this absorptive process, helping to avoid pathological dampness.

If, as we suggest, the triple warmer is the fascial system throughout the body, it too will be centered at the gravitational center where the source, the yuan, resides. This is possibly why the source was also known as the "source of the triple warmer." Since the source is the electrical and magnetic center of the body, the triple warmer may also be conceptualized as the biodynamic field itself.

Dantian

We have examined possible relationships of the fields of the body to the source and the triple warmer. We examined the relationship of this area to the lower dantian and noted that many authors identified this area as the lower dantian. Based on these discussions, it is reasonable to presume that the lower dantian is also related to the center of the body's field. It is actually a complex relationship. Each of the three dantian have anatomical locations corresponding to magnetically and electrically active centers.

Many, if not most, activities in the body generate an electrical or magnetic field. We have discussed only the sum of all these fields, the general biodynamic field. However, several important areas and organs generate substantial fields of their own within the flux of the general field. The heart generates the strongest electrical and magnetic fields in the body; the eyes generate the next strongest fields.[60] Thus, the upper dantian lying between the eyebrows is also located in the center of significant natural electrical and magnetic fields. Middle dantian, which lies over or near the heart, relates directly to the natural electrical and magnetic fields of the heart. There are apt energetic correspondences for these locations. Consider for example the relationship of the open point theory of Xu Wen Bai to the wei qi theory of the *Ling Shu* (LS 76). If the wei qi issues from the eyes upon

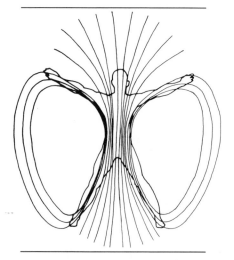

Figure 8.28 Until we have adequate equipment to visualize the entire biodynamic field at once, we can only surmise its appearance. This drawing is a rough conceptualization.

awakening to flow down all the yang meridians and eventually return to the eyes, the natural electrical and magnetic fields of the eyes may be the biological mechanism that drives this phenomena. Just as the circulation of the wei qi is governed by the apparent movement of celestial bodies vis-a-vis the rotation of the earth around its axis, the natural electrical and magnetic fields of the body also respond to the biorhythmic fluctuations of environmental magnetic fields. Like all such fields these active areas would have the capacity to trigger actions through the transmission of signals in response to changes in the larger, exterior fields.

The natural magnetic and electrical fields of the heart are very strong. Their locational relation to the middle dantian is significant, but there are no other correspondences to energetic phenomena immediately apparent. The electrical field is possibly quite significant in that the field can be measured at any part of the body's surface in a routine ECG procedure. The significance lies in its obvious conductivity throughout the body and the implication of the systemic conduction of any electrical signal, however large or small, throughout the body. Since electrical signals produced anywhere in the body can be conducted throughout the body, then the notion of the total body electrical and magnetic fields, the sums of all the component parts, is clearly evidenced. These correlations provide further evidence for our interpretation of the triple warmer and its source as representing the total body field and its epicenter.

Lower dantian relationships may be even more complex. Aside from its location in the center of the general field, and thus its relationship to the source, the moving qi between the kidneys, and ming men, it may also be related to the electrical and magnetic activity of the various nerve plexii in the abdomen. Because it is located roughly where the *Swadhistana Chakra* is found in Indian energetic anatomy, it may share a relation to the sacral plexus and to a lesser degree the solar plexus with the Indian energetic concept.[61] It could also be related to the center of gravity of the body, which lies in roughly the same place in the abdomen. It is known that the magnetic, electrical, and gravitational vectors affect each other.[62] Each of these areas has relatively strong biological fields and a significant place in classical energetic theory. All are worthwhile subjects for research.

Relationships to Physical Principles

The relationship of the triple warmer to the concept of "no form" predates the modern theories of energies and particles that exist at the border of quantum physics and the physics of matter. While this is a fascinating source of theory and speculation, it is the classical Chinese concepts of the source and triple warmer and their correlation with modern concepts of matter and energy that is most practically essential to our discussion.

The idea of energy in Western acupuncture literature is very vague. In some cases, it is nothing more than a buzzword that indicates the author intends something different than a symptomatic or anatomophysiolgical principle. It is used, yet unexplained. In other cases it is a concept that indicates functional sets, grouped functions known by some emblematic characteristic. For other Western authors (e.g., Yves Requena), the relationship of qi to modern ideas of potential and kinetic biochemical and bioelectrical energies is quite clear. In some modern Chinese work, the opposite is true and the emphasis seems to be on the results of qi. It is explained as "an untranslatable word in the Chinese medical lexicon. . . .a tendency, a movement, something on the order of energy."[63] Certainly, there are instances in the medical literature that can be referenced for each of these ideas. Thus, qi must precede and include all these functions.

Considerable research has been done on the implications of quantum physics for biological systems. One interesting view proposed by the Polish scientist Wlodzimierz Sedlak incorporates both Burr's view of the biodynamic field and the quantum properties of such a field.[64] Many ideas he describes mirror classical Chinese concepts of the body's energetics and its functions. Sedlak has researched the works of numerous scientists and performed his own experiments. He proposes:

> . . .The organism may be considered as an oscillator-emitting biological field with a large-band spectrum.[65]

He further proposes, "The biological oscillator belongs to self-regulating systems."[66] That is, it regulates and protects itself. He also discusses the conductive properties of many biological tissues:

> The biological semiconducting oscillator may be considered as physical plasma.
>
> This plasma possesses its own information through longitudinal and transverse magnetohydrodynamic waves. The biological field transfers itself inside the living organism by means of magnetohydrodynamic impulses.[67]

Magnetohydrodynamic impulses are electrical impulses generated by the effects of the body's magnetic field on the biological or physical plasma of the body. The term plasma refers not to the blood plasma, but to an energetic state of matter where there is a high degree of ionization and conductivity. This is sometimes known as the "fourth state of matter."

Sedlak is particularly interested in examining the quantum nature of biological systems. Albert Szent-Gyorgyi's research concerning the energetic nature of living tissues provides a bridge by which we may posit the mechanism of interaction between these fields and a biological plasma. Szent-Gyorgyi's work teaches us that the highly conductive and interconnected connective tissues have properties that are ideal as the ground substance of the fields described by Sedlak. In effect, the connective tissues are the carrier by which the internal and external fields connect and interact.

The biological field model does not lack for support and the idea that the triple warmer, as the system of fasciae and their connective tissues, is capable of performing the functions assigned to it in classical Oriental medical theory through these "quantum" processes is theoretically justified. To reiterate this model, the fasciae and thus the connective tissues are the physical manifestation of the triple warmer. The general field is the energetic manifestation of the triple warmer.

☐

Since modern scientists have theorized that the connective tissue system is energetically active and that we can consider it as capable of extending beyond the physical body,[68] the subtle electrical, ionic, and magnetic forces in the general and cosmological environment are capable of triggering events and effecting processes within the body. Since the physiological and neurological processes of the human system are affected by the body's nervous system and the other control and regulation sub-systems at work in biological life, significant effects are possible from very small influences. Since this model is in no way dependent on special qualities or unknown processes, the energetics of Oriental medicine need not be divorced from the biochemical effects observed by Western medical scientists.

Meridian Systems

An explanation of the origin of the meridian systems is a corollary thesis of interest. Unfortunately, the meridians, unlike the organs or the fasciae, have no analog in Western theories. Consequently there is a paucity of available research. If the meridians are measurable lines of lowered electrical resistance and greater electrical conductivity, what factors may have influenced their evolutionary development? How did these longitudinal and vertical pathways, the jing or meridians, and the luo, the horizontal vessels, develop? Were similar factors involved in the development of each? Are the extraordinary vessels the result of the same processes?

There are two aspects to this question: internal factors and external factors. Internally, we can look at the development of "cleavage lines" or "Langer's lines" as a model of the possible development of the meridians. These lines of tension in the skin resulting from internal forces have been mapped and studied by tissue sampling and the experience of surgeons. Externally, we must consider the effects of electrical and magnetic fields, in particular, the earth's electrical and magnetic fields.

In the 1860's Professor Langer of Vienna studied the discovery of Dupuytren in the 1830's, that puncture of the skin with a conical instrument sometimes produced oval holes instead of the round holes that were expected. He mapped the surface of the body where this phenomenon occurred.[69] These are what we now call Langer's lines. In adults these lines are seen in Figure 8.29.

These lines are individually different. They are important for surgeons, since incisions along these lines tend to heal more easily and with less scarring than cuts that cross Langer's lines. These lines are potentially of great import to the study of Oriental medical principles, since histological study has determined that they correspond with an orientation of connective tissue matrix fibers.[70] If, as the classical texts suggest and modern research is beginning to show, the meridians lie in the fascia and connective tissues, we might surmise that there is some structural alignment in the fascia that is related to the meridians.

On first examination, many of these lines do not closely correspond with the pathways of the meridians. Many are more horizontal than vertical. While some lines are vertical, specifically those on the limbs, head, and portions of the back, the alignment is not sufficiently clear to propose

□

that the meridians are directly related to Langer's lines. Yet, when we look at the embryological development of Langer's lines, the vertical alignment is much more obvious.[71] This is most obvious in the developing limbs.[72]

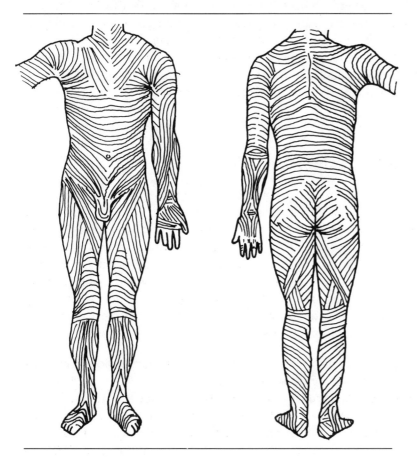
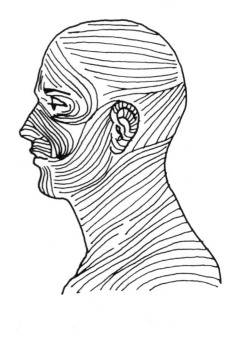

Figure 8.29 Langer's lines in an adult.

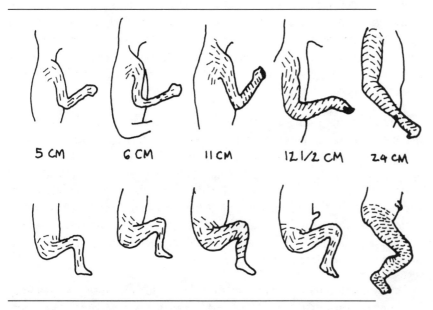

Figure 8.30 The embryological development of Langer's lines on the upper and lower limbs.

To a lesser degree, the lines on the front and back portions of the trunk are also vertical:[73]

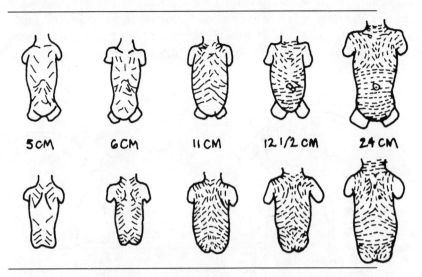

Figure 8.31 The embryological development of Langer's lines on the trunk.

In the fetus these lines are found to be associated with a "preponderance of collagenous and elastic fibers" that follow the lines.[74] These fibers develop according to Wolf's law along the lines of stress or tension on the surface of the body as the fetus grows. The internal stress causes a shift in the arrangement of the lines: "During the development of the collagenous fibers, existing internal forces of the growing fetus determine the manner of their distribution."[75] Since the early growth of the limbs is outward and the early growth of the torso is longitudinal, the lines are parallel to the axis of this growth. Since we know that the electrical currents emanating from the polar axis of the embryo are thought to be associated with and at times to predict the position at which the limb buds develop, we may postulate that the earliest fibrous alignments are also stimulated by these currents. Then, as the embryo develops and the tensions and stresses of the growing mass increase proportionally, the alignments are directed toward the adult pattern of horizontal lines by the growth of the body. The greater the force of growth, the more the physical tension and stress effectively overwhelms the subtle directive force of the field currents.

There is no exact correspondence of the alignment of these Langer's line fibers with the meridians in either the fetus or the adult. However, there is a developmental parallel strong enough to suggest the possibility that the meridians might be alignments of collagenous fibers in the dermis, instead of, or in addition to, being lines of electrical conductance. It is also possible to consider that it is because the Langer's lines are material, fibrous structures that they rotate toward the horizontal with three-dimensional growth. The meridians may be more electrically induced and thus retain a relationship to the field currents. Since the *Ling Shu* informs us that the meridians do not circulate until birth (*LS 10:104*), perhaps the forces of the immense growth of the fetus are sufficiently lessened and enough of the adult form is established at birth, that the growth forces do not change the vertical and horizontal alignment of the meridians after birth.

□

Is the development of the meridians and Langer's lines substantially similar? Are both initially induced by the same electrical stimulus? These questions must be answered by further research. In searching histologically for the cleavage lines, it is possible to find them only if the incision is made at the right angle to the line. Other incisions easily miss the lines. If the meridians are also related to alignments of collagenous fibers, a similar precision may be required.

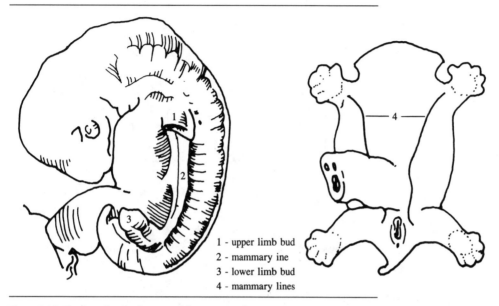

1 - upper limb bud
2 - mammary ine
3 - lower limb bud
4 - mammary lines

Figure 8.32 The frontal and side views of the mammary line.

An interesting parallel to the cleavage lines can be found in the developing breasts. The site of breast development occurs on what has been called the "milk line," "mammary line," or "mammary ridge." This is an ectodermal thickening that first develops during the sixth week of development. It extends from the base of the upper to the base of the lower limb buds on both sides.[76] This line thickens along its length and then recedes so that only a small portion in the pectoral region remains. Here, the ectodermal thickening grows down into the mesoderm, finally giving rise to the breasts and nipples. In some cases, this line does not recede normally and supernumerary breast formation occurs. In this condition a number of nipples, some with accompanying breasts, develop along these lines from the armpits to the upper thighs.[77]

There is little discussion of how or why these ridges first appear. We can postulate that they may develop in response to tensile stresses along the ectoderm in response to limb bud growth, as Wolf's law predicts. Since endogenous electrical currents enter and exit at the sites of limb bud development, and are believed to predict these sites, we may further postulate that there is also an electrical component as well as the mechanical stress factors.

The interesting parallels here are the very close proximity of this ridge or line to the stomach meridian pathway on the front of the body. There has always been question as to why the stomach meridian is the only yang meridian on the front surface of the torso. If the stomach meridian is related to the mammary ridge and the forces that gave rise to it (given that

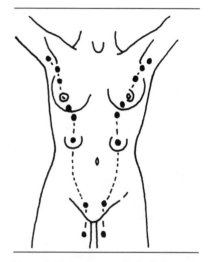

Figure 8.33 Supernumary nipple formation. Notice the approximate correlation of these lines to the stomach meridian pathways.

this ridge is of ectodermal tissues which we have already described with reference to the yang areas), then it is possible to see why the stomach meridian develops on the torso. Also, if the stomach meridian is related to this ridge, we can see an example of how the physical forces in embryological development can give rise to the meridian pathways.

Electrical and Magnetic Field Effects

The external factors that may figure in the development of the meridians are the electrical and magnetic fields associated with the earth itself. Presman's hypothesis, that through the process of evolution, electrical and magnetic fields were used by living organisms to obtain information about changes in the environment,[78] is a likely starting point for investigation of meridian development. It promises associations with the chronobiological principles of Oriental medicine, the electrical nature of the meridians, and the electrodynamic model of the human body.

In a uniform electric field small electrical currents are induced. The direction of these electrical currents is roughly parallel to the field itself. In a uniform magnetic field small currents are also induced, but these currents flow roughly perpendicular to the magnetic field. These are summarized in the following manner by Presman:[79]

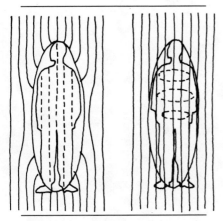

Figure 8.34 The direction of induced currents in electrical and magnetic fields.

Thus, since a human body is moving in an essentially vertical electrical field, the Earth's electrical field, there is a tendency to induce vertical currents in the body. Are these currents related to to the jing, the vertical meridians? Since the body moves through a more or less vertical magnetic field, there is also an influence towards the induction of horizontal currents. However, the Earth's magnetic field is neither absolutely vertical nor horizontal. Depending on the geographic location, the Earth's magnetic field strikes an upright body at an angle. Thus, if the Earth's magnetic field is related to the horizontal luo vessels, the developmental process is not as simple as the potential relationship of the Earth's electric field to the jing.

Research into the relationships and interactions of biological systems and fields is on the frontier of the biological sciences. The Russian scientist A. P. Dubrov has written a fascinating and farsighted book on geomagnetic fields and their functions in biological systems.[80] He concludes that the geomagnetic field is one of the most important factors in determining biological rhythmicity, in determining the symmetry of biological systems, and in producing profound effects on the endogenous weak magnetic fields of living organisms.[81]

Given the subtle electrical nature of the human system it is reasonable to propose that in some way the geomagnetic fields play an important role in determining the evolutionary development of the meridians and their interaction with the environment, or how the organism senses environmental changes and reacts or adapts to those changes. The extent to which the electrical and magnetic fields of the earth participate in the development of the meridian system and the extent of the influence of integral forces such as those influencing the development of Langer's lines is an open question. There are scientists who feel that these general fields must participate in the informational processes of the human being. Their hypotheses are strongly reminiscent of the Oriental medical ideas of rhythmicity and response.

Becker suggests that the meridian systems are part of a primitive direct current electrical system which is important in communication and healing. He proposes that the meridians developed before the evolution of the secondary electrical system, the nervous system.[82] Over evolutionary time, it is easy to consider subtle fields as major influences on the development of a direct current electrical system. Because of the increasing body of evidence that shows the fundamental importance of magnetic fields and the Earth's magnetic field in particular, Becker has proposed:

> [There is] a constant relationship between all growth processes as regulated by the internal direct current system, and the Earth's normal magnetic field parameters.[83]

Recent experiments have shown that weak magnetic fields can affect the mitotic division of cells and DNA activity. Other experiments have shown that weak magnetic fields induce changes in the embryological development of chicks.[84] Becker cites these and other fundamental effects from weak magnetic fields when he proposes, "The earth's normal magnetic field provides a timing signal for all aspects of biological cycle activity."[85]

Researcher Frank Brown has found correlations that demonstrate in all organisms greater and lesser degrees of rhythmic alterations in behavior and physiological events with the lunar cycle. He has correlated the lunar cycle with changes in the earth's field.[86] Most of the evidence for these conclusions is quite recent, but is slowly becoming tested and accepted. Although these are lines of inquiry not often followed, such research may be very fruitful for those interested in understanding Oriental medical theory.

Of course, any theory or research into the development of the meridian system must include the extraordinary vessels. If our theory is correct, the meridians are located in the planes of fasciae and develop in response to internal and external forces, fields, and currents. After birth they circulate and further develop relative to the natural fluctuations of the fields and forces of the external environment. The fact that the medical literature has explicit statements about the circulation of qi starting after birth *LS 10),* and the circulation of this qi being determined in part by the movement of the astronomical bodies *(LS 15),* tends to suggest that the Chinese had in mind what we call field effects. Perhaps it is best to say that the Chinese had observed phenomena, and patterns of phenomena, that they attributed to qi, and other concepts, that we are able to label as field effects. It is neither necessary nor important (yet totally fascinating) whether the classical Chinese had conceived of a field. It is possible and reasonable to see all these phenomena as field effects. Thus, the twelve meridians are a product of complex interactions between internal and external forces.

The extraordinary vessels are different than the twelve meridians and their related organs. Their functions are different. This is quite clear in the embryogenesis of these different systems. Because they may be related to the germ layers and tissues and particularly the axes of the body, the extraordinary vessels are more "of the body." They are conditioned by the geometry and structure of the body. The state of being a three-dimensional living being with relative symmetries and asymmetries is a major determining factor. Yoshio Manaka's brilliant insights into the extraordinary vessels, examining their topological nature, seeing them as related to the various structural axes of the body in his octahedral model, and describing them with reference to the various symmetries and lost symmetries of the body, provides access to the genius of the Chinese authors who first attempted to describe these energetic entities.

Modern geometrical theory has developed sophisticated models of the relationship of material objects to space and time, as is evidenced by the theory of relativity. Examining the topological geometry of the body describes not only abstract entities and relationships, but provides the foundation for fruitful research into the nature of energy and energetic relationships in the body. In biological terms it is becoming possible to consider and describe the function and properties of the body and parts of the body relative to the structure of the whole. While such models have yet to be fully described, the structural basis of the extraordinary vessels is evidenced in their use by practitioners such as Yoshio Manaka and Osamu Ito, where quite obvious structural changes can be clinically observed.[87]

In thinking about the geometry of the extraordinary vessels, it may also be possible to see the nature of the "oceans" of yin, yang, the twelve meridians, the yin and yang organs, and blood. This could refer to their nature as reservoirs rather than as pathways in which energy circulates. In reference to the fields, they could refer to the whole field rather than specific aspects.

The Chinese disposition tended to express observations philosophically. Nature was observed quite clearly and these observations applied to medicine. That their observations were sufficient and thoughtful is evident, if only by the fact that modern observations using different means and methods may be so frequently related. While this is a great resource for our interest and study, the philosophical expression is itself a source of understanding. The distinctions that differentiate five-phase cycles and their relationships to the branches, stems, meridians, and organs, from the yin and yang, eight trigrams, and extraordinary vessels relationships allow us to develop a theory of the extraordinary vessels.

One scholar and researcher feels that a distinction of the systems of eight and five can be traced to the *Yi Jing* and the *Lao Zi*.[88] The system of the *Yi Jing* may be presented thus:

The one —— the two —— the four —— the eight

Tai Ji

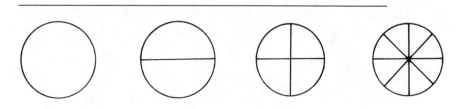

Figure 8.35 The one gives rise to the two; the two give rise to the four; the four give rise to the eight — exemplified in the *Yi Jing* philosophy.

The system of five can be traced to *Lao Zi*:

The one —— the two —— the three —— the myriad things (five)

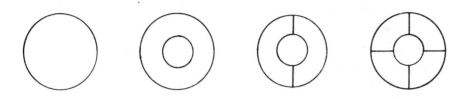

Figure 8.36 The one gives rise to the two; the two gives rise to the three; the three gives rise to the five — exemplified in philosophy of *Lao Zi*.

If we understand these differences of naturalistic philosophical origin more clearly, we can gain greater insight into medicine. We must not presume that one system is more profound than the other, both have a common origin in the body, the moving qi, the tai yi, tai ji. Both manifest in profoundly different ways and affect the body differently.

Through their distinct natures we are able to use them to address and correct different problems in the body, as their differences focus on varying components of the body. In Japan, a practitioner who describes his treatment as addressing the "root" of the problem generally means that he is treating by five-phase principles or through the extraordinary vessels. One is able to treat at the tai yi by treating through either route.

Summary

If our arguments about the nature of the meridian systems are correct, the meridians are a product of the interaction of internal and external environments and are related to bioelectric phenomena. Thus, there are some essential functions that we may assume. These assumptions follow classical ideas of the nature and function of the meridians. The meridian systems will have an adaptive role and act as a medium for adaptation to all environmental changes. This adaptive function manifests in several ways:

Protective: receiving information from the environment and processing this information; closing it out if harmful (external invasion) and transmitting it if useful (chronobiological stimulae).

Biorhythmic: communicating environmental changes and fluctuations to the rest of the body so that the body can adapt, resonate, or harmonize with these natural changes and fluctuations.

Communication: communicating internal information concerning bodily phenomena from the interior to the exterior.

Maintenance: allowing communication between different aspects and systems of the body, thus promoting regulation.

Energetic: acting as energy channels. This energy is both passive (informational) and kinetic (performing work).

Healing: supporting the healing process and health in general, particularly the process of self-healing.

These processes thus cover the full range of biological control and regulation. As well, they indicate a further understanding of the nature of qi. While it remains "untranslatable," we can see that the quandary between the substantive, energetic, and functional aspects of qi are more easily synthesized by considering the informational attributes of biological energy. It is only if we consider qi substantive, kinetic, or metabolic that there is difficulty with the concept. If for example, we consider the meridians as only the electrical wiring of the human body, the paths by which "doses" of active electrical energy are circulated, we are faced with the problem of explaining how a single stream of current is able to perform so many functions, respond to so many stimulae, and to create responses that require much more powerful currents than are typically found. On the other hand, if we consider qi, and all the vessels, meridians, and "oceans" of its function, to be a set of informational signals by which very slight stimulae act as "signals" and "data" that regulate metabolism and other biological process, we can take advantage of all the modern research that demonstrates the systems nature of life.

We have described some of the likely anatomical relationships of the organs and meridians through the various systems and planes of fasciae. In light of this, one could reexamine the internal pathways of the meridians and retrace everything through the fascial planes associated with each structure related to these trajectories. We have shown the possible development of these relationships at various stages of embryogenesis and have traced the probable electrical and magnetic nature of these relationships to an origin in the natural electrical and magnetic fields inside and outside the body. In proposing a biodynamic model of the human energetic system we have examined the embryonic axes and the tissues developed around these axes and proposed the probable topological nature of the extraordinary vessels relative to these axes.

In short, we have attempted to demonstrate that the classical Chinese anatomical, physiological, and energetic descriptions have feasible corollaries in Western research and that these physical analogs are capable of performing as the Chinese medical authors proposed. There are still many stones unturned and a plenitude of insufficient answers. However, it is only through initiating a multi-disciplinary inquiry into the nature and origins of Chinese medicine that Oriental practitioners may take advantage of the mass of Western research and their Western counterparts may come to understand the value of Chinese medical theory.

Chapter

- 9 -

Science

Revisited

Science Revisited

During the last few decades much research has been done to elucidate the mechanisms by which acupuncture affects the human body. Discovery of the neuropeptides, the encephalins, and the endorphins has opened up new and exciting areas of neurobiological research. At the same time it has demonstrated the validity of analgesic acupuncture as an alternative to chemical anesthetics or analgesics in surgery or pain control. While attracting less attention, research into the properties of the meridians and acupuncture points has done much to explain how acupuncture and moxibustion produce profound effects on the body function.

The observations that have emerged from this research postulate a set of ideas that link ancient Chinese descriptions of the meridians with modern concepts of physiology, biochemistry, and the biophysics of cells and tissues.

Other areas of scientific inquiry have also contributed to a consensus of ideas about biological life and its relationship to the environment that parallel and confirm the observations of the Chinese medical thinkers. Both modern and ancient science, Western and Oriental thought, are based on observation. Much of any science deals with analogies and models proposed to explain what we cannot absolutely measure or observe. All scientists must assemble sets of observations that are too complex to relate in a controlled experiment. Much of the natural world can only be examined in this manner. Thus, practically, the modern physicist and the ancient philosopher are often working with an identical and primary tool, the ability to imagine and propose.

There are other important points of similarity. As recently as the 1950's Western scientists exemplified a faith in their own methods of observation that was nearly religious in its intensity. Only phenomena that could be verified within the limited context of the controlled experiment, and related to quantified hypotheses, were permitted to enter the sacred books of scientific dogma. Today, the limits of these tools are more apparent, and unshakable faith in a quantified reality is more the domain of a religious devotee. In some very real ways, the physicist of the twentieth century shared with the Han dynasty scholar a need to see beyond the capacities of their instruments. In this they share the single most powerful tool of scientific inquiry: speculation. We need not be surprised that they could reason in similar fashion.

In this chapter we will explore various ideas that have the potential of explaining the function of acupuncture, and provide evidence supporting each idea. Rather than attempting to put forward a definitive theory, we would hope to show one way that information can be organized. The

□

intention is not to insist that these ideas are valid or correct, but to provide a basis for further thought and research. The evidence does seem sufficient to consign the idea that there is no possible justification for Oriental medical theory in Western thought, to the museum of nearly forgotten scientific oddities, chauvinisms, and short-lived scientific errors.

Electrical Properties of Acupuncture Systems

As proof of the existence of the meridians, many researchers in China and elsewhere cite what is called "propagated sensation of the channels."[1] In general, this idea comes from the observation that a certain percentage of any population is very sensitive to stimulation of the meridians. Yoshio Manaka notes that roughly one in eight hundred people exhibits this sensitivity strongly and a larger number exhibit it to some lesser degree.[2] During acupoint stimulation, these individuals can feel a sensation propagating along the pathways on the surface of their body; sometimes fast, sometimes slow, and often directly along the classical pathway. This phenomenon is often cited as an important factor in the development of meridian theory. As we will see, it may be related to electrical changes brought about by the application of acupuncture.

Manaka anecdotally reports experiments with a meridian-sensitive person. He found that the pathways of sensation change if a magnet is placed next to the point being needled. This suggests and supports the idea that the phenomenon might be electrical or magnetic in nature.

Other researchers in China have presented striking evidence for the existence of the meridians.[3] Chinese dermatologists have studied and photographed many instances where certain skin diseases were found to occur along the pathways of the meridians. This phenomenon is convincing evidence for the existence of the meridians in some form. While it does not necessarily help explain the characteristics of the meridians, it does present striking visual proof of what can otherwise only be measured with various devices.

With the development of electroacupuncture and numerous electrodiagnostic devices, it has become possible to make measurements of the electromagnetic characteristics of the meridians and their points. Most research focuses on the electrical characteristics of the acupoints; however, some research has focused on the electrical characteristics of the meridians themselves. Essentially, the meridians and their points have been found to be lines or sites of lowered electrical resistance relative to the surrounding skin. Where the meridians are said to be, there is a lesser resistance than found at sites where the meridians are said not to traverse.[4]

Thus, the concept described in the medical texts as "energy" or qi circulation throughout the body through the meridians can be seen to have at least in part a biophysical, bioelectric basis. The potential pathways for such a circulation or movement can be clearly seen in the lines of lowered electrical resistance and greater electrical conductivity. Similarly the concept of the acupoint, at which energy is seen to converge or pass and can thus be affected, becomes a more clearly comprehensible concept. According to the measurements of many scientists, these acupoints coincide in large part with points on the surface of the body where there is lower electrical resistance. Not only have these electrical properties been documented, but variations and fluctuations of resistance levels in various functional states have been measured and observed.

Essentially these variations can be summarized as follows:

> When pathological changes take place in the viscera, concurrent changes are found in the cutaneous resistance of relevant meridians and acupuncture points. Similar changes are also reflected by the unbalancing resistance of the bilateral acupuncture points.

> When changes were found in nerves, viscera, and organs before or after sleep,[5] meals, urination, childbirth, or physical exercise, resistance changes would also take place in the acupuncture points of the relevant meridians.

> A change of electrical resistance in the points could also be brought about by changes of external environment, temperature, season, time of day.

> Following acupuncture or moxibustion or after changing the function of nerves by blocking or cutting, corresponding changes would also occur in the cutaneous resistance of acupuncture points.[6]

As we would expect, the points reflect and exhibit changes as a result of pathological occurrence. The points also respond to environmental changes. This is just as we would expect, and partially confirms our thesis concerning the electrical and magnetic nature of the meridians and their relationship to a fluctuating electrical and magnetic environment.

The resistance of the acupoints also varies with many physiological changes, including those initiated by acupuncture and moxibustion. It has been proposed that since the meridians are pathways of electrical conductance, they might serve as information channels, since electrical signals can function as information. Becker and his colleagues theorize that since acupuncture is able to play such a strong role in the relief of pain, the meridian system is able to act as an "information transfer system." This system would be important in the transfer of DC electrical current information produced, for instance, by an injury. The injury signal could be routed to, and interpreted by, other areas of the body as the stimulus that would initiate processes to facilitate healing and regrowth.[7] Such an electrical system would act as the medium for the propagation of signals around the body that would function to control and stimulate growth and healing within and throughout the whole body. In other words, it would function as an integrative system, helping coordinate a vast matrix of physiological events.[8]

In his book, *Electromagnetism and Life,* Robert Becker proposes that such an electrical signaling system is a fundamental, primitive electrical information network. This system is important not only in communicating injury to the rest of the body, but as well for detecting changes in the environmental electromagnetic field.[9] Obviously, this capacity would be an important feature of a system capable of biorhythmic change.[10]

□

Becker's work also led him to suggest that the perineural cells are the medium of this information transmission.[11] The perineural cells are composed of connective tissues in a relatively regular pattern. We have already shown that the fascial planes and the connective tissues are able to conduct electrical energy, and could be the biophysical basis of the integrative and informational electrical system that Becker and his colleagues describe. This idea is reinforced by the vast permeation and diversity of connective tissues throughout every tissue, with fibers extending into every cell in the body. This nearly universal distribution provides the potential for an integrative electrical system.

Some research even provides tentative evidence that the meridians retain their electrical characteristics after death, further supporting the idea that they must have a biophysical basis.[12] By proposing that the meridian concept contains the possibility of such an integrative system, Becker and his colleagues provide further evidence that supports the classical ideas of the meridian system in relation to the fascial systems.

The importance of these fascial systems to body energies and healing is becoming more apparent. There is even research evidence that the meridians do lie in the superficial fascia. Two leading researchers in Japan, Yoshio Nagahama, M.D., and Hiroshi Motoyama, PhD., have independently concluded that the meridian system lies in the connective tissues and more specifically in the superficial fascia. In his book, *Shinkyu no Igaku (Western studies of Acupuncture and Moxibustion)*, Nagahama summarizes research completed by himself and by other scientists. His own conclusions about the nature of acupuncture and moxibustion are that they serve to restore the normal functioning of the connective tissues. He has coined the expression, "connective tissue therapy" to describe acupuncture.[13] A clearer statement of the relationship of acupuncture and moxibustion to the connective tissues probably cannot be found. Many of the studies and research described in his book have profound practical implications.

Nagahama notes that over years of research into needle insertion and the depth at which the *teqi*, the obtaining of the qi or stimulus occurs, he has found the strongest teqi occurs when the needle touches the superficial fascia.[14] In Japan, needles often are not inserted very deeply, only a matter of a few millimeters. In China, and consequently many other places, needles frequently are inserted more deeply, as much as one-half an inch and deeper. Either way, the superficial fascia is stimulated. However, with deeper insertion the underlying myofascial and nerve structures (among others) are also stimulated. Deeper insertion thereby presents the possibility of affecting different systems to greater and lesser degrees. Correspondingly different physiological responses will result, a possibility that figures in other research.

Nagahama has found that when the needle touches the superficial fascia as it is inserted, electrical potential changes that generate small electric currents occur.[15] This is what he sees as the teqi, the small electrical current having a therapeutic effect. He feels that reflexive acupoints may indicate pathologies in the body, and that if such a reflexive acupoint is needled, the electrical potential changes that occur are different from the changes that result from the needling of a non-reflexive point. These electrical potential changes subsequently generate what he calls "abnormal electrical currents" that will be transmitted to the place of origin of the pathology and thus help treat it.[16] This could be related to, and explain, the "propagated sensations" studied by other researchers. In Nagahama's opinion, it is essential to locate, select, and treat the reflexive points.[17] This theory helps explain the importance of palpation in diagnosis and correct treatment. Palpation is a safe and simple form of diagnosis that often provides the groundwork for straightforward treatments.

Hiroshi Motoyama has also completed considerable research concerning the electrical nature of qi, the meridian systems, and the biophysical counterparts in the body that might account for the electrical effects and provide an appropriate medium for their transmission.[18] He too has concluded that the meridian structures lie in the dermal connective tissues, the superficial fascia.[19] In addition he has attempted to define what the flow of qi energy may be, demonstrating that it cannot be the simple drift of ions through the tissues, but must be a flow of electrons, since ions move too slowly.[20] These two scientists corroborate the findings of other scientists concerning the electrical nature of the meridians, and the electrical properties of the connective tissues, helping to further substantiate the classical theses concerning the meridians and the triple warmer in relation to the connective tissues and fascia.

Nagahama feels that the generation of small electrical currents from the electrical potential changes caused by needle insertion results from the interaction of the needle (inserted into the connective tissues) with the interstitial fluids that bathe and nourish the connective tissue fibers. These fluids surround the fibers and contain a vast array of chemicals, ionically charged particles, molecules, and atoms. These interstitial fluids also provide an interface with the lymph and capillary systems, since the fluids are constantly interchanged between the capillaries, lymph system, and the connective tissues.[21] Nagahama proposes that this constant interchange of blood and lymph fluids with interstitial fluids is actually what the ancients meant by the *luo*. He feels that this proposal is capable of explaining all implications of multiple meanings given the term in classical medical literature, by providing a generally more inclusive interpretation.[22]

The importance of this idea is furthered by the innovative theories of the Swedish researcher, Bjorn Nordenstrom. He has discovered an electrical system that transmits current from different areas of the body through the circulatory system. These currents are initiated by ionic transfer and differences of electrical potential in the tissue-capillary bed.[23] This has been shown to have profound effects throughout the body. Recent work from Yoshio Manaka and his research assistant Kazuko Itaya at the Oriental Medicine Research Center of Kitasato University in Tokyo, provides very clear evidence for the cardiovascular effects of acupuncture, showing how Nordenstrom's and Nagahama's theories of bioelectrical effects are very pertinent in acupuncture.[24]

Their research demonstrates that acupuncture can produce an increase in vasomotion throughout the body, and that the insertion of a needle to any point can produce the effect. This phenomenon is thus a "baseline" effect of acupuncture that occurs regardless of the points needled and techniques used. The importance of this research is manifest at several levels. Increases of microcirculation and vasomotion will increase oxygenation of the tissues (which has important ramifications for bioelectrical energy transfer in living tissues), and will help flush toxins, waste products, and other accumulated particles and chemicals from the tissues, improving their overall function. The bioelectrical currents demonstrated by Nordenstrom will also be dramatically affected by microcirculatory and vasomotor changes, producing further biological effects. While research of this phenomenon continues, it is immediately apparent that the implications are enormous.

This might help explain why some patients show little improvement at the time of treatment, but a marked improvement by the next day. The effect also suggests that gentle treatment around the sequellae that result from contusions, sprains, bone fractures, and other trauma will help reduce the swelling. Manaka reports good success treating sequellae in this manner. Since this is a "baseline" effect produced by needling, some interesting speculative questions are raised.

The most interesting speculation is that the needle effect is not the result, but a part of a chain of results. That small electric currents can have beneficial, regenerative, and healing effects is something that has been scientifically demonstrated. In 1967 Becker and his colleagues, while studying fracture healing in frogs, discovered by accident that red blood cells at the site of the fracture underwent a process of "dedifferentiation," eventually becoming bone cells. After studying this phenomenon, they theorized that the tiny currents generated by the bone fracture might be the operative stimulus. They conducted experiments and found that tiny currents are able to transform or dedifferentiate nucleated red blood cells into other cells.[25] Later experiments and research have confirmed this phenomenon.[26] With his colleague, A. A. Pilla, Becker further found that "appropriate pulsed magnetic fields" are able to create the same effects.[27] Although these effects have only been demonstrated in amphibians, we should not rule out the possibility (or more likely, probability) that similar processes occur in humans. As Becker says:

> Therefore, in at least this one-cell system, the nucleated erythrocyte, specific effects of low-level current have been observed and part of the mechanism involved in producing the effects has been determined. The effect is a most profound one, involving the basic machinery of the cell and resulting in major alterations in cell function.[28]

Pilla further proposes an electrochemical model showing how electrochemical information, small currents in living tissues, can cross the cell membrane to effect functional changes in the cells.[29] He feels that any change in the environment of the cell that causes changes in electrical potential across the membrane of the cell will cause modifications of cell function, and that this is the mechanism by which functional changes in the cell, particularly those of repair and maintenance, can occur. He also proposes that a cell can be "stimulated, inhibited, or exhibit passive response, depending upon the frequencies and amplitudes of the signals employed."[30] Becker also proposes, based on experimental evidence, that the strength of the current passing through a tissue is a factor determining varying responses.[31] We can extend this by saying that different tissues will respond to different frequencies and amplitudes of current. Adey calls this a "window effect." Different tissues will have different windows, which we may call "signatures." Thus, differences in currents produce different physiological effects.[32]

The mechanisms, both direct and indirect, of these effects can be considered from different physiological perspectives. The electrical potential changes brought about in the cellular environment could result from changes in ionic concentrations, or from direct current passing through the tissues or the extracellular matrix fibers. These changes in potential could act on the cell by lateral electrophoretic[33] or electroosmotic[34] rearrangement of cell membrane structures. They could act by depolarizing the cell membrane or by producing extracellular ionic concentration changes which would transmit information to the cell by electrochemical transfer.[35] They could also act by transmitting electrical information through extracellular fibers directly through the cell membrane-bound proteins (such as fibronectin) with which they are bound to the intracellular matrix fibers — microfilaments, microtubules, and microtrabeculae.[36]

These various routes can affect cell metabolism in a number of ways, one of which is to cause changes in the natural ionic currents of the cell, such as the calcium currents. They could do this by rearranging the membrane-bound molecules responsible for the currents, or by causing a release within the cell of bound calcium ions. The rate of calcium ion efflux and influx could also be increased or decreased. Changes in the calcium current can cause structural changes within the cell, since calcium ions can breakdown and disassociate the microtubules,[37] cause contraction of the microfilaments,[38] and rearrange the structure of the microtrabecullar lattice.[39] Changes in cell shape can initiate changes in cell function and DNA activity.[40] The changes in the calcium current could also affect many other biochemical processes within the cell, producing many other functional changes.

Becker suggests a global model of how these small currents are transmitted around the body effecting specific responses in specific tissues at specific locations. He feels that since cells are sensitive to these currents, the direction, magnitude, and force of the current serves to identify a location within the body and accordingly effect specific physiological responses.

> The direction (polarity) plus the magnitude and force of current could serve as a vector system giving a distinct value for every area of the body. The electric field surrounding continuously charged cells and diminishing with the distance from the nerve would provide a third coordinate giving each cell a slightly different electrical potential. In addition, a magnetic field must exist around the current flow, possibly adding a fourth dimension to the system. Together these values might suffice to pinpoint any cell in the body. The electric and magnetic fields, varying as the current varies with the animal's state of consciousness and health, could move charged molecules

wherever they were needed for control of growth or other processes. Since currents and electromagnetic fields affect the cell membrane's choice of what ions to absorb, reject, expel, this system — in concert with the chemical code by which neighboring cells recognize each other — could precisely regulate the activities of every cell. It could express the exact point along the limb at which new growth must start, distinguishing between right and left, top and bottom.[41]

The electrical potential changes and currents needed to initiate such changes and effects are generally very small.[42] Certainly those created by the administration of acupuncture therapy are sufficient.

These models, where tiny variations in the electrical environment of the cell can initiate functional changes and cell shape changes, are similar to Manaka's topological model of the body. If these bioelectrical, biochemical, and structural changes are, as Becker suggests, responsible for left-right, up-down differentiations, the topological model would be an effective summary of the cumulative function of the system. On a smaller scale, there is also an implicit relationship of structure and function, and a potential relationship to time-varying factors that might initiate and control some of these variations.

Indeed these models could help explain how the geomagnetic field acts on all cell membranes, potentially altering their permeability, affecting cell function in a most profound manner:

> By altering the permeability of biological membranes, the GMF [geomagnetic field] can affect the whole organism.[43]

A.P. Dubrov believes that changes in the permeability of biological membranes in response to the GMF and other fields is a universal feature of biological membranes and a "perceptive response" to those fields. Citing the suggestion of other scientists, Dubrov states:

> . . . Acupuncture points are sites of connection of the living organism with the terrestrial air - ion, electrical, and magnetic fields. . . . We must consider the possibility that these points are sites of connection of the earth's magnetic field lines with the intrinsic biomagnetic field of the living organism.[44]

Becker also states that the acupuncture points and meridians play a significant role in the body's interaction with the regulatory effects of the geomagnetic field on the living body.[45]

The conclusions of these authors tend to support our interpretation of the stem—branch cycles, their correlations to astronomical phenomena, and the "cycling of the qi in the meridians." The temporal components of Manaka's topological theory can be seen here also. More work is required to elaborate these mechanisms, but we can say with confidence that different electrical (and possibly magnetic) signals arriving at the cells can produce very different responses within the cell. Physiological activity can be increased or decreased by the small electrical currents stimulated by acupuncture. The small electrical currents believed to be generated by the insertion of a needle into the fascia or connective tissues can indeed have beneficial effects.

Because of the nature of the connective tissues, it is quite plausible that these effects could occur both locally, at the site of needle insertion, or at a distance from the acupoint. The currents can be conducted away by the connective tissues to other parts of the body. Other work examining the electrical properties of the skin, specifically of the guinea pig, demonstrates some remarkable properties of the skin.[46] The glabrous (hairless) skin of guinea pigs and humans was found to generate relatively powerful electric currents around small incisions. Hairy areas were found to be much less electrically active. The researchers, Jaffe et al., theorized that the glabrous skin contains a "battery" and that this battery is the product of the properties of the "live" tissues of the skin (the superficial fascia), not the more superficial "dead" skin. They feel that this battery has the function of, or is important in, wound healing.

Shallow incisions did not generate much battery effect, but incisions to the depth of the live tissues caused a peak of the battery effect. Beyond this depth, the effect decreased substantially. Perhaps this effect may be what Nagahama was observing. The current is produced by a "cross-circuiting" or "short-circuiting" of this battery in the skin as the needle passes through the skin and battery layers. Either the needle or the thin layer of fluid that coats the surface of the needle as it is inserted will act as the medium of this electrical cross-circuitry as it connects the two electrode layers in the skin.

While it cannot be said that an exact mechanism, an exact functional description, or a precise Western description of acupuncture function has been discovered, it can be said that many phenomena that could play a part in such a definitive description have been demonstrated. Certainly, there is no lack of material for further research and we can begin to postulate that the insertion of acupuncture needles at specific locations is theoretically able to act as a signal that can be transferred to nearly any area of the body where it may be interpreted at the cellular level.

Electrical Properties of Moxibustion

Many large molecules in the body are semiconductive. This is particularly true of the proteins, and thus the entire connective tissue matrix. These semiconductive properties are dependent on the degree of hydration and oxygenation of the tissues.[47] The connective tissues are thermoelectric.[48] If heat is applied to them, small electrical currents will be generated. Thus moxibustion, like acupuncture, will generate small electric currents that can potentially have the same effects as the currents generated by the insertion of needles into the superficial fascia. Theoretically one could practice something close to acupuncture using only moxibustion. Thus, the thermoelectric properties of the connective tissues provide a theoretical model that can account for another aspect of the classical medical concepts.

Physiological Effects
of Finger Pressure and Massage

The primary focus of this text is on palpation, particularly of the abdomen. Palpation is useful both diagnostically and therapeutically. Scientifically it produces profound changes in the body. Because connective tissues have piezoelectric properties, the application of pressure anywhere on the body will generate small electric currents.[49] These currents will have numerous physiological effects, just as they do in acupuncture. This is aside from the effects of mechanical stimulation of muscular tissues, blood vessels, and nervous tissues that are known to have beneficial effects on stress and blood circulation.

Pressure applied to living tissue can actually transform the tissues. Work done on organic gels, part of the cytoplasm of cells, shows that pressure will cause the gel to become a sol (solution). Thus, particle accumulations trapped in the gel state may be released at the same time the gel becomes more hydrated.[50] Hydration makes the tissues more energetically conductive. Massage will not only induce small electric currents that will be conducted away from the point of pressure, but will also help rearrange the tissues, actually making them more conductive. It becomes obvious looking at only these two properties of pressure stimulation that massage and shiatsu have enormous potentials.

These effects will also show to some degree in the process of diagnosis by palpation. The diagnosis itself can often have therapeutic value and is often relaxing for the patient. It will also, to some degree, prepare the tissues that are treated, making them, in their temporary sol state, more energetically active. This can only enhance the effects of the acupuncture or moxibustion. This may in part explain why the classical texts discuss the application of pressure to a point before needling.[51]

Clinical Perspectives on Abdominal Palpation

In Oriental medical literature emphasis was, and still is, put on the treatment of reactions on the abdomen found by palpation. Treating patients to rid the reactivity of the abdomen with the intention of treating disease is not a subject of Western interest. We have found one interesting discussion from Nayoshi Edagawa, a Japanese physician. Edagawa was trained exclusively in Western medicine and had no prior training in Oriental medicine. However, he noticed that very often diseases were accompanied by unusual patterns of tension in the musculature of the body, particularly on the abdomen. He further noticed that when the patient's disease receded and was symptomless, these unusual patterns of tension remained in some form, causing continuous irritations that frequently led to a recurrence of the original problem. Having noticed this, he theorized that treatment of the tense areas of the abdomen should help treat the problem and prevent recurrence.

He began by injecting small amounts of a very dilute solution of dexamethasone into the tight muscles. This caused the muscles to relax, and helped relieve the symptoms. Based on these original observations he treated many patients and obtained excellent results with a wide range of diseases. He summarized these results in a book, *Doctor Nao's Chiryo Jiten:*

Depending on the disease, one can often find pressure pain or
tension in one of the segments of the rectus abdominis muscles. Treating this can cure many of a patient's symptomatic
complaints.[52]

Although he used injections, he felt that acupuncture or finger pressure
could achieve the same results; however he attempted no trial of this idea.
He felt that treating diseases internally with medications would only treat
the internal manifestations of the problems. Contrary to what had been
common practice in the West since the nineteenth century, Edagawa suggested attention to the external manifestations of the problems.[53] He cited,
as an example, patients with recurrent stomach problems. Though treated
with medications to relieve the symptoms, the symptoms would often
recur. When the tense areas of the abdomen were also treated by his
method, the cycle was broken and the problems no longer recurred. He
also noticed that when the problems recurred, no pathologies could be
found by Western analytic methods, and eventually the problem was
labeled psychosomatic or psychological. In these cases, treatment of the
abdomen would often prevent recurrence. He felt that injections into the
tendinous intersections, sites where connective tissue sheaths join the muscle segments of the rectus abdominis muscles, were particularly effective.
Inspired by his initial results, he has also begun palpating and treating tension of the neck and back.

Since first noticing this phenomenon, Edagawa has surveyed the
modern medical literature, but has found no reasonable answers. He is
currently studying the classical medical literature in search of an explanation of the phenomenon. There, we think, he is more likely to find an
answer.[54]

Applying Edagawa's observations and experiences to the clinical
experience of practitioners who diagnose the abdomen by palpation, we
can derive a possible anatomical and physiological explanation. Naoichi
Kuzome, whose entire diagnosis and treatment focuses on the abdomen,
finds that most common reactions lie on the linea alba, along the lateral
edges where it joins the bands of the rectus abdominis muscles, along the
lateral edges of the rectus abdominis muscles, or at the aponeuroses of the
internal and external oblique muscles and along the tendinous intersections
of the rectus abdominis muscles. In other words, it is common to find
tight, hard, tense, sore points or areas on the abdomen that lie on the
aponeuroses or connective tissue sheaths that bind the various muscles
together. Edagawa's clinical study supports the same idea.

The number and location of these aponeuroses and junctions is not the
same for everyone. For instance, the rectus abdominis muscles often have
three, four, or five tendinous intersections, depending on the person. If
these areas are where the pathological tension occurs, we could see these as
areas of prenatal weakness, tendency, or susceptibility. Areas on the abdomen are thought to have phase-organ correspondences and to cause problems of the corresponding phase-organ. Perhaps, the areas where these
tendinous intersections and aponeuroses lie act as stress points or areas of
weakness that make the person more susceptible to specific problems.

Integration

It is apparent from all these researches that an enormous number of physiological changes may be brought about by the insertion of needles and the application of heat or pressure to acupoints. More commonly cited research shows the numerous effects of acupuncture on the nervous and blood systems. The simple act of inserting a needle into a point on the surface of the body produces an enormous variety of change. It is no surprise that there are many theories of the function of acupuncture, and its correct practice. Quite probably some of these effects are seen to a greater degree in one kind of application, to a lesser degree in another, and to some degree in all styles. To understand this, we need the largest, most unified perspective.

By considering the "fields of life," as Burr calls them, or the DC electrical current communication system proposed by Becker, in conjunction with the nature, functions, and properties of the connective tissues, significant aspects of the classical Chinese medical model may be given reasonable hypotheses. Many of the ideas in the classical texts may be justified by Western theories and methods.

The meridian system can be seen as the physiological functions of the field. The meridians are probably a network of integrative communication channels that result from the field-tissue interface. The acupoints on the meridians are thus "nodes" on these channels. The triple warmer and the source are the entire system, the medium, the center of the network created by the tissues and their fields. In dramatic contradistinction to the most common operative concept of the energetic body, the meridians are not the main point, nor the central functional entity, but the branches of the source. Energetic pathology can be understood as disruptions of the tissue field that create pathophysiological changes in the body. The reaction of the body to external and internal environments can be understood as alterations of the field and energy flow that (depending on the intervention) can have either beneficial or harmful effects. All the physiological effects of acupuncture, moxibustion, and massage can be understood within this model.

The fields and their tissues represent a single entity, a unity, capable of far more than the sum of their numerous parts. It is little wonder that the ancient Chinese strove to describe a single unity, a unifying principle. They called this qi and classified it according to how and where it manifest and what it appeared to do. Whatever we call it, in clinical practice many of the physiological events occur simultaneously, often indistinguishable from each other.

Chronobiological Effects

Regardless of each individual's constitutional tendencies, weaknesses, strengths, and life style, certain acupoints become active in all people, in the same time zone, at the same time. The mechanism behind such universal actions cannot be individual. The pattern must be environmental. A number of environmental variables could account for these biological rhythms.

☐

Light — electromagnetic radiation — plays an important role in the chronobiological processes and spatial organization of living organisms. It is well known how important light is to the growth of plants. The phenomenon of phototropism is well documented.[55] Animals also exhibit light-sensitive cycles.[56] In people the cyclic release of adrenal hormones has been demonstrated.[57] Likewise, the cyclic fluctuations of sex hormones may be in part controlled by cycles of light and dark.[58] The effects of gravity on living organisms has also been demonstrated. The phenomenon of geotropism, the response of plants to gravity, is well documented.[59]

When we discuss chronobiological or biorhythmic phenomena it is the interaction of the gravitational, magnetic, and electromagnetic fields (particularly the geomagnetic field) that produce the observed results. Not only plants are sensitive to gravity; both animals and plants are sensitive to gravitational fields. Considerable research demonstrates these multiple effects. One researcher, in discussing the effects of gravity on all living organisms, argues that it is because they are "colloidal systems in a state of unstable dynamic equilibrium" that all living organisms must be sensitive to gravity.[60] Similarly, the endogenous fields of the body (electrical, magnetic, electromagnetic, and gravitational) are highly sensitive to external fields and the slightest change in these fields may be sensed. Living organisms in general are very responsive to changes in the fields of the earth. As one researcher states:[61]

> Spatial orientation and temporal organization of biological objects . . . can be attributed to the different interactions of the physical vectors of the inertial and rotational gravitational fields, the geomagnetic field (GMF), and the vectors of the intrinsic biological magnetogravitational field of living organisms, which are different in right-handed, left-handed, and symmetric organisms.

There is a constant interaction of the intrinsic fields of the organism and external fields. That they are different in right and left-handed or symmetric organisms is significant. The same author, A.P. Dubrov, a leading Russian researcher, has developed a theory concerning the relative symmetry of all objects ranging from molecular isomers to whole organisms. He presents evidence showing that the relative symmetry of all organisms (their topological nature, in Manaka's terms) is primarily conditioned at conception by these fields.[62] The topological structure thus determined controls the manner and extent of their interaction with the fields.[63]

His notions of "functional symmetry" and "functional dissymmetry" are close to Manaka's, because these ideas refer not only to the actual symmetry of the objects, but as well to their rhythmicity and temporality. They manifest, for example, as differences of response to the GMF in a group of presumably healthy people. As an example Dubrov cites research where the same GMF events produced increased tonus of the parasympathetic nervous system in some subjects and increased tonus of the sympathetic system in others.

Essentially, the GMF and the gravitational fields have been found to be of enormous importance. Dubrov states:[64]

□

The GMF and gravitation is of a special nature in that it is unselective and acts on *all cells* of the organism *directly,* on the organism as a whole and thus on *all* living organisms. . . . We believe that the combined effect of the GMF and gravitation may be a common denominator for all vital activity in the biosphere, and for non-living matter too.

In support of this claim he describes a large and mounting body of evidence that the interaction of the varying fields, the GMF and gravitational field in particular, plays a significant and often essential role in biological processes. One of the more significant discoveries by the American scientists F.A. Brown Jr. and Y.H. Park[65] was that:

> . . . the GMF in its action on biological objects, interacts with other vector forces, particularly the gravitational effects of the moon. . . . The combined effect of the GMF and gravitation is responsible not only for the spatial, but also the temporal organization of biological objects.[66]

In other words, the earth's magnetic and gravitational fields, and those of the moon, act on each other and on all living organisms to produce structural and functional effects and chronobiological rhythms.

Because all these fields vary in a cyclic fashion, chronobiological effects are found in living organisms. The earth's rotation around its axis produces cyclic variations in periods of lightness and darkness. It also produces local exposure to differences in the geomagnetic field. Further, the geomagnetic field is not uniform around the earth. Because of the effects of solar winds and interplanetary fields, the earth's field is slightly compressed on the side facing the sun and slightly expanded on the other.

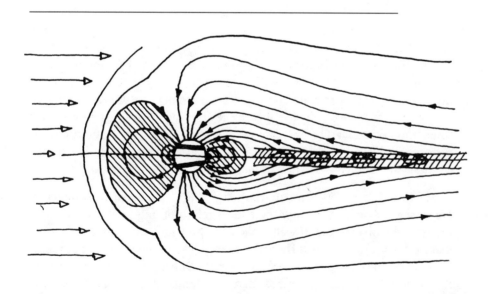

Figure 9.1 The geomagnetic field is compressed by the solar wind closer to the sun and shot out into space on its other side.

As the earth rotates within this field, the magnetic field in our immediate environment will fluctuate daily such that on a quiet day, the angle of declination of the magnetic field to the surface of the earth will vary: While the magnitude of the variable GMF field is small, less than two percent of the general strength of the constant field, its biological significance is actually much greater.[67]

The magnetic field is also affected by lunar movements. The rotation of the moon around the earth produces both geomagnetic and gravitational changes. The geomagnetic changes might, at least in part, result from the action of the gravitational vector of the moon's gravitational field on the geomagnetic vector. Both the GMF and gravitational changes manifest in cycles, which in turn produce chronobiological effects. The rotation of the earth around the sun produces cyclic variations in the intensity of light and temperature as the seasons pass their course. This in turn has specific chronobiological effects on living organisms. As the earth rotates around the sun it is affected to greater and lesser degrees by the gravitational fields of the other planets in the solar system, in particular that of Jupiter, which produces perhaps the third strongest gravitational effect on the earth, second only to the sun and moon.

These gravitational changes also produce cyclic changes in the earth's gravitational and magnetic fields and thus on living organisms. Sunspot activity, which peaks approximately every eleven years,[68] and solar flares, have also been found to produce biological effects and may also affect chronobiological processes.[69]

As we have seen, the stem and branch cycles and descriptions seem to correlate well with the relative movements of the Earth, Moon, Sun, and Jupiter. We can see that the biological importance of these correlations may be that they parallel the normal variations and fluctuations of the geomagnetic field. Thus, these correlations relate the sixty-year, twelve-year, twelve-month, daily, and bihourly correspondences of the stems and branches with geomagnetic field fluctuations resulting from these planetary movements. This is particularly interesting in light of the Chinese emphasis on the importance of the stem and branch cycles, which, we have postulated, are geometric coordinate systems that define the relative position of the Sun, Moon, Earth, and Jupiter to each other at any time. As such these correspondences can be used to map specific biological effects and cycles. As Dubrov sees it, this is "of great importance, since the natural-gravitational-magnetoelectric complex has its own characteristic features in each period of time."[70] Thus, there are specific biological effects for every given period of time.

Not only does the natural gravitational-magnetoelectric complex produce specific effects at specific times, it is particularly important at the moment of conception:

> Thus, we find that the initial instant at which the living organism begins to function (moment of conception, moment of formation of embryo in animals and plants, moment of soaking of dry plant seeds, etc.) is of great importance.[71]

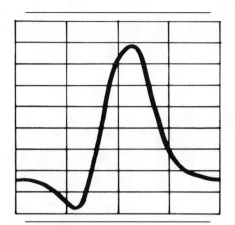

Figure 9.2 A typical daily variation of the angle of declination of the geomagnetic field.

This can be seen in the work of other scientists investigating the effects of gravity on very early development[72] where the initial restructuring of the egg immediately after sperm entry is affected by gravity. Dubrov states this concept quite clearly in relation to the functional biosymmetry of living objects and the essential role and significance of biosymmetry:

> We can conclude that the GMF determines the biosymmetric status of a living object. This probably occurs in the period of fusion of the gametes and coincides with the moment of untwisting of the chromosomes, when there is a favorable opportunity for action on single stranded DNA. The template enantiomorphic characteristic of the DNA molecule formed at this moment subsequently determines the direction of asymmetric synthesis and stereoisomeric configuration of all the subsequent replicating molecules. The enantiomorphic characteristic of the object formed in this way becomes the decisive factor in the functional response of the living creature to the action of the GMF and the other physical factors.[73]

Various authors feel that the moment of conception is an important moment in the life of all organisms, setting the scene for much of what follows.

Some evidence also supports the theory that there is at least indirect field influence during embryological development, as well as at the point of conception.[74] This moment and the ensuing drama can be seen in the Chinese cycles of the branches, where embryonic development figures as part of the overall cycle of life. It can be found again in various theories and descriptions of embryonic development that are documented in both medical and non-medical literature.

Recent experiments have demonstrated that weak magnetic fields play vital roles in growth, development, and the normal regulation of life processes. Becker has postulated that:

> . . . direct electrical currents normally generated within living organisms and time-varying components of the earth's normal magnetic field play pivotal roles in the control of biological growth processes.[75]

Becker has specifically researched the electrical nature and function of the acupuncture meridians and points and has theorized that they are an important component of the body's intrinsic DC electrical system, which is important both in healing and our ability to adapt to environmental changes.[76] He also describes roughly fifteen-minute rhythms in the current strength at the points measured, a fluctuation that while different in periodicity from those described in the classics, is probably important in its contribution to those rhythms.[77]

That the organism manifests a constant relationship among all growth processes as regulated by the internal direct-current system and the earth's normal magnetic field is very similar to our understanding of the rhythmicity and probable field effects that we feel the classical Chinese authors were trying to describe in their own inimicably obscure and symbolic manner. It may also be important to our understanding of how the physical body structurally adapts to the earth's gravitational field. If the body is physically out of balance, its center of gravity will shift, possibly producing physiological, electrical, or magnetic field changes in the body. Likewise, if the center of gravity of the earth is rhythmically changing according to lunar and other celestial movements, this will also produce changes in the body. This could underlie some of the energetic effects observed by structural therapists who address the structural posture of the body.

Dubrov's ideas of "functional symmetry" and "functional dissymetry" are quite important here, as are Manaka's ideas about topology and isophasality (see later chapters), which clinically demonstrate some of these effects. The biological significance of the GMF can be seen in other clinical perspectives as well. Two examples should suffice. Statistical research has demonstrated significant links between psychiatric disturbances and variations in the GMF due to phenomena such as magnetic storms.[78] Recently a Japanese researcher, Kyoichi Nakagawa, postulated an interesting theory that provides a more Western clinical viewpoint on the significance of the earth's magnetic field. During several decades of research regarding the causes of nonspecific ailments, Nakagawa discovered an intriguing phenomenon. If the body is not exposed long enough, or to enough of, the earth's magnetic field, as occurs in many working and living environments, a wide range of symptoms can develop. Nakagawa describes this as the "Magnetic field deficiency syndrome."[79] He feels that part of our normal function is due to our interactions with the normal magnetic fields of our environment and has devised a number of ways to treat the syndrome using magnets.

Once again, there is a high degree of congruence between the systems and patterns described by the Chinese theorists and the processes described by the most advanced Western research. The greatest difficulty is not the association of the two culturally determined medicines, but in the major habits of thought commonly found in the exponents of either discipline. Western researchers are clearly involved in an age where functional explanations are composed of complex networks of slight, often miniscule, subtle forces. The predominant Western viewpoint is primarily biomechanical or biochemical. Oriental medical practitioners are commonly taught to focus on complex, subtle phenomena and to think in categorical units, patterns, and groups of patterns. Yet an idea such as the flow of qi in the meridians cannot be well stated by either of these perceptive viewpoints. Perhaps the concept of an extremely pervasive, multi-dimensional network of bioelectrical, biomagnetic, biochemical, biogravitational, and field effects would provide a fuller image.

Models of Environmental Influences

We have already seen how the body interacts with fluctuating environmental fields to establish biorhythms; and we have theorized that these interactions produce the biorhythmic cycles described in the classical texts. However, the biorhythmic aspects of acupuncture theory are not commonly taught in the West, due in part to their fluctuating influence in China. In general, these ideas are more difficult to consider because their symbolic and categorical content is very high. Yet, even the most basic

□

aspects of fundamental Oriental medical theory — pathogenic influences, climatic influences, environmental influences — are impacted by modern research.

If, as we have posited, the meridian systems lie in the superficial fascia, so that the qi "circulating" within them is in fact the bioelectric energies associated with the connective tissue structures of the fascia, then it is clear how climatic conditions can affect this qi. If areas of the body are exposed to temperature changes, these areas will respond. The systems of the body will attempt to retain a homeostatic biofield and a constant temperature. The communications system based in the fascia and connective tissues will be activated.

If these tissues are exposed to heat, this could create a greater flow of bioelectricity or even facilitate the flow of bioelectrical signals through increased conductivity, "battery effect," or biochemical reaction. There should be some measurable increase. Conversely, if the tissues are exposed to cold, the flow of bioelectricity would be reduced or the ground substance would become less active. As may be expected, these responses would be complex and multi-dimensional. If an area of the body becomes exposed to cold, the blood circulation at the surface decreases to prevent a loss of heat from the exposed area of the body. This change in blood flow will also contribute to the lowering of the tissue temperature and the fascia will become cooler, further decreasing the flow of energy.

Also, as the flow of blood to the tissues decreases, the degree of oxygenation of the tissues will decrease in some proportional relation. Szent-Gyorgyi and his colleagues have shown that the rate of electron and proton flow along and through proteins is dependent on both the oxygen and water content of the proteins.[80] The opposite can be seen to happen in response to heat. Either way, these mechanisms offer a modern viewpoint of the ideas in the classical texts that speak of the invasion of heat or cold and their consequent pathological effects.

We can look at wind in a similar manner. That is, wind might make the body more open to thermoelectric changes in the fascia. Though it is hard to see how wind itself could affect the tissues, scientists have found that the surface of the body is surrounded by a miniscule layer of stationary air. This thin layer of air is thicker in hairier animals as it is maintained in part by pilo-erection, a phenomenon less marked in humans because of their relatively lesser covering of body hair.[81] This thin layer of air acts as an insulator, helping to maintain and regulate the body temperature; it is one of the body's thermostatic mechanisms.[82] When some part of the body is exposed to wind, this thin insulating layer of air will be displaced, disrupting its thermostatic properties. This in turn will increase the probability of temperature changes through the loss of heat via convection, and loss of the insulation effect.[83]

Ionized particles will also be contained in this thin layer of insulating air.[84] The work of the Rumanian scientist Dumitrescu, who has photographed what seem to be the acupoints by a process called "electronography," which essentially images the movements of ions in the area just above the skin, tends to support the notion that this thin layer of air is ionized.[85] It will also be humid, another condition that will be affected by disruption of both the thermostatic layer and the field itself.

□

We can use the same logic to view dampness and dryness, the two other classic external factors. Dampness is known to reinforce the effects of both cold and heat, creating a greater likelihood of temperature gain or loss.[86] Likewise, very dry or hot weather that leads to dehydration will cause the body's temperature to rise.[87] In response to heat the main factors that are important for temperature control are increased circulation to the skin and loss of heat by radiation and sweating. In response to cold, the operative response is decreased circulation to the skin to minimize heat loss. When a person sweats, ionized particles such as sodium ions are lost. With the loss of radiant heat, electrical and magnetic changes occur at the surface of the body. Both these factors must influence the meridian systems.

The Polish scientist, Wlodzimierz Sedlak, describes similar functions in the body's resistance to environmental influences.[88] He feels that the biological field has the function of screening noxious environmental influences. More specifically, he posits that the surface potential of the field, the surface concentration of electrons (electrostasis, ECS in his terminology), performs this function:

> At every level of structural complexity, the organism reacts by a change of potential to both external and internal stimuli. The organism sends out ECS electrons to meet the environment.
> . Electrostasis is the border between the organism and environment. . . . the ECS screens the biological system from the noxious influence of environmental radiation.[89]

His work concerns the quantum and plasma nature of biological systems, so he is particularly concerned with electromagnetic radiation. However, it is probable that the same principles, the conditioning of the interface between the organism and the environment, apply when we speak in non-quantum terms such as the thermoelectric properties of this interface.

Maresch, the Viennese physicist who found "electrically superior points of the skin," feels that these are important points for detecting environmental changes (such as changes in atmospheric conditions that result from changes in temperature and humidity) and communicating these changes to the body.[90] Bischko summarizes the basic theory:

> Disturbances in the field of atmospheric electricity on certain small areas of the skin can cause measurable changes in the electrical values that are demonstrable. These points are called electrically superior points of the skin and are congruous with acupuncture points. [The points] must be considered receptors.[91]

This matches the descriptions of the electrical properties of the meridians and their fluctuating electrical characteristics. It further matches the theoretical discussions founded on the thermoelectric properties of the connective tissues and very clearly fits the theory by providing a basis for measurable observations.

Just as it is possible to see how external factors, such as temperature variations, can affect the flow of qi or bioelectricity in the body, it is also possible to see how internal fluctuations in the flow of energy can result in temperature variations. When palpating the body, one significant sign is temperature variation. Because of the thermoelectric properties of the connective tissues, if the flow of qi or bioelectricity is decreased at any point (flow changes resulting from internally generated problems), noticeable temperature changes can be potentially produced. For example, the feeling of cold would relate to decreased activity, and the feeling of heat to increased activity. Of course, the relative flow of blood can produce these changes, as we noted above. Perhaps, the interdependence of blood flow, bioelectrical flow, and temperature is simply another way of stating what the Oriental classics describe as the interdependence of qi and blood.

While exogenous and endogenous pathological entities are easier to discuss because their qualities and relationships are well within the general experience of consensual reality, attempts at explanation are complicated by their multiple meanings. In some cases cold and hot, for example, are relative qualitative expressions; in other cases they are empirical measures, and in still other uses they are symbols for sets of phenomena that are related by quality. For example, flushed cheeks, rapid pulse, red tongue, and thirst are related to "hot" by virtue of their qualitative similarity to "hot," not because they are the result of a single mechanism. It does not follow, however, that the set of things that are "hot" in Chinese medicine cannot be approached theoretically; only that any potential explanation will have to take into account that the relationships never were based on some single, causal mechanism. It is for this reason that most attempts to explain Chinese medical theory with biochemical or biomechanical theories fail. It is one particular advantage of the biodynamic field theory that it attempts to explain how an immense variety of biological events can be coordinated and interrelated.

Sensorial Correspondences and Possible Field Effects

Another area where Western research has been completed and where more is being initiated all the time, is the area of perception. Researchers are seeking to learn how perceived sensations, such as sound, alter the electrical and magnetic fields of the body, particularly those that surround the head. The sense organs of taste, touch, sight, smell, and hearing, send electrical signals to the brain where they are interpreted. This interpretation we then "perceive." We "see" the results of the chain of electrical signals that arrive at the brain. It is also this chain of events that leads to our "feelings" or emotional experiences of the "outside world." Once the sensory signals enter the brain, they produce changes in the electrical fields of the brain. These changes are measurable as EEG's and also cause changes in the magnetic fields around the head, that are measured as MEG's.

Much work has been done measuring these electrical fields and their changes.[92] EEG's have been measured in many different organisms under many different conditions.

Work is also being done to calibrate the changes in the magnetic fields relative to specific sensory inputs: auditory, visual, and somatosensory stimuli.[93] Though these field changes are slight, they are sufficient to change the field of the whole body. Changes anywhere in the field will probably effect changes throughout the field, much in the same manner that the heart's electrical field can be measured anywhere on the surface of the body in the ECG.

It is possible that as the fields around the head change, they effect changes throughout all the fields of the body. However, it is more likely that these changes affect the body's tissues directly. The brain in particular will be sensitive to these changes and initiate responses within the nervous system. These responses too are able to affect the body's fields. There is already experimental evidence showing that tissues are sensitive to a changing electrical environment.[94] Further, brain structures are sensitive to electric and magnetic fields of similar frequency and amplitude to those produced by normal brain activity.[95] This strongly suggests that the nervous system is also sensitive to the electrical and magnetic fields evoked within itself by sensory or other stimuli. Such high degree of sensitivity is felt to be due to the modulation of calcium ion activity at the nerve cell membrane surface (similar to the models we briefly examined earlier).

These changes are very slight, but remember that biological systems are extremely sensitive, being able to sense tiny changes and to amplify those changes to effect larger responses.[96] Considerable speculation has accompanied discussion on the role of this sensitivity and what interactions it might initiate. Certainly, it can initiate quite profound changes, either behavioral or metabolic. For our purposes, however, the importance of the measurement of field changes in response to sensory input is that if the fields change, then so too will the flow of energy within the body. Thus, not only are endogenous and exogenous events from the microscopic to the cosmic capable of influencing the state and function of the meridian system, so too are perceptual stimulae.

In the classical Chinese medical literature, the different senses were classified in fives according to the five phases.[97] There are the five sapors, the five odors, the five colors, the five notes, and the five tones. This ancient philosophical system, *wu xing,* is analagous to the "base mathematics" of binary or decimal arithmetic. In the practical context of understanding the various correspondences of each phase, it is best to regard the five phases as a classification system. However, it is not the classification system that concerns us here. Rather it is the perceptions themselves and how the classical authors understood human responses to these stimulae. In some cases, as in *ba fa,* or eight-principle diagnosis for example, colors, odors, and tones are clues observed by the practitioner. The inference is that each observation indicates that the patient belongs to a specific class. In other cases, Oriental physicians propose that sensorial inputs affect the condition of the patient. Manaka has described the sounds in reference to the organs and possible uses in healing:[98]

Organ	Sound
Liver	Xu
Heart	Ke
Spleen	Hu
Lung	Si
Kidney	Chui
Triple Warmer	Xi

This idea is well developed in regard to the five sapors; there are explicit passages where the body's responses to a particular flavor is documented. Indeed, sapor is one of the major qualities of Chinese pharmaceuticals and foods and appears in almost all classical and modern pharmacopoeia. Though there is some disparity among the various classical sources,[99] on the whole they imply the same thing: a person's energies are altered and different organ or meridian systems are affected according to the sapor consumed.

There are a number of options for examining this idea. With taste, a quality belonging to comestibles, we could consider the entire corpus of information as an early attempt to explain nutritional physiology. This would not be completely justified because there are other passages that clearly describe a nutritional theory. Or, we could think of these ideas as simply extensions of the five phases from observation to philosophical or conceptual unity. In general, we describe the working of these sensorial correspondences as energetic effects, again, without too much attention to just what this energy might be.

As with the other elements of the Chinese medical paradigm that we have discussed, field theory has the advantage of a more explicit idea of energy and effect. We need only to show that perceptual stimulae can alter the various fields to which the body is sensitive to propose that there is some sense to the Chinese ideas of sight, sound, and taste. Another advantage of the theory is that it permits the simultaneous extension of the functional hypotheses to the idea of mental and emotional states affecting the body's energetics.[100]

There are clear statements where emotional and mental states were thought to result from specific energetic disorders. There are also clear statements of emotional and mental states creating energetic disorders. As with the Chinese medical literature, our Western ideas of how color or music effect change, even heal, imply some method where very small stimulae have pronounced effects. Of course, when considering emotional and energetic states, we are dealing with complex physiological phenomena. But these, as well as the related perceptual stimulae, also result in changes in the electrical and magnetic fields around the head and thus the rest of the body.

Mental and emotional states are often seen in relation to muscle tension. Overly tense muscles can affect the flow of energy in the body, creating abnormalities in the electrical and magnetic fields because of the increased motor neuron stimulation involved in the tensing of muscles, the increased rate of depolarization of the muscles, and the sustained state of such nervous stimulation in tense muscles. Again, field theory explains how these conditions can affect the relative flow of the energy within the fields and the meridians.

It is thus not so unrealistic that the Chinese creators of phase theory chose to classify perceptual, mental, and emotional phenomena according to the five phases. They were ordering their observations, using a synthetic and emblematic logic to order complex phenomena in a useful way. Obviously, they were not discussing calcium ions and motor neuron stimulation. However, they were very clearly attempting to express their observation that the human responses to these stimulae were consistent and orderly. Theorizing that the local electrophysiological or magnetophysiological effects that result from each phenomena have more general effects, and that these effects are patterned and orderly, is really very much the same attempt.

Each electrophysiological and magnetophysiological event will yield specific results and sets of results — a signature. This is at least superficially analogous to the windows Adey describes.[101] In short, any perceptual or emotional stimulae will have specific local effects on different areas and functions of the body. Each local effect will be signalled to a specific general class of areas and functions, and thus will have a consistent "sphere of influence." Thus, the habit adopted in Western literature (we include ourselves) of speaking of "correspondences" is to some extent misleading. The relationship of "fire," the heart, small intestine, rapid pulses, red coloration, hot herbs, the emotional response to warm colors, rapid musical phrases, or certain notes, is not only their qualitative similarity, or some magical energy, it is also the consistent and routine response of humans to these stimulae through the subtle changes in the biodynamic fields. Later in this discussion, we will note some practical examples of phasal relationships in Western and Eastern research.

Note that the biodynamic model allows many of these observations and theories to be integrated. We have already discussed the nature of the geomagnetic field, its variability, and its ability to instigate biorhythms. One author we cited, A.P. Dubrov, has further developed the GMF model to include conditioning of the relative symmetry or lack of symmetry of biological objects. He also presents information demonstrating that symmetrical, asymmetrical, left-handed, and right-handed organisms interact differently with the GMF and other fields.[102] Organisms of different shapes and orientations will respond differently to the GMF and other fields. Since these fields are always fluctuating, the frequency and amplitude of the signals will vary in specific phases. These variations also manifest as specific signatures with the capacity to effect to a greater or lesser extent organs of a specific shape, size, or orientation.

This is another method of accounting for the correspondences of specific organs and meridians to each of the general phases. Each organ — lung, heart, liver, spleen, kidney — has a specific shape, specific position within the body, and an individual relative symmetry. If each of these factors (among others of course) conditions an organ to respond to a specific field signature, then these traditional correspondences (heart with fire, lung with metal, etc.) are also descriptions of sequenced, repeating, and consistent patterns of response. In short, the phases are phases in the sense of regular progression. At specific phases of GMF activity the heart or lungs will manifest a level of activity that is maximal, minimal, or somewhere between. The timing of these phases, fire around mid-day and summer, metal around late afternoon and fall, etc., will be the result of the same celestial mechanics. Organ sensitivities or responses to endogenous field signatures would behave in the same manner, with, of course, different mechanisms.

□

The elegance of considering phasal relationships in this fashion is that it moves the idea of a correspondence from a fairly ambiguous idea of symbolic and semantic similarity, to a specific theoretical construct. That is, in Oriental medicine the phases are sets of biological events that are linked by the response of body-specific fields to environmental fields via an interchange of subtle bioelectric, biochemic, and biomagnetic signals. Further, the timing and intensity of these signals, and their progression from one to another phase, are determined by the regularity of patterns in the microcosmic and macrocosmic environments. Unlike theories that depend on symbolic relationships, this approach sacrifices none of the essential qualitative tone of the Chinese idea itself.

Certainly, it is possible to see most, if not all facets of the five-phase theory within the multifield model. The association of the color white, the spicy taste, the emotion of grief, and the season of fall to the lungs and the emblem "metal" is the consistent function of the endogenous and exogenous fields associated with these phenomena, their similar signatures. Thus, we can draw on the conceptual richness of the modern Western model for such demonstrable and useful ideas as resonance, harmonic frequencies, and information exchange.

Considering these phenomena, we can postulate that the following factors are all important in determining the resonant signature of a specific organ, tissue, or body area.

-- The relative symmetry, asymmetry, left or right handedness, and shape of the object.
-- Position within the body.
-- Relative mass and density.
-- Degree of hydration.
-- The normal physiological electrical and magnetic activity of the object.
-- The relative pathological state of the object.

Were we able to determine the specific signature of an area of the body, we would be able to predict the results of perceptive and mental states. Electrophysiologically such a model is quite plausible. That the Chinese seem to have understood this, mapped its clinical consequences, and attempted its practical application, is truly amazing. Although this model is purely theoretical at this time, it is helpful for understanding more advanced models, such as those of Yoshio Manaka.

Phase Effects in a Field Model

Manaka has arrived at a very sophisticated model of the five phases. It is clearly stated in the context of the acupoint—phase relationships for the jing, yong, shu, jing, and he points, and can explain many aspects of the five-phase theory.[103] His theories are based partly on a topological understanding of the body and partly on biorhythmic cycles. He wanted to understand the elemental relationships among meridian points and to have a means for experimentally testing and demonstrating these relationships. He suggested that points classically ascribed the same phasal quality might be "isophasal," i.e., they manifested similar properties at the same time. Thus, if one earth point is said to be active or "open," then all earth points might be active. If a patient visits at a certain time of the day, for instance, three to five p.m., corresponding to the bladder meridian, and if some imbalance of the earth phase is evident, then treating the earth point of the bladder meridian should help. Similarly, via the tai yang—shao yin relationship, treating the earth points of the heart, small intestine, and kidney meridians should also affect the condition. In short, if his theory were to be correct, and if what the Chinese physicians had observed and labeled as phases were to correspond to this isophasal pattern, then those points traditionally considered active or open at a particular time should be effective in treatment.

As the indicators of change for his experiments, Manaka chose the presence or absence of reaction on palpation of points on the abdomen. Reaction is easily confirmed, both by the patient and the practitioner, and is easily repeatable. Thus, it is a more objective measure than the pulse or the patient's subjective perception of their symptoms. As well, it is a very direct measurement. The palpatory response identifying the problem with a specific phase is reassessed to measure improvement. For therapeutic stimulae Manaka chose the application of magnetic polarity. Such stimulae have the advantage of being so small that there can be no implication that a central nervous system response is at work. The stimulus levels are not sufficient to trigger a nervous system event. Further, the stimulae are polar and permit testing the polar qualities of the classical system.

Using this methodology, he has demonstrated that isophasal relationships exist, and suggests that they are part of what is classically described as five-phase theory. These relationships demonstrate both properties pertaining to polarity (yin—yang), and the phase relationships of the meridians. Indeed, these isophasal properties are very probably definable by mathematical relationships[104] as is Manaka's topological octahedral model of yin—yang the extraordinary vessels:[105]

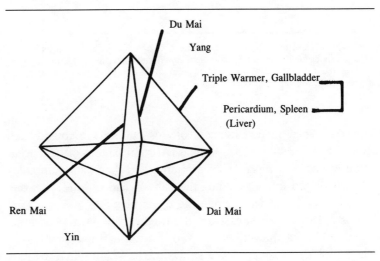

Figure 9.3 The extraordinary vessel octahedral model.

The lines that define the triangles of each area are yin—yang boundaries. These eight areas can also be seen in the work of Kentaro Takagi, who studied the "pressure perspiration reflex."[106] Manaka cites this work because it clearly demonstrates an octahedral response in the body.[107] As

□

well, superficial lymph drainage also follows this pattern. From the surface of the body lymph drains into the inguinal or axillary lymph nodes. On the front, and less obviously on the back, this drainage is quadrantally patterned, with the navel as the central point.[108]

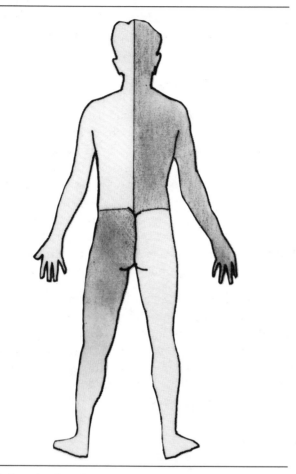

Figure 9.4 If the body is placed in a hot, moist environment, it should sweat evenly on its surface. However, if pressure is applied to the upper left mid-axillary region, and simultaneously to the region of the right iliac spine on the mid-axillary line, sweating will occur on the lower left and upper right quadrants only, easily visualized with an iodide salt solution.

There are also other, rarer, evidences of this pattern. In roughly ten percent of newborn babies there is a peculiar left-right pattern of discoloration for several weeks after birth. This is often called the "harlequin color change" or "particolored infant." When the baby is laid on one side, one side of the body clearly reddens, while the other blanches. This occurs along very clearly demarcated lines from the forehead down the midline, even along the midline of the genitals,[109] and is a non-pathological condition of unclear etiology that graphically shows the left-right, yin-yang pattern of symmetry/asymmetry.

A serious, yet rare, familial disorder called "familial rectal pain" or "familial painful harlequin flushing" also demonstrates the octahedrality. This syndrome manifests as severe pain in the rectal region and occasionally the ocular and submaxillary regions, with accompanying flushing. The flushing demarks left-right, superior-inferior, anterior-posterior quadrantal patterns with the umbilicus as the center. Symptoms can be instigated by bowel movement, a fall, probing in the anal region, coitus, or childbirth, and are very debilitating. It appears to be transmitted by an autosomal dominant gene and affects a large percentage of the family.[110] While this, and the other conditions cited, are rare, they demonstrate patterns that are useful for the explanation of the common yin—yang relationships described by Chinese medical theory.

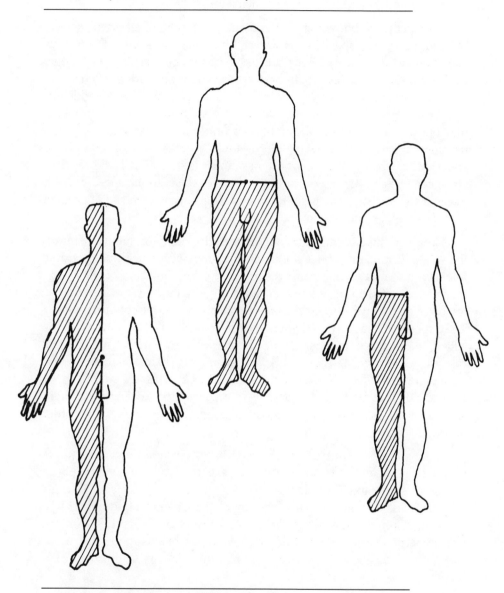

Figure 9.5 In this disease, flushing is most commonly seen in the above three patterns, which clearly lie in quadrantal relationship to the umbilicus.

Phasality and octahedral patterning give us regular, even mathematical, predictable and confirmable models of point and meridian relationships. These relationships further support the concept of the "energetic body" as a field capable of generating, transmitting, and responding to very small signals.

Summary

Manaka's work has been a true inspiration in the writing of this text, not only for his remarkable theoretical and clinical ideas and procedures, but for his open-ended patterning of ideas. His theory of human energetics and healing permits us to synthesize most, if not all, of the information derived from Eastern thought and Western experimentation in a general theory.[111] His ideas set us on a path of discovery leading to a greater theoretical understanding of Oriental medicine.

Essentially, the body is an extremely complex field of electrical, chemical and magnetic capacities. However, there are rules that describe its operation. Order and harmony are the dynamic, but regular case. Some rules are known and described; these are the "explicate order." Others are unknown, hidden or poorly described; these are an order that is hidden or "implicate."[112] Just as laws and rules require specific conditions in which they operate, there are specific conditions under which the order of things becomes apparent. For example, Newton's general laws of gravity are applicable to objects of mass whose movement is substantially slower than the speed of light. On acceleration to velocities closer to the speed of light, Einstein's relativistic laws begin to apply and gravity is seen as the product of the space-time continuum.

However, this ordering does not require relativistic conditions. Beneath the soil, a germinating shoot will invariably grow with a negative geotropic orientation — away from the forces of gravity. Yet, once out of the soil in the presence of light, it can be persuaded to grow in the same direction as the force of gravity. Certain chemicals under specific, set conditions show a set speed of reaction, yet when a catalyst (such as platinum black) is added, their speed increases, without an accompanying change in the catalyst. Generally the urinary bladder is impervious to water, yet under certain conditions, such as extreme heat and lack of fluids, water can be reabsorbed through the bladder. As circumstances change, different aspects of the order of things become apparent, different facets of order unfold.

Much of the scientific literature cited in this section describes aspects of the explicate order. However, there are aspects that have not as yet been unfolded. This can be seen in both classical theories and in Manaka's clinical examples. His illustration of the topological nature of the body, the rules implicit in this model, the clinical law of isophasality, and the concept of symmetry lost through growth are all examples of this hidden or implicate order. Manaka cites two clear examples of symmetry lost through evolution.

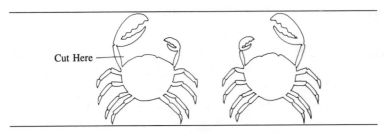

Cut Here

Figure 9.6 Claw regrowth in the fiddler crab occurs asymmetrically.

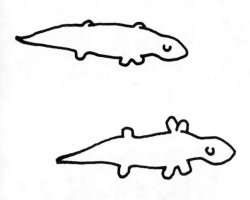

Figure 9.7 When transplanted at the correct stage of development, the extra limb stimulates the growth of a sixth limb to retain some approximation of symmetry.

If the larger claw of a fiddler crab is removed, the claw will grow back, but as a small claw; while the smaller claw will enlarge to become the larger claw. If an extra leg is implanted into the side of a developing salamander, another leg will grow in contra-symmetry to the added leg. There is a hidden or lost symmetry that directs these phenomena, just as the pressure perspiration reflex of Kentaro Takagi makes a certain octahedral symmetry in the body unfold. Manaka feels that the general laws of acupuncture utilize these hidden laws. Ancient people observed or understood these and other hidden laws and used them in healing. Somehow, ancient peoples were more attuned to nature and observed patterns that our concentration on cause and effect has overlooked.

An important component of the hidden order is its existence in time. Generally these hidden orders arise and become manifest through evolution. At certain stages of evolution, these various orders played more obviously significant roles. They were then absorbed or enfolded, made implicit, almost vestigial (much in the same sense that the appendix is seen as a vestigial structure in carnivores). Perhaps Sheldrake's idea of morphogenetic fields is important here,[113] but it may not be necessary to invoke a field of unknown physical qualities to explain how evolutionary traits manifest.

There are also new developments in physics that can help us better understand these phenomena. The notion of "atomic memory" is one that has been invoked and used since the 1940s. Theoretical and experimental evidence shows that things are able to retain a memory of former states and under the right circumstances can be made to revert to those states.[114] Provided that the correct stimulus is used, things can be made to revert to former states. Perhaps these states remain as hidden orders that become apparent with the correct stimulus. If the large claw is removed, the smaller claw enlarges. If a north-facing magnet is placed on left or right ear large intestine points, tension and pressure pain at LI-4 can be shifted from left to right. The same stimulus, when placed on SP-3, makes both left and right LI-4 less tense. These stimulae access former states or relationships that arise during evolution and remain implicit or enfolded within the body. Each can be made to "stand out in relief."[115]

Such a view of the body and energetic anatomy brings us to consideration of the origin of the universe and matter, the multiplicity of the states of being and their relationships, the wholeness of nature. These are precisely the views expressed by the Chinese classics, the centrality of the tai yi. All are images of each other, holograms as it were, memory patterns of what was and is and its evolution. In this context it is worth noting the use of the holographic concept both in physics,[116] and in the realm of acupuncture.[117]

Given the theoretical basis described by the Chinese classics, Manaka's clinical observations of implicate order become extremely valuable for clinically testing the principles found in the Chinese medical classics. It provides us with a unified interpretation of qi in all its various forms and manifestations. Manaka is very cognizant of the seeming simplicity of these ideas and the corresponding immense complexity of which they are capable. The notions of yin and yang and their multiplicity of actions,

□

reactions, connections, and descriptions become an infinite regression when they are used to explain one another. Thus, he is striving continually for a simpler means of description that does not sacrifice their conceptual ability.

In this task he synthesizes modern information theory and the theory of biases or "biasology." This a major development of general theoretical approach. Essentially, his theory states that it is possible to view a biological organism in terms of specific information and as a system for the transformation of this information through time. In Schoffeniels' work[118] this is expressed mathematically as:

$$dI = diI + de\text{-}I + de\text{+}I$$

Where content (I) is a variable information state (dI) that is equivalent to the sum of informational inputs (de+I) and outputs (de-I) and the information degraded by the organism (diI). A biological organism exists within a specific environment (the earth, solar system etc.), receiving energy and matter as information (de+I = air, food, fluid, bioenergetic stimulae). Some energy and matter are output as information (de-I = urine, stool, impact on environment and culture). The organism also degrades a certain amount of information (diI = metabolic use, "lost" signals). In very general terms, and in a relatively simple equation, the total energetic state of the body at any time may be summarized with reference to its inputs, outputs, and transformations.

The unspecified or undefined manner in which these informational contents refer to input, output, and change in the organism mirror many of the unspecified descriptions in Chinese medical theory. The transformations of the stems and branches, for example, are quite poorly defined in the medical literature. Some of the effects are noted, but the mechanisms are left almost undefined. In modern Chinese medical practice we often define a patient's condition as "vacant liver" without referring to, or further specifying, any particular function or component of the liver. Indeed, the term is used where there is not even a conceptual vacancy, simply a state relatively less pronounced than that of some other organ or function. Components such as liver yin, liver yang, liver qi, or liver blood are defined and specified, but compared to the Western approach of identifying a specific infection, or biochemical malfunction, these too are poorly defined and remain generalized concepts.

In this terrain Manaka's theory of biases offers particular usefulness. The word "bias" refers to a slope, an inclination to one side. In general terms, it can refer to a disposition, a prejudice, a mental inclination or leaning, a slanting or diagonal line, the force or weight on a ball causing it to roll in a curve; in radios it is the fixed voltage applied to an electrode. In Manaka's terms it is the cause of a physical, structural, energetic, or functional imbalance in the body (which we could call a pathological bias), or the stimulus required to correct this bias (the corrective bias). Diagrammatically we can represent this in a simple topological model. This idea is not unique; when summarizing the effects of markedly reduced magnetic fields relative to the normal geomagnetic field, one author describes this effect as "visualized as equivalent to the *loss of a favorable bias* in a complex sequence of cellular events . . ."[119]

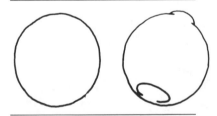

Figure 9.8 The bump may be visualized as the disease and the dent as the bias (problem) that led to the formation of the bump. A circle would represent a healthy body state.

□

We can talk about favorable and unfavorable biases in general biological terms and pathological and corrective biases in medical terms. The slow leakage of mercury from amalgam fillings can present the body with a slowly developing unfavorable bias, one that can cumulatively disrupt many of the body's control systems. The removal and replacement of these fillings is then the removal of the unfavorable bias, such that the normal favorable biases of the body can be restored with therapy. The slow cumulative effects of poor diet, excessive alcohol consumption, and constant stress can cause a series of unfavorable biases that eventually may cause a pathological liver condition. The dietary and lifestyle factors are unfavorable or pathological biases, as they predispose the person toward certain symptoms. The application of a "liver tonification treatment" through five-phase or ion-cord techniques applies a favorable or corrective bias. However, without changing the diet, alcohol consumption, or stress problems, the unfavorable bias will return. These circumstances are, unfortunately, evidenced all too often in clinical practice.

The topological properties of the body — the up-down, left-right, front-back, internal-external, yin-yang polarities and asymmetries — the normal fluctuations of the body — temporal-topological rhythms — and the hidden patterns of the body, all generate specific clinical rules. These manifestations represent generalized information flows that Manaka has called the "X-signal system." He summarizes this idea providing a theoretical basis for a relatively simple but profound clinical approach:

> There is a rudimentary information system in the body that seems to underlie the theories of classical acupuncture and has the following characteristics:
>
> 1. It requires only a very small stimulation to give input to the system.
>
> 2. The points of input and output of the system demonstrate patterns not definable with current knowledge of neurology.
>
> 3. The points, lines, and areas of the system compose integrated functional structures, a topological-geometrical system [i.e., the octant view of body structure].
>
> 4. Each part of the total figure can reflect the whole [is holographic].
>
> 5. This fundamental system is hidden or enfolded into the body and obscured by the more recently developed information systems [central, parasympathetic, and sympathetic nervous systems, etc.].
>
> 6. As something original and essential it can be made to manifest with profound consequences; this gives rise to clinical laws.[120]

This idea of the X-signal system has more than just the obvious merit of incorporating the implications found in modern information theory and systems theory. It mirrors rather neatly the first line of the *Dao De Jing*: "The way [dao] that can be spoken of is not the constant way"[121] Remembering what Needham says of the dao, this parallel is even clearer:

In a way, the whole idea of the tao was the idea of a field of force. All things oriented themselves according to it without having to be instructed to do so, and without the application of mechanical compulsion *(S&C 2:293)*.

In Manaka's terms, the signals are of unknown nature — X-signals — yet we can surmise their existence. While the natural order of things is often hidden from us, we can observe its effects. Just as the ancient Chinese observed the field of force of the earth, the geomagnetic field, with the earliest developed compass *(S&C 2:293)*, they observed the body and its relations and could derive clinical rules that provided the basis of the medical classics transmitted to us today.

Chapter

- 10 -

Integration

and

Differentiation:

Clinical Precautions

Integration and Differentiation:
Clinical Precautions

One goal of this text is to present a series of treatment systems that provide common applicability, and an additional series of systems that can provide more specialized applicability. As Manaka has pointed out, no practitioner should limit themselves to just one system, for no single system will be effective in every instance.

Because of this, we will be presenting quite a wide range of systems, each of which has its own logic, theory, diagnosis, and treatment. Although there are many overlaps, each system has its own specific applicability; each is like a specific lens that can focus on certain things at certain times, but not all things at all times.

Applying all the theoretical and practical models described in this volume will require considerable thought and work. To help with this process, we would like to outline a theory of systems models, showing how to best understand and use these various paradigms.

When we set out to look at and understand something, an enormous number of potential perspectives present themselves. For instance, when a patient goes to the hospital, a vast array of diagnostic systems might be employed such as X-rays, CAT-scans, blood-cell counts, blood chemistry tests, urine tests, stool tests, pap smears, bacterial cultures, neuro-muscular tests, psychological tests, etc.. Each of these is able to examine some specific aspect of the patient's make-up and condition. Each is necessarily limited by its inherent focus and by the procedural restrictions built into each test. All the pieces of the picture gathered by the various diagnostic systems must be considered if we are to perceive the inherent unity of the whole. In theory then, applying as wide a range of tests as possible will enable us to look more fully or 'holistically' at the person.

Of necessity, every perspective from which we look at the body offers a restricted perception. This is because we have to construct paradigms, theories, and models that will enable us to make the perceptions and then to classify the information perceived. Without conditioning our perceptions, we are unable to classify them so that we can understand them. From our learning and observing we construct perceptions of reality; we create the means for observing and for understanding what we observe. By our ingenuity and inventiveness we continually expand and enhance our modes of perception and it is in large part because of this that we can evolve as a species and come to observe and describe things and perform actions to change or remedy these perceptions.

For instance, it is by the system of upper gastrointestinal barium meal X-rays that we are able to diagnose an obstructed portion of the intestine and perform some remedial activity, such as surgery, to correct the problem. Each system of diagnosis is designed to clue us into and help confirm specific aspects of the patient's condition. We can apply this idea more generally.

When we use a microscope, we use low magnification lenses to see the grosser anatomical structures. When we speculate that things are composed of smaller or finer units then we use stronger and stronger lenses to see those finer and finer structures. Although each lens gives focus to the same thing, each lens allows us to access different information. The more we alter our lenses, the greater the range of information that can be accessed.

We can think of each system of analysis and perception as a different lens. Each one gives us access to different aspects of the thing being studied. Behind these systems or lenses is a raison d'etre that helps us determine the applicability of one system of lenses over another. This raison d'etre is the thing itself that is being studied. When we observe nature we notice order, structure and most of all patterns. These patterns condition the formation of the systems so that the systems can easily recognize the patterns. We developed microscopes of certain power to observe certain microscopic structures in things. Similarly, we developed X-ray apparatus so that we could study the internal structures of the body. When someone fractures a bone, there are certain signs and symptoms that accompany this. These clue one into the use of the X-ray apparatus to confirm that there is indeed a fractured bone. It would generally be considered poor procedure if one were to order a stool test or pap smear when a patient presents signs of a fractured ulna.

As these illustrations suggest, we develop systems of observation, analysis, and interpretation as means of gaining access to certain information about things. The things themselves help determine the nature of the system we use to observe them. The patterning of the things being observed and our observations of those patterns play major roles in determining these two factors. Thus our continuous testing of the systems prove the applicability of the system.

These systems are just as relevant to the theories of Chinese medicine. Even though we generally don't use sophisticated measuring devices, they still apply. The Chinese of two millenia ago certainly were not ordering up the same tests as our modern doctors do now. They were probably basing their systems theories entirely on natural observation and their own speculations, but the same kind of processes did occur.

Thus within the specific field of medicine where patients may present with an enormously complex range of symptoms, specialists throughout history observed patterns within this range of symptoms and proposed systems models which enabled them to observe, diagnose and treat. In so doing, they observed models that matched the energetic changes and patterns.

□

In such fashion, the biorhythmic ebb and flow of energy was observed in the body. These ebbs and flows were described as various energies seen to circulate through pathways, for instance, the twelve meridians and eight extraordinary vessels, the fifteen luo vessels, etc. Certain symptom patterns were observed in relation to each of them. It is natural that all these things would be seen within the philosophical background of the time, thus theories of the five phases, yin and yang, the relationships of stems and branches to the biorhythmic changes, all became important. Each development involved the same continuous testing. Those that didn't work or weren't useful would be abandoned.

Through observation and practice different models arose; those surviving the test of practice are still found today. Each system was probably developed to address problems not addressed directly by other systems, just as different lenses were developed to attain greater ranges of perception. Thus, each system retained a built-in limitation and specific applicability, determined by the presenting symptom—pattern complex.

For instance, the idea of yin and yang helps classify problems into areas and general nature. Organ functions and five-phase theory helps pin down the more exact location of the problem. The five phases also help us understand the seasonal changes and influences in relation to the patient's problem as well as the specific dynamic organ relationship. The extraordinary vessels help classify and treat a wide variety of symptoms, including structural changes and imbalances. The Chinese clock and the branches help identify daily and seasonal variations and patterns. The six stages of the *Shang Han Lun* help determine the depth and location of an externally generated problem. Each system is an intellectual construct that was felt to describe some basic energetic process. Inherently, each system addresses specific problems and patterns. It would be inappropriate to try to squeeze the presenting patterns of all patients into one diagnostic paradigm; no matter how broad the paradigm, there would be too many exceptions.

For instance, if a patient presents what is clearly a pattern fitting the system of biorhythmic disturbances, it would be inappropriate and doing the patient a disservice to apply an eight-principle treatment. Similarly, if a patient presents a pattern that matches an extraordinary vessel disturbance, it would be inappropriate to apply a five-phase treatment.

These are not just theoretical speculations, but are born out in the many years of practice of many practitioners.

> We must choose the method that works best. . . . It is important that we be aware that not all methods work at all times; thus we must have other methods we may use in special cases, and be flexible to change our methodology based on the response of the patient.[1]

The responses of the patient can be many and varied and come at many different times, and treatment must be adaptive to the responses of the patient. If palpation and diagnosis do not strictly match the details of a described pattern, we must be flexible in our diagnosis and treatment, moving on to check out the whole condition and any specific points.

□

According to Yoshio Manaka,

> This approach is very different from Western medicine where individual symptoms have specific treatments. Many times the question is asked, for example, what is a good point for asthma. Yet one point is not always unchangeable. In fact for each patient, these points continually change. There are daily changes in the points, which are based on the daily biorhythms, biological changes, or changes after an infection, etc. When a stimulation comes from the external environment, the response and attitude of the patient is quite changed. There is an adaptation and the condition becomes complicated. Of course, the treatment of acupuncture reports certain groups of points that are effective for certain symptoms, and this has been statistically verified. Ultimately the treatment should depend on the condition of the patient. So if one were to say that a certain combination of points were good for asthma for 50-60% of the patients, by modifying the technique and points used the results might be much, much better. Thus ancient acupuncturists always observed the response to certain techniques or procedures and obtained feedback from the patient. Just as one modifies their technique in a chess game or fencing match, based on the reaction of the opponent, the ancients looked for ways to be flexible in changing their technique when dealing with the patient.[2]

He regrets that many practitioners limit themselves to only one system, and neglect the many great systems developed by the Chinese throughout history. Today we only use a few of these great theories and treatments, because we have difficulty understanding and applying many of them. But this is no reason to abandon them. We should not forget them, for nothing is perfect and thus we should always try to understand all of them.

This is a basic premise of Manaka's practice. He is continually working with and testing ideas and systems, so that he has many tried and tested systems to choose from if a patient does not respond to a usual therapy. He feels that teaching one system as though it were the only one can only retard the development of the student. It is very much in the nature of Chinese medicine and medicine in general that practitioners need to be conversant in many things and have many perspectives. Abandoning or ignoring the many useful systems that have developed over time in the tradition of Oriental medicine, in order to focus on only one, cannot provide adequate training, understanding, or clinical accomplishment. This is the main reason why Manaka's teaching reflects a diversity of systems and perspectives, stressing probabilities and not certainties. He prefers to encourage his students to keep an open mind and differentiate the system that will work best for an individual patient.

The statements and ideas of practitioners throughout the tradition of Oriental medicine tell us that yin and yang are necessarily different from the five phases,[3] that these systems analyze and process different information; that when the twelve meridians are replete, they spill over into the extraordinary vessels, never to return *(NJ 28:16);* that the twelve meridians, and thus the five phases, are energetically different from the extraordinary vessels, or that the five phases are different in nature from the six stages of the *Shang Han Lun*[4] and that these six stages are different from the six pairs of yin and yang meridians given the same name.[5]

Thus, for each of the diagnostic and therapeutic systems described in this volume, there are specific symptom patterns that help us with the differentiation. Some, as we will see, have very wide applicability and can be used often with many patients; others have specific limited applicability and are useful for the exceptional cases.

Diagnosis can be of utmost importance. From a broad spectrum of systems and paradigms we must select one system that can offer the appropriate treatment, or achieve the desired benefit. It is here that palpation as the main diagnostic tool is invaluable. The patterns and conformations made apparent from hara dignosis can be remarkably specific. Often palpation of secondary points or areas and taking of the pulse will enable the practitioner to quicky confirm or negate the applicability of a treatment strategy.

If a patient presents with patterns that do not match any of the patterns described in the book, or presents with patterns from several systems at once, initial treatment should be directed at a simple and generalized treatment procedure, such as hara shiatsu. There are often cases where even though the diagnosis seems straightforward, the treatment selected does not change the condition. It should be remembered that no two people have the same medical history nor the same background. Given the same signs, symptoms etc, two patients may respond differently to the same treatment, perhaps because one patient might have had some surgical procedure performed several years before, such as an appendectomy or a hysterectomy.

Manaka stresses this point over and over again: no matter how much confidence the practitioner may have for the determined diagnosis, sometimes the treatment will not succeed. It is appropriate at such a juncture to proceed with another diagnosis and treatment. Thus it is important that we be familiar with and able to use as many diagnostic and therapeutic paradigms as possible. To do this we must study widely and give particular emphasis in our studies to the *sho* or conformation of the patient, the key signs, that will help us pick out one system over another.

To determine the conformation of a patient, start with one identifiable sign, gathering information that provides differentiation to aid in identifying the pattern. Often the conformation will not involve symptoms per se, but instead evince more subtle signs, such as pulse strength, reactivity to pressure, etc. When treatment is appropriate, these signs will change. The practitioner can determine an immediate assessment of the efficacy of the treatment, and begin to formulate a prognosis, of central importance in treatment.

Preliminary to introducing diagnostic and therapeutic procedures in the specific clinical systems that follow, it is important to arrive at a description of a healthy hara. There are a variety of ways of describing and mapping out the abdomen; the following diagrams show the basic areas referred to in various places throughout the text.[6]

□

The big abdomen/hara belongs to tai yin. Around the umbilicus belongs to shao yin. The small abdomen/hara belongs to jue yin. Commonly, pain of the big abdomen is usually caused by congested food, or outside pathogen. Pain around the umbilicus is usually caused by congested heat or phlegm fire. Pain of the small abdomen is caused by congealed blood, phlegm or stagnant urine.[7] The leg yang ming (stomach) meridian comes into the lining of the abdomen. The leg tai yin (spleen) meridian rises up and comes into the abdomen. The leg jue yin (liver) meridian comes into the small abdomen. A branch of the ren mai disperses to the abdomen and the ren mai goes around the lining of the abdomen.[8]

In the words of Todo Yoshimasu,

> The hara is the basic place of the living energy. Therefore the root of all diseases are here. When you diagnose the disease you have to diagnose the hara.[9]

In particular, it is important to be able to feel and diagnose the moving qi or the source qi below the umbilicus.

> Takeshi Sawada palpated the hara of all his patients, and always checked the source qi below the umbilicus. Even if the disease didn't look severe, yet the source qi below the umbilicus was vacant, he always said that this problem would be slower to heal. If the patient looked very sick, yet the source qi was healthy, he said that recovery would be easily achieved.[10]

The Healthy Hara

The descriptions following are taken from the works of Sorei Yanagiya.[11]

In general, the area below the umbilicus around CV-6 should have a certain springiness or resilience on palpation. As one palpates up the abdomen towards the sternum one should find it becomes looser, for instance, around CV-12 and CV-15. The abdomen should have a uniform temperature, or if there are temperature variations, it should be slightly warmer below the umbilicus and slightly cooler above the umbilicus.

The only pulsing or palpitation one should feel is a very tiny pulsing on deeper pressure around and below the umbilicus. This is the moving qi between the kidneys. The heartbeat should not be too strong or visible.

The abdomen should be uniformly elastic and not tense. There should be no visible or palpable lumps on the abdomen. In comparing the left and right sides of the abdomen, the left side should feel slightly stronger than the right. If one does find some problem on the left side, it generally is not as severe as finding one on the right side.

When palpating from below the sternum, around CV-15, down to the umbilicus, there should be a slight depression in the middle around CV-12 and one around the umbilicus.

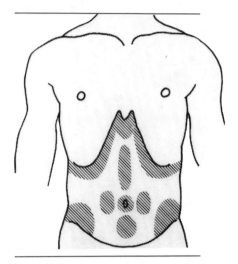

Figure 10.1 The most common and significant reflex areas on the abdomen.

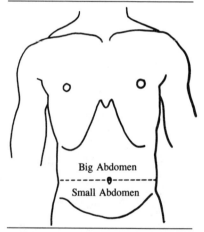

Figure 10.2 A traditional delineation from the Yixue Rumen.

The ren mai should be slightly depressed and lower than the lines of the stomach and kidney meridians.

The umbilicus should be uniform in shape and indent smoothly into the abdomen and not be too close to the surface.

If one feels elasticity and strength below the ribs, this is a sign of good lung qi.

The skin of the abdomen should be slightly moist, it should be relatively elastic and pinch up easily, it should not be too thin or too thick. It should be relatively smooth to the touch.

Over age sixty, there is a tendency for the yin and yang to become weak, so one will find some abdominal changes, especially in those over seventy years old, where below the umbilicus can be softer and weaker. These are normal and to be expected.

In general, the woman's hara will be a little softer than a man's. In a pregnant woman,[12] one should use the pad of the finger and not the tips to palpate the pulse of the moving qi between the kidneys. It should feel floating, soft, and round. (If it is sinking, hard, and tight, blood stasis may be indicated.)

Clinical Approaches

The finding of abdominal reactions that differ from those described above by Yanagiya will clue the practitioner to a possible problem or pathology. Various interpretations and treatments associated with the different patterns of these reactions can be found in the ensuing chapters, which cover the following information:

Systems of shiatsu from Naoichi Kuzome & Shinsai Ota;

Breathing exercises and several other muscle relaxing exercises;

General and specific uses of the ion pumping cords;

Manaka's meridian—mu point diagnosis and treatment principles;

Specific diagnosis and treatment of the extraordinary vessels using ion pumping cords;

Five-phase diagnosis and treatment;

Chinese clock and other biorhythmic diagnoses and treatments;

Other specific treatments including some dermatome therapy and palm acupuncture.

□

Chapter

- 11 -

Hara Diagnosis

in Practice

Hara Diagnosis in Practice

Our focus throughout this text is on palpation. It is the single thread that runs throughout the various systems and theories that we present.

The procedures of diagnosis by palpation can be complex. Because the different systems of diagnosis and the specific sets of treatments that accompany each are based on the concept of confirmation, rather than a system of "one sign - one problem," it is necessary to keep a variety of signs in mind. Failing to do so leads to the most common problem beginners find when learning abdominal diagnosis. The attempt to associate a particular abdominal finding with a single symptom or state, forgetting the overall context, results in the sense that one sign has contradictory indications. Since all the systems overlap to some degree, it is important to develop a good sense of patterns. A good general procedure is of considerable value and will enable a practitioner to obtain almost all the diagnostic information needed for both simple and differentiated diagnoses.

Naoichi Kuzome's diagnostic procedure is an excellent start. He is a shiatsu therapist in Japan, with over sixty years of experience. His diagnoses and treatments are conducted almost exclusively using abdominal confirmation. His emphasis on shiatsu has developed the concentrated sensitivity and experience that create the best teaching materials. The techniques he has proven and developed are perfect for teaching patients to treat themselves.

Differentiation of Abdominal Findings

There are essentially two parts to the diagnostic procedure. The first, palpating the abdomen, is followed by the palpation of other points, checking the pulse and other significant diagnostic symptoms to confirm the abdominal diagnosis. A complete diagnosis and a treatment plan will follow from this procedure, regardless of the treatment system used. Practitioners with vast experience, such as Manaka or Kuzome, need to question the patient only briefly, making sure the patient has had the opportunity to express any concerns.

In the simplest case, differentiation of abdominal findings may be reduced to a series of easy steps. If for example one finds tenderness or tightness on the area around the umbilicus, particularly around KI-16, look for other significant indications:

Step One: Palpate KI-3, the kidney meridian, and GB-25 to confirm or eliminate a diagnosis of kidney meridian imbalance or kidney dysfunction.

Step Two: Palpate ST-11, SP-4, and PC-6, to confirm or eliminate the chong mai as a treatment target.

Step Three: Palpate ST-12, ST-9, KI-8, KI-6, and LU-7 to confirm or eliminate the yin qiao mai as a treatment target.

Step Four: Palpate GB-41, TW-5, and the gallbladder meridian to confirm or eliminate the dai mai as a treatment target.

Step Five: Palpate SP-3, SP-21, LV-13, and the spleen meridian to confirm or eliminate the spleen meridian or spleen function as sources of the problem.

Remember that a complete procedure could include all reactive areas or points on the abdomen. For each confirmation there are usually specific treatments with specific methods for evaluation of the treatment in process. When these treatments involve points on other areas of the body, such as the back shu points, check these points for reactiveness as well.

In evaluating a patient's condition, it is also valuable to keep in mind that a complete medical intake and monitoring is not without significance. The body is an intricate entity. All available sources of further information need be considered. While it is often easy to obtain a clear diagnosis, it is as often difficult to select the best acupoints and techniques to treat the condition.

Significant Reactions

Observation of point reactiveness is important in treatment as well as in diagnosis. By monitoring any changes in palpatory response during treatment, a practitioner may immediately assess the effectiveness of the treatment. If the reactiveness improves during the treatment, the body's healing has been activated. An improvement of reactivity is a trustworthy positive sign, and holds greater significance than patient report of improvement during treatment.

Instances of contradictory signs also occur. As a start, it is advisable to assume that what you sense with your hands is significant. In some systems of diagnosis, such as kanpo yaku, the very contradiction of the practitioner's observation and the patient's report may suggest a pattern. Usually fashioning the various reactions into a suitable harmonic for your diagnostic system presents the most difficulty. Not only do you need to gain a sense of the range of reactions between "reactive" and "very reactive," but you also need to distinguish between "no reaction" and "lack of reaction."

Both Manaka and Shudo say that reactions fit two categories. The first category is oversensitivity; on palpation the patient will report sensations. This tends more to indicate a condition with accompanying repletion. The second category is lack of reaction, undersensitivity. This is an advanced vacancy condition, where the patient is unable to report anything, as distinguished from a normal, healthy response.

☐

Significant Findings

While some treatment systems pay greater attention to one set of findings, and less to others, the most significant abdominal reactions are consistent across all systems. Kuzome has said that if a patient is motivated to come for treatment, regardless of what the reported problem, one will always find something significant on the hara. If initially you can't find anything, go back and check again. These are not empty words. He has palpated and treated over two hundred eighty thousand patients! At the very least a second look will increase your sensitivity.

Temperature variations

With the hand parallel to and just above the surface of the abdominal skin, check for any significant heat differences. A sensation of qi might be felt at a certain point, perhaps as the sensation of an updraught striking the hand or fingers, like a wind or a gentle breath. This updraught may be cool, cold, warm, or hot. A sensation almost like electricity might be noticed, or a pressured sensation as the hand passes over an area on the surface of the patient's abdomen. All these sensations have significance, depending on the points or areas affected.

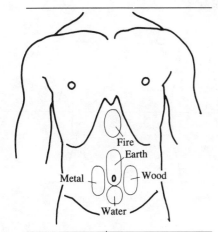

Figure 11.1 Traditional five-phase reflex areas.

When feeling the patient's skin surface with the hand, one should check the five areas of the abdomen that correspond to the *Nan Jing* five-phase areas, the three areas of the torso that correspond to the three heaters, the chest, the area above the umbilicus, and area below the umbilicus. One should also feel the four quadrants of the abdomen. Temperature variations in these areas are significant. As one begins to palpate the abdomen, superficial temperature differences and temperature variations at different depths can be noticed. For instance, one may find:

> Warm on the surface, warm below.
> Warm on the surface, cool below.
> Cool on the surface, warm below.
> Cool on the surface, cool below.

The significance of these findings can be seen within the eight-principle diagnostic construct, as hot, cold, internal, and external. Generally, heat tends more to reflect repletion and cold to reflect vacancy.

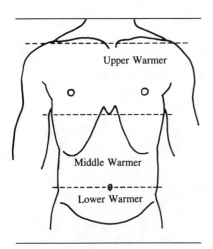

Figure 11.2 The three warmers.

The skin surface on many patients will be observed as warmer above the umbilicus and cooler below. This is a general indication of counterflow qi, or vacancy below and repletion above.

Tension

Tension or lack of tension of the muscles on the abdomen should be closely observed, particularly in the area below the rib cage and along the rectus abdominus muscles. Although tension may be perceived as a replete condition, it usually stems from an underlying vacancy, and thus more accurately reflects this vacancy. Some practitioners, among them Sorei Yanagiya, simply think of it as a vacancy sign.

Lack of tension in the muscles is generally a good sign that indicates an elastic, healthy abdomen. (Remember that lack of tension does not mean soft or loose muscles.) Tension is often found on the abdominal muscles. ☐

In the many years of experience of such practitioners as Manaka and Kuzome, it is considered propitious if the muscles of the abdomen relax, establishing an equal tension of left and right sides, during treatment or over a course of treatments. Once this tension is released, the body's natural healing powers take over. This is equally true for the other signs that may be found on the abdomen — pressure pain, tightness, hardness, lumps.

Pressure pain

Pressure pain found on palpation points is almost always significant. It may be found superficially, or deeper with stronger pressure. Severe or sharp pains are often more significant than dull, achy pains. Generally, all painful focii are important (Kuzome confirms this). When pressure pain is found, regardless of depth or severity, other reactions should be observed. It is important, for example, to watch the patient's face and body. If the face or body flinches, the pain is probably more severe than the patient might report. Watching the patient also enables you to judge what pressure to apply to the reactive areas; it is important to not cause too much discomfort for the patient. Usually the patient will not flinch if the pain is dull or achy. Some patients flinch no matter what points one palpates. In these cases, think of checking areas of the body that tend to become reactive with stress or emotional problems. Psychological conditions may be indicated by this type of sensitivity. Kuzome suggests that one might check around SP-10, ST-36 to ST 38, and between the third and fourth toes. If there is reactiveness on any or all of these points, shiatsu would be an appropriate therapy. These points and areas can relax the abdomen, making it less sensitive, so that you may return to your diagnostic procedure.

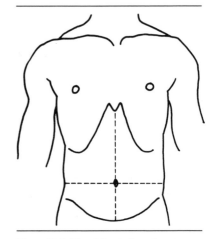

Figure 11.3 The abdominal quadrants.

Pressure pain tends to manifest in specific focii that can reflect specific organs or meridians, and easily provide more precise diagnoses. Remember that pain is generally thought of as a repletion sign *(NJ 48)*. If the pain is relieved by touch, or pressure, it might be more a sign of vacancy. Conversely, if pressure will not relieve the pain, it might be more a sign of repletion.[1]

Fluid sounds

When palpating the abdomen and subcostal region, sounds of unabsorbed liquid, such as sloshing or gurgling, may be detected. Since the stomach is the organ most usually affected, this finding is commonly termed fluid stagnation in the stomach. It may be found below the sternum and above the umbilicus, though it can occur anywhere in the abdomen.

Traveling or reactive sensations

On palpation, either superficially or, more frequently, with deeper pressure, the patient may report sensations or reactions that travel to certain areas of the abdomen, or elsewhere in the body. Kuzome reports that these reactions may also be felt elsewhere in the body, running up, down inward, almost anywhere. They may even be felt in the shoulders, arms, hands, neck, face, head, back, legs, or feet. The most significant of these findings may radiate to the areas of the body where the patient's problems are located, or to the organs or meridians that are the source of those problems. For instance, there might be an area on the abdomen that with pressure elicits a sensation that runs to or is felt in the lower back. If the patient has a chronic low back problem, this point might be prioritized in the diagnostic assessment. Similarly, a pain might run into the liver, where the patient has some problem; or to a certain area on the head, where the patient experiences severe headaches.

These reactive areas of the abdomen are viewed by Kuzome as the root of the problem that manifests in the affected area of the body. This is easily understood in context of the internal pathways, fascia, and energetic centers and functions that exist in the hara. In these instances, a more effective treatment will be based on a more detailed understanding of the theoretical phases of energetics. Finding areas that have traveling or reflective responses, even if they do not reach to an area where problems are known to exist, is nevertheless important.

Strength and weakness of abdominal musculature

Strength or weakness of the muscles of the abdomen can be diagnostically significant. Generally, the muscles should have a good strength, and some resilience or springiness. Too much strength may be a sign of repletion. Weak, flaccid muscles, or lack of strength, tonus, or resilience, may indicate vacancy.

Tightness — hardness and softness — looseness

Tightness differs from tension. With muscular tension there will be some rebound, some springiness to the muscles, and the muscles will be clearly defined. With tightness, the muscle feels hard and there is much less or no springiness or rebound. Tightness is generally something that is more exacerbated and harder to treat than tension. It is usually seen as some kind of vacancy. Softness and looseness may appear similar to weakness, except that some springiness remains in the muscles. Though a sign of vacancy, softness does not indicate as great a vacancy as does weakness.

These indications may also be found at different depths. For instance, there may be superficial tightness that is so hard, one cannot press any deeper. Or one might find:

> Hardness on the surface and hardness below.
> Hardness on the surface and softness below.
> Softness on the surface and hardness below.
> Softness on the surface and softness below.

Palpation around the midline will often reveal softness on the surface and hardness below. This pattern is also common around the spine.

Kuzome reports that if the hara is weak or soft (signs of vacancy), some hard, tight, or tense spot will always be found elsewhere. This hard or tense spot is a good area to treat with shiatsu. Careful attention should be given to the condition and indications of a patient with a vacant hara.

□

Lumps

The significance of lumps on the abdomen may vary with their location, size, and quality. Lumps may be soft or hard; stationary or mobile. Moving lumps, more yang in nature, are easier to treat. Stationary lumps, more yin in nature, are thus more difficult to treat (NJ 56). Often, lumps may be only stools or gas in the intestines. If so, they will pass after application of shiatsu or some other treatment. It is important not to jump to diagnostic conclusions too early. If with passage of stools or wind, the lumps remain, then it is important to determine their cause. Persistent lumps need be reexamined by a qualified specialist to assure that no tumor is present.

Most lumps are not tumorous, but consist of knots of muscle or other tissues. Sometimes peculiar lumps can be found that evince no particular pathological cause. Again, the location and qualities of such lumps determine their diagnostic significance. Lumps may be found with superficial pressure and with deeper pressure. Some elicit pressure pain or reflective sensations. Generally, it is advisable not to palpate directly on the lump, but rather on the edges.

Pulsing or palpitations

Pulsings or palpitations on the abdomen are usually signs of vacancy. Their significance varies with their relative strength, depth, and location. Sometimes these pulsings or palpitations are visibly obvious, indicating greater vacancy. Sometimes the pulsing may be palpable with slight pressure, sometimes only with deeper pressure. The pulsing or palpitation can be very gentle and mild, or it can be very strong.

Generally, there should be no pulsings on the abdomen, except a very slight pulsing around or below the umbilicus found with deeper pressure. This can be the moving qi between the kidneys, and is viewed as a positive sign when it is the only pulsing found. Though most practitioners feel that the pulsing in the abdomen is the descending or abdominal aorta, Tohaku Ishi disagrees with this idea. He states that a pulsing felt with superficial pressure is the superior mesenteric artery, whereas the pulsing felt with deeper pressure may be the aorta.[2]

Skin qualities and textures

Skin that is loose and creased may indicate vacancy; skin that is tight may be a sign of repletion. When healthy, the skin will "pinch-up" easily between the thumb and forefinger, and evince some springiness. If the skin is tight, it will be difficult to pinch the skin; if the skin is loose, the skin will easily pinch, but will have no springiness and might not at once return to its original shape or position. In cases where the skin is tight there is a general sense of having to pinch the underlying tissues as well as the skin. In cases of extreme vacancy, when the skin is pinched it remains pinched and will not return to flatness.

Other differential sensations that may be observed using the skin-pinching technique include pain or tightness, tension, small lumps, and sometimes vague sensations that aren't readily described other than as "there's something here." This technique may be used as a means of diagnosing obviously reactive points and those points where the patient is undersensitive. Pinching is the most useful method for differentiating non-reaction from lack of sensitivity. Some practitioners, such as Denmei Shudo, use pinching with great dexterity and skill, being able to diagnose the entire hara and the lengths of the meridians in just a few minutes.

Remember to note the textures of the skin:

> If the skin is dry, it can be a sign of vacancy.
> If the skin is too moist, it is generally not a good sign.
> If the skin has some moisture, but not too much,
> this is normal.

The roughness or smoothness of the skin can also be significant, as can the color tones, paleness, or redness. The areas affected generally indicate the significance of the findings.

Swellings and indentations

If there are areas on the abdomen that are swollen or indented, and these differ from what one might expect in a healthy hara, these can be accorded significance. Swellings or indentations are usually palpable. Swelling tends to be a sign of repletion, indentation a sign of vacancy. It should be noted that when we speak of repletion on the abdomen (tension, tightness, swelling, etc.), it is generally associated with a vacancy. This is termed false repletion. Any signs, whether palpable or visible, that deviate from a healthy hara, are diagnostically significant.

Diagnostic Procedure

Just before initiating the diagnostic routine, it is advisable to increase one's level of sensitivity. Tsugio Nagatomo, a Japanese practitioner who attained the distinguished age of more than ninety years before his recent demise, often recommended the following procedure for developing finger sensitivity:

> When palpating, the most important thing is to develop finger sensitivity. To cultivate this sensitivity, try the following: Sitting with legs crossed and hands placed together, palm to palm, fingers to fingers, empty the mind and do only slow deep breathing. After 10 to 30 minutes (depending upon the individual), one can feel sensations in the ends of one's middle fingers, and one can see a white, translucent, thin thread between the fingers. When the thread is seen clearly, the sensitivity should be sufficiently developed. When palpating the body, one should not miss anything. This practice needs to be repeated.[3]

Nagatomo recommends a further method to facilitate this development. If one places small magnets between the fingers before this meditation, the thread may be seen and felt more readily. With sufficient practice, more specialized procedures may be adapted to suit an individual practitioner's ease or need.

☐

Most practitioners feel that it is important for the patient to lie supine, with legs outstretched and arms by the sides, during the diagnostic procedure. If this position is too uncomfortable for the patient, bend the legs, even up to a ninety degree angle, until they are comfortable. In these cases, the practitioner must be much more sensitive and attentive, as it is easier to miss diagnostic signs on the abdomen, for the muscles of the abdomen will be looser and less obviously reactive.

The patient should relieve any urgency of bowel or bladder before palpation. It is important to keep the patient relaxed and comfortable. In particular, the rectus abdominus muscles should be relaxed. Some patients seem to have initial reservations about having their abdomen palpated. To this end Kuzome advises that as one begins diagnosis, only the gentlest pressure need be applied over the abdomen — that is, just depressing the skin gently to touch the underlying muscles. This serves two purposes, to reassure and relax the patient, and to gain an indication of what may be found and where. Gentle pressure should be applied with finger tips, vertically or perpendicularly. This gentle pressure diagnosis should be applied as follows:

Step One: First, palpate along the ren mai line from the sternum to just above the pubic symphysis. One should avoid pushing the umbilicus itself.

Step Two: Palpate down the left kidney meridian line, from just below the sternum to just above the pubic symphysis.

Step Three: Palpate down the left stomach meridian line, from just below the ribs to just above the pubic symphysis.

Step Four: Palpate down the left spleen meridian line, from just below the ribs, to just above the pubic symphysis.

Step Five: Palpate up the right kidney meridian line, from just above the pubic symphysis, to just below the sternum.

Step Six: Palpate up the right stomach meridian line, from just above the pubic symphysis, to just below the ribs.

Step Seven: Palpate up the right spleen meridian line, from just above the pubic symphysis to just below the ribs.

Step Eight: Palpate under the ribs from the sternum out to the left side.

Step Nine: Palpate under the ribs from the sternum out to the right side.

Step Ten: Palpate from the anterior edge of the left iliac spine, down to the right, along the top of the pubic symphysis, and up to the right iliac spine. Finish at the same spot on the right as one started from on the left.

Step Eleven: Palpate the area just above and around the anterior and superior edges of the left iliac spine.

Step Twelve: Palpate the area just above and around the anterior and superior edges of the right iliac spine.

☐

This order serves two purposes. Palpating down the lines on the left will help move stools through the descending colon. Palpating up the lines on the right will help move stools up the ascending colon. Thus, the movement of the large intestines is stimulated. Since the left side of the body is yang and the right side is yin, palpating downward on the left will help curb the tendencies of yang to move upwards. Palpating upward on the right will help curb the tendencies of yin to move downward.

Thus the procedure should be performed as indicated by the numerical sequence in Figure 11.4.

Kuzome notes that in steps one to seven, following the "meridian lines," should not be taken too literally. This instruction refers to the general areas each line passes through, and should not be restricted to just the meridian trajectories themselves. Having followed this procedure with gentle pressure, repeat the round with slightly firmer pressure. In most cases, this second round will be sufficient to locate the more reactive areas and points. When palpating any point, and particularly a point on the abdomen, pressure should never be applied suddenly; it should always be applied smoothly and evenly.

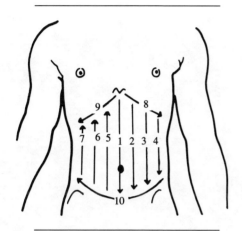

Figure 11.4

Kuzome talks about five depths or degrees of pressure:

The first is touching the skin.
The second is pressing into the muscles.
The third is pressing harder to just touch the organs.
The fourth is pressing into the organs, or to touch the deeper organs.
The fifth is pressing as though you were trying to touch the spine.

This does not mean that one should go through five rounds of diagnosis at each increasing level of pressure. Rather, it is an indication of the relative depths that pressure may be applied to the abdomen, and a gauge of where reactions are found.

For people with tense or tight abdominal muscles, reaching the fourth of fifth degree of pressure or depth without causing considerable pain will be difficult. Kuzome recommends applying pressure to the depth at which the reactions are found.

When palpating a vacant hara, though very little pressure is applied, the hands sink in easily even to the point of touching the spine. This is the fifth degree. Someone with tense rectus abdominus muscles, a traveling sensation, or severe pain, would experience significant discomfort at the second to third degree of pressure, just touching the organs. If a first, then a second round of palpation gathers little diagnostic data, a third round may be initiated, with firmer pressure.

In general, when tense, tight, loose, tender, or traveling reactions, or lumps, are found, it is advisable to make a second, confirmatory palpation. Again, as Kuzome comments, where an abdomen is weak and vacant, lacking muscle tone, the fingers will sink in easily; there will always be a tense or tight area within the weak area. Locating this area should be given special attention. Compare the left and right rectus abdominus muscles, and give close scrutiny to the areas around the umbilicus, particularly KI-16 and ST-25, and to the whole ren mai trajectory on the abdomen. Other areas

□

that are generally seen to be of greater significance are CV-12 and CV-6; the subcostal regions; the areas at the sides of the abdomen, between the ribs and the iliac spine; and the areas at the anterior and superior aspects of the iliac spine. Completing this procedure should produce a clear "map" of the abdomen. Good record-keeping is a help.

Now the diagnosis may be expanded. Depending on what was found and the possibilities of correspondence, parts of the diagnosis may be confirmed or eliminated. Based on the information in the following chapters, one can determine the phases, the extraordinary vessels or meridians, organs, or functions that may be affected, and the associated points to treat. Other relevant points on the front of the body, the chest, and the abdomen may then be palpated, with special attention given to the mu points. Next, the points on the arms and legs may be examined. Have the patient change position to examine the back, paying special attention to the back shu points. Finally, feel the points on the head and neck, all the time noting the points that are reactive.

This procedure is a simple, thorough, and systematic approach to hara diagnosis. It can be performed on virtually anyone who can lie down. It should, for the sake of thorough monitoring, be performed each time you see the patient.

If a clear diagnosis has been obtained from this procedure, then the correct treatment should be easy to ascertain. If the diagnosis is not clear, information from the pulse, looking, listening and smelling, and asking will be necessary to complete the diagnosis. Remember that diagnosis is always relative to the state of health. Your comparisons are to the healthy hara. It is also important to remember, as we have discussed, that acupoints are not stationary. They are said to have a location, but it is more useful to think of these locations as starting points for palpation.

The case history given below is illustrative of the options available in a single case.

Patient: Male, age 29.

Main complaints: Intestinal problems; gas with occasional cramping; tendency towards constipation; some fatigue and mild low back pain.

Abdominal findings: Hardness and tightness from CV-13 down to CV-10; mild tension around the umbilicus, mild sensitivity at KI-16; laxness below the umbilicus, especially soft around CV-6 to CV-4; mild palpitation around the umbilicus.

Treatment Selection - General: Kuzome's shiatsu therapy may be selected, treating on the area above the umbilicus (CV-13 - CV-10). Or, the anpuku massage techniques might be preferred. If the patient's breathing were noticeably weak and shallow, the patient could be shown corrective breathing exercises.

Treatment Selection - Specific: The following indications are clear and require further differentiation and confirmation: *Spleen vacancy:* Symptoms of intestinal problems and fatigue; reactions in the periumbilical and supra-umbilical regions. *Yin qiao mai-ren mai connection:* intestinal problems; fatigue; low back pain; tightness above the umbilicus and laxness below; some periumbilical reactions.

□

Further palpation reveals tightness at ST-12 and LU-1, softness at SP-3, and pressure pain at LU-7 and KI-6. The patient in clear light shows some darkness below the eyes, an indication of possible kidney patterns. The pulse reveals weakness in the kidney (left deep chi position). These further findings would tend to favor selection of the yin qiao mai-ren mai with ion-pumping cords, though the existence of a spleen vacancy would still remain a possibility, since many signs and symptoms, excluding the pulse, are present. For this patient, a good treatment plan might be to apply the ion-pumping cords to yin qiao mai-ren mai for 10 to 20 minutes. Then Kuzome shiatsu might be administered to resolve any remaining tightness in the supraumbilical region. The patient could also be instructed to perform this same shiatsu technique at home. Corrective breathing techniques would be additionally useful as regular home practice. The remainder of the treatment would focus on treatment of, for example, relevant back shu points and then appropriate local symptom-control points.

The suggested treatment here is not requisite; any of the available options could be selected for focal treatment, choosing from any of the procedures described. Further, needling an open point first might well have preceded all possible steps as a method of clarifying the symptoms to arrive at an accurate diagnosis.

Common Patterns of Abdominal Reactions

Based on the clinical view of the authors whose works are described in this text, the following series of drawings illustrate common patterns of abdominal reactions. Some are general, some very specific, and some require differentiation because of many overlapping possibilities. Treatment procedures and therapeutic principles will be described throughout the remaining chapters of this text for these patterns.

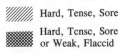

Hard, Tense, Sore

Hard, Tense, Sore or Weak, Flaccid

Figure 11.5

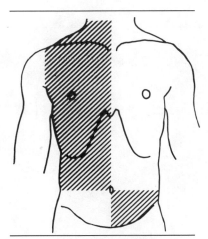

Figure 11.5a The abdominal quadrant areas can be expanded to include the chest region.

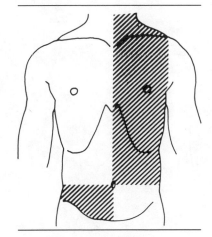

Figure 11.5b The abdominal quadrant areas can be expanded to include the chest region.

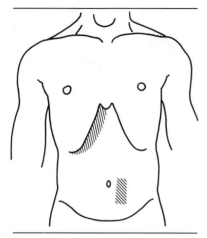

Figure 11.6 Liver vacancy.

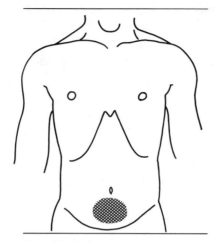

Figure 11.7 Kidney vacancy.

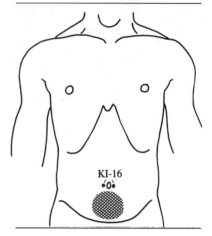

Figure 11.8 Kidney vacancy.

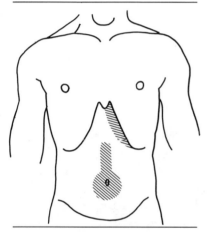

Figure 11.9 Typical spleen vacancy.

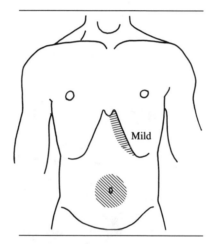

Figure 11.10 Spleen vacancy.

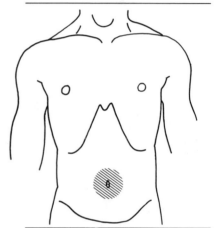

Figure 11.11 Spleen vacancy. Sometimes small intestine problem.

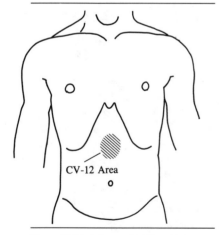

Figure 11.12 Spleen-stomach problems.

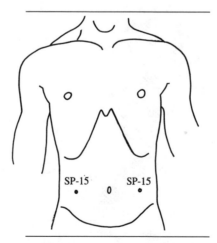

Figure 11.13 Sometimes spleen problem.

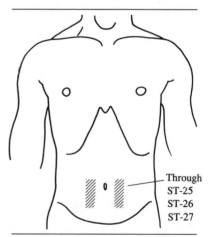

Figure 11.14 Intestinal problems. Digestive problems.

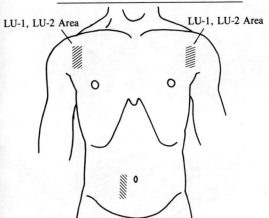

Figure 11.15 Lung vacancy.

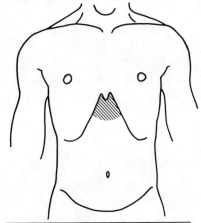

Figure 11.16 Heart problem.

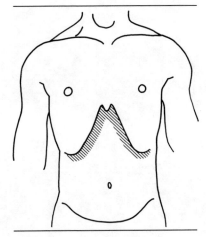

Figure 11.17 Yin Wei-Chong Mai (Possibly liver and spleen related).

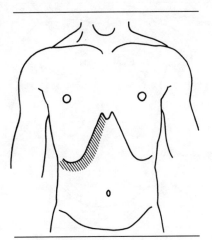

Figure 11.18 Yin Wei-Chong Mai. (Possibly liver vacancy)

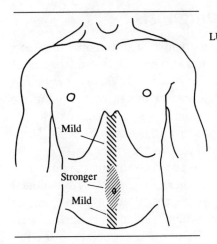

Figure 11.19 Yin Qiao-Ren Mai.

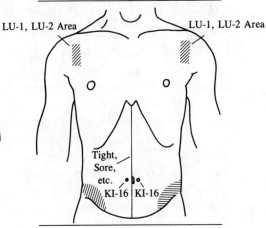

Figure 11.20 Yin Qiao-Ren Mai.

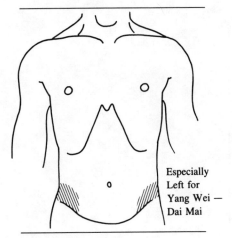

Figure 11.21 Yang Wei-Dai Mai. Yang Qiao-Du Mai. Yin Qiao-Ren Mai. Gallbladder.

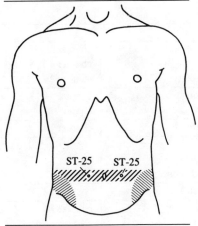

Figure 11.22 Yang Wei-Dai Mai.

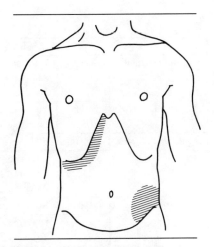

Figure 11.23 "The Cross Syndrome": Right Yin Wei-Chong Mai. Left Yang Wei-Dai Mai.

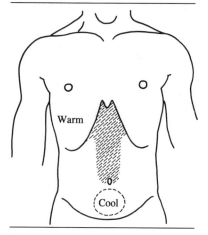
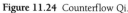

Figure 11.24 Counterflow Qi.

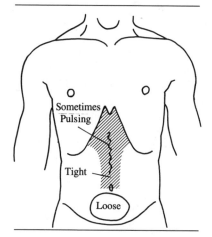

Figure 11.25 Counterflow Qi.

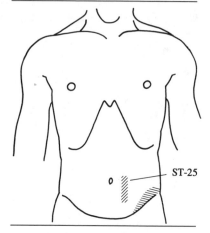

Figure 11.26 Blood stasis.

Abdominal Differential Diagnosis

The following tables describe the possibilities of differential diagnosis and treatment for the most significant and common areas and points of abdominal reaction. Each area or point is described with chapter references for both "General Treatments" — shiatsu treatment following the style of Naoichi Kuzome (chapter 12); anpuku massage treatment (chapter 13); and abdominal breathing therapy (chapter 14) — and "Specific Treatments" requiring further confirmation and pattern identification — extraordinary vessel treatment (chapter 16); five-phase treatment (chapter 15); and other specific treatments patterns (chapter 17). As briefly mentioned above and described in greater detail in chapter 18, open points can be used at any time and thus can function in both general and specific treatment. Hence no specific reference is made to the open points in the following examples.

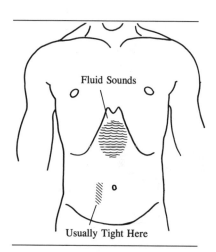

Figure 11.27 Fluid Stagnation in the stomach.

Subcostal reactions			
Bilateral reactions	General	Kuzome treatment	chapter 12
		Anpuku treatment	chapter 13
		Poor breathing ability	chapter 14
	Specific	Yin wei mai-Chong mai	chapter 16
		Liver vacancy (possibly spleen too)	chapter 15
Right side reactions	General	Kuzome treatment	chapter 12
	Specific	Liver problems	chapters 15, 16, 17
		Yin wei-Chong mai	chapter 16
		As part of "Cross syndrome"	chapters 16, 17
Left side reactions	General	Kuzome treatment	chapter 12
	Specific	Spleen vacancy	chapter 15
		Yin wei-Chong mai	chapter 16

Substernal reactions		
General	Kuzome treatment	chapter 12
Specific	Heart problem	chapter 15
	Yin wei-Chong mai	chapter 16
	Biorhythm fire-phase treatment	chapter 18
	Palm therapy	chapter 17
Supra-umbilical midline reactions		
General	Kuzome treatment	chapter 12
	Anpuku treatment	chapter 13
Specific	Spleen vacancy	chapter 15
	Spleen-stomach problems	chapter 16
	Yin qiao mai-Ren mai	chapter 16
	Biorhythm phasal treatment	chapter 18
	Palm therapy	chapter 17
Periumbilical reactions		
General	Kuzome treatment	chapter 12
Specific	Spleen vacancy	chapter 15
	Kidney problems	chapters 15, 16
	Yin qiao mai-Ren mai	chapter 16
	Yin wei mai-Chong mai	chapter 16
	Yang wei mai-Dai mai	chapter 16
	Taiji treatment	chapter 17
	Biorhythm water-phase treatment	chapter 18
	Palm therapy	chapter 17
Sub-umbilical reactions		
General	Kuzome treatment	chapter 12
	Anpuku treatment	chapter 13
	Poor breathing ability*	chapter 14
Specific	Kidney vacancy	chapter 15
	Yin qiao mai-Ren mai	chapter 16
	Taiji treatment**	chapter 17
Left of umbilicus reactions		
General	Kuzome treatment	chapter 12
	Anpuku treatment	chapter 13
	Exercise therapy	chapter 14
Specific	Liver problems	chapters 15, 17
	Intestinal problems	chapter 16
Right of umbilicus reactions		
General	Kuzome treatment	chapter 12
	Anpuku treatment	chapter 13
	Exercise therapy	chapter 14
Specific	Lung vacancy	chapter 15
	Intestinal problems	chapter 16
	Liver problems	chapter 17

*   If weak, cold
** If frail and distraught

Anterior superior iliac spine reactions		
General	Kuzome treatment	chapter 12
Specific	Gallbladder meridian	chapter 16
	Yang wei mai-Dai mai*	chapter 16
	Yang qiao mai-Du mai	chapter 16
	Yin qiao mai-Ren mai	chapter 16
	Part of Cross-syndrome*	chapters 16, 17
KI-16		
General	Periumbilical Kuzome treatment	chapter 12
Specific	Spleen vacancy	chapter 15
	Kidney vacancy	chapter 15
	Kidney meridian problems	chapter 16
	Chong mai-Yin wei mai	chapter 16
	Yin qiao mai-Ren mai	chapter 16
	Dai mai-Yang wei mai	chapter 16
	Biorhythm phasal treatment	chapter 18
	Taiji treatment	chapter 17
ST-25		
General	Kuzome treatment	chapter 12
specific	Left - liver problems	chapters 15, 17
	Right - liver problems	chapter 17
	Right - lung vacancy	chapter 15
	Triple warmer meridian problems	chapter 16
	Dai mai-Yang wei mai	chapter 16
LV-14		
General	Kuzome treatment	chapter 12
specific	Liver vacancy	chapter 15
	Liver meridian problems	chapter 16
	Yin wei mai-Chong mai	chapter 16
	Part of Cross-syndrome**	chapters 16, 17
LU-1		
Specific	Lung vacancy	chapter 15
	Lung meridian problems	chapter 16
	Ren mai-Yin qiao mai	chapter 16
CV-12		
General	Kuzome treatment	chapter 12
	Poor breathing ability***	chapter 14
Specific	Spleen vacancy	chapter 15
	Spleen-stomach problems	chapters 15, 16
	Ren mai-Yin qiao mai	chapter 16
	Biorhythm phasal treatment	chapter 18

* Typically left
** If on right
*** Tight with looseness below navel

CV-6		
General	Kuzome treatment Anpuku treatment Poor breathing ability	chapter 12 chapter 13 chapter 14
Specific	Kidney vacancy Ren mai-yin qiao mai	chapter 15 chapter 16
Fluid accumulation in stomach		
General	Kuzome treatment Anpuku treatment	chapter 12 chapter 13
Specific	Treat accompanying reactions Especially to right of umbilicus	chapters 15, 16 17

If reaction is found in one of the above areas, no further confirmation is necessary for general treatment therapy. There is also the option of further differentiating and confirming the diagnosis to formulate a specific treatment plan. The above information describes the most common options when using this book. In most cases treatment focuses on the general or specific treatments. In difficult or advanced cases it may be better to select from both to accelerate the recovery process. Ultimately selections need be made according to the practitioner's judgement and preference.

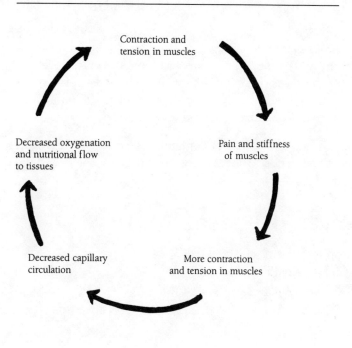

Figure 11.28

As a final summary of palpatory diagnosis and to show the most significant abdominal areas in relation to other body areas where reactions manifest, we would like to examine the concept of *kori,* a common Japanese term referring to the tight, stiff, tense areas of the body. The term kori also refers to pain, stiffness, and other secondary problems that result from the initial build-up of tension.

It is generally believed that lifestyle is the main cause of the tensions that accrue in the muscles, factors such as poor diet, stress, bad posture, and incorrect exercise probably being the most common. These cause a build-up of tension in the muscles which then feeds into a vicious cycle where the resultant pain and stiffness causes further contraction and tension of the muscles. This leads to decreased circulation at the capillary bed level, which then causes decreased oxygenation and nutritional flow to the tissues, resulting in further contraction and tightening of the muscles, fascia, and connective tissues causing more pain and stiffness, etc.

We can envision this kori, or build-up of muscle tension, as causing energy blockages. Physiologically we can argue that the increased tension accompanying muscle swelling affects at least four systems, with physiological changes in each. It can be seen to compress the lymph vessels, weakening the immune system. Compressing the venous system, it causes build-up of carbon dioxide and other waste materials such as lactic acid with increased pooling of blood (stagnant blood). Compressing the arterial system, it decreases oxygenation and flow of nutrition to the tissues. Compressing the nerve branches it causes irritation, pain and "error signals" — misfiring of nervous impulses. All these affect organ functions quite profoundly.

Through the experiences and lineages of many traditions and practitioners, release of the areas where kori occurs has more than just the effect of relieving local pains or tensions associated with them. It also affects the general levels of immunological function, regulations of tissue and organ function, and feeding and cleansing of the tissues and organs.

The following are some of the most commonly seen areas where kori develops, each of which tends to be associated with particular or general symptomology.

around GV-20
in the occipital region, BL-10, GB-20 area
around GV-14
around GB-21 on the tops of the shoulders
on the sternocleidomastoid muscles
around ST-11, ST-12
around SI-11
around BL-38
around TW-15
around LU-1
down the bladder meridians lateral to the thoracic and lumbar vertebrae
in the PSIS regions
at the sides of the sacrum
around the center of the buttocks
in the subcostal regions

☐

along the rectus abdominus muscles
along the linea alba
in the ASIS regions
along the superior surface of the pubic bone
in the inguinal joint
around LI-10
around LI-4
in the cubital crease on the palmar side
around GB-31
around LV-9
in the popliteal crease
around the "eyes of the knee"
around ST-36, ST-37
around the gastrocnemius muscles
anterior to the medial and lateral sides of the Achilles tendons,
    posterior to the malleoli

Summary

In part of his commentary on *Nan Jing 8,* Sosen Hirooka gives us a reminder of the forces we are investigating when we palpate the abdomen. Simple in outlook and description, it refers to an elegant idea:

> On pressing below the umbilicus, the hand will feel a tiny moving response [pulsing]; the numbers of this movement are the same as the numbers [of the pulse] at cun ko [radial pulse]. If one is slow, the other is slow. If one is rapid, the other is rapid. Using this pulsing, we know how many beats the radial pulse beats. This is truly caused by the original movements of the kidney qi [moving qi].

> Press below the umbilicus. If it is tight deep inside [prison] or causes pain, this is a sign of kidney disease. Press this place, if it is not tight deep inside and it is not painful, but is full, has quality, harmony, and moderacy, and the hand feels a tiny movement, response, this is healthy. If the person is oversensitive and is easily affected by the environment, it will be hard to feel this tiny movement. This is the rule of abdominal diagnosis.

> It is difficult to diagnose people of high position or women [who won't allow their abdomens to be palpated]. Therefore by watching, listening, and smelling constantly and very attentively and not being lazy about it, the mysterious shen will come into your body [one will begin to feel the moving qi without touching].

> Bian Que, the writer of the *Nan Jing,* did this. Below the umbilicus is the dividing earth of dantian, qihai, and yinjiao [dantian, CV-6 and CV-7]; these are the places where one can feel this tiny movement.[4]

We hear in this quotation the encouragement to develop our observation and intuition. As Sosen Hirooka says, we should not be lazy.

□

Chapter

- 12 -

Hara

Shiatsu

Hara Shiatsu

Naoichi Kuzome, a shiatsu therapist living in Kotohira, Japan, has practiced for over sixty of his eighty-five years. His case reports include two hundred eighty thousand patients. The author was honored and fortunate to have gained the opportunity to study with him. The information herein presented is a summary and compilation of his many years of experience and represents most of his written work on hara diagnosis and treatment.[1]

Kuzome's diagnostics and treatments are straightforward and extremely effective. They may be used in a clinical setting or as home treatments. His diagnosis is almost exclusively abdominal with attention to hardness, tightness, tension, lumps, looseness, weakness, and reactions or sensations that move with pressure. The latter are particularly noteworthy in Kuzome's system. Almost exclusively his treatments are simple shiatsu techniques performed on the reactive areas found, thus providing a range of home treatment techniques that complement clinical practice. The results obtained by these treatments are well known; the acupuncturist should not fall victim to the prejudice that only needle treatments are "professional." Over the course of clinical practice, there will certainly be cases where these treatments alone are all that is required.

The information in this chapter differs from the usual acupuncture literature as there is no separation of the diagnostic and therapeutic phases. The procedures are actually very simple to use and require no further diagnostic confirmation. The treatments themselves are almost entirely oriented to patient self-involvement in the healing process. Practitioners of this therapy act as teachers, using their skills to show patients how to treat themselves. Coupled with breathing exercises, exercise, and the use of moxa at home, many problems are relieved without further clinical visits. Other problems respond best to home treatments in conjunction with clinical procedures. This style of treatment helps relieve the financial burden associated with many chronic conditions. The psychological and spiritual benefits of a patient becoming more "in-touch" with themselves through active involvement in their healing process are now becoming more generally recognized. Kuzome's work is a practical step toward this ideal.

Many people tend to limit the application of shiatsu to use as a method of relaxation, rather than as a method of treating disease. Kuzome comments that he treats everything from the abdomen, even knee pain or toothache. He stresses the importance of home treatments and patient involvement in their healing process:

> Explain to the patients that even if their symptoms go away, they should not stop treating themselves until the lump or tightness on the hara has completely passed away as well. The symptoms can easily return from this lack of self-attention.

He also notes that many patients are lazy, not following through with their treatments. These people don't get as good results as those who are diligent. Whether the patient is diligent or not, the self-treatment techniques reinforce clinical treatments, providing a firm base of consistent improvement. This becomes clearer, not just in practice, but also in the analysis of these techniques. Many of the abdominal patterns relate to the diagnosis of internal medicine and acupuncture. In large part, much of the material is rooted in classical medical ideas.

Kuzome offers specific indications that help determine the effectiveness of hara shiatsu for particular patients. If, when the patient lies down, the rectus abdominus muscles appear raised, tight, or clearly defined, this shiatsu therapy will be effective. With the patient lying down, palpate along the upper edge of the abdomen below the rib cage. If there is swelling or tightness, particularly if the fingers are not able to slide up and under the ribs, these techniques would be of use. If an examination of the umbilicus reveals raised muscle or skin around the edges of the umbilicus, this too may indicate problems that can be ameliorated with his treatments. Pulsing or palpitation that is visible on the abdomen, or vascular spiders and other visible circulatory problems on the legs, are indications for this therapy. Kuzome notes that these problems can be treated quite effectively. If the areas around CV-21 or CV-20 are painful or reactive in any way, use these treatments. Kuzome reports that pain in these areas is due to tension of the rectus abdominus muscles which strains the rib cage.

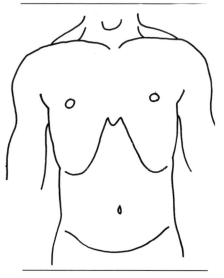

Figure 12.1 A healthy spread of the rib cage.

Another manifestation of strain on the rib cage is the physical displacement of the ribs themselves. Generally, the wider the spread of the ribs the more likely that the person is healthy. Ribs that are more closely spaced may be the result of a natural predisposition, but are often due to excessive tension of the rectus abdominus muscles. Kuzome has noticed that people with closely spaced ribs often develop problems of the stomach or fluid stagnation. These problems can result from such contraction of the rib cage. Shiatsu therapy would be a useful treatment methodology for contracted ribs.[2] If the rib shape is not a natural predisposition, it will respond to treatment by becoming more opened and raised. This change is most often seen in children; their response is quick and obvious. Also, in such cases of contraction of the ribs, if there is tension or pain anywhere on the rectus abdominus muscles, especially near the pubic symphysis, these areas should be treated as well. Since it is very hard to tell if the rib shape is a natural predisposition or a clinical indication resulting from excessive tension of the rectus abdominus muscles, it is important to try treating the condition.

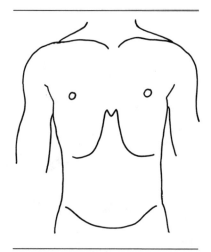

Figure 12.2 A narrow costal arch - an unhealthy spread of the rib cage.

Reactions such as pain, tension, tightness, or lumps that are observed in the areas palpated are good indications for the use of hara shiatsu. Reactions found on the abdomen may be categorized as follows:

    Anatomical locations
    Most significant reactions
    General comments
    Common associated symptoms

Though primarily a practitioner, and only secondarily a theorist, Kuzome nonetheless offers notes and comments that provide an understanding of prognosis and of the diagnostic process. Since he is not afraid to treat people whom he diagnoses as soon to die, nor to admit his occasional mistakes, close attention to his cases is valuable. For example, in his experience people who have had a particular abdominal surgery (especially of the lower abdomen) tend to have some certain pulsings on the abdomen, usually the upper abdomen. He also notes those indications where, before jumping to diagnostic conclusions, we should wait to see if the reaction decreases with passing of gas or the initial application of shiatsu. He adds that in certain cases, the patient might pass very strange stools after regular massage.

Stressing the importance of a very thorough and complete diagnosis, Kuzome suggests that too close attention to areas of the abdomen most easily and commonly found to be reactive need be avoided; When applying his techniques, follow these guidelines:

Use the tips of the fingers.
Apply pressure with the fingers perpendicular to the abdomen.
First touch the skin level, then press to deeper levels.
Keep the patient relaxed, the patient's legs stretched.
The patient should have an empty bladder.
Keep at the same level as the patient.
Use no pillows, or only a head pillow.
Have the patient lie face up, arms at the sides, legs extended.

It is easy to miss diagnostic signs if the patient's legs are bent, as the rectus abdominus muscles become less tense and thus less reflective. When treating, keeping at the same level and height as the patient ideally centers your movements for both diagnosis and treatment, and facilitates the use of your own energies from the hara. When Kuzome treats patients who are bedridden in hospitals he hops onto the bed and works kneeling next to the patient.

Kuzome comments concerning important things to remember. For example, when palpating a fist-sized area around CV-12, should the fingers sink in with no resistance, this is a sign of no stomach qi, a relatively serious condition. This situation may be found in patients just before they die. Great care should be taken in treating a person with such a condition. In another instance, when palpating below the sternum, should the area prove hard like a board with only light pressure, this too may be a sign of impending death, and of particular concern if the rest of the hara were very weak and vacant. Again, great care should be taken in treatment. Kuzome has noticed that patients who have chronic problems may go through what we would call a minor healing crisis. In these instances, symptoms that occurred through the years during the development of the problem can recur. The recurrence is usually mild. He describes the development of the problem as similar to climbing a mountain. The healing process is like coming down the mountain. At certain heights, when either climbing or descending, the same experiences can occur.

□

At height 1, the symptom might be excessive tension or aching;
at height 2, mild low back pain;
at height 3, mild digestive problems;
at height 4, more severe digestive and low back problems;
at height 5, severe low back and digestive problems.

If many areas of the abdomen elicit shooting reactions, particularly reactions over all the body, an infirm hara is indicated. This strongly suggests a psychological component. Often patients with this conformation seem emotionally upset or disturbed, or have poor concentration. Treating these reactive areas can have profound effects on such patients.

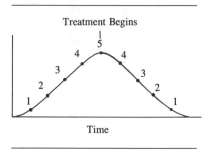

Figure 12.3 Disease process.

Kuzome found that certain patients who practice intensive meditation and breathing techniques can manifest exaggerated abdominal reactions. This might occur when adverse abdominal conditions are extant prior to undertaking such a discipline. Meditative techniques or breathing practices have a catalytic effect. He has often recommended that individuals commencing such disciplined activity first take cleansing or preventive treatment to address any hidden conditions.

Children, having greater sensitivity and more fluent energy, he has found to be very responsive to therapy. They are often able to change more quickly and more permanently than adults. As well, Kuzome has found this system to be quite applicable to treatment of animals. It works well with smaller animals, such as dogs, cats, chickens, ducks. On larger animals, especially on cows and horses, he has found the abdominal muscles too strong for him to have any success. He reported that during the initial diagnosis and treatment the animals would be restive and need restraining. After the initial treatment, the animal would lie on its back as soon as it espied the doctor.

While working with Kuzome the author asked what he understood by the moving qi between the kidneys. Kuzome replied that when one presses with a deeper pressure around or below the umbilicus on the ren mai line, usually above qihai dantian, one can feel a slight pulsing. He then told this story:

> One day a neighbor came running into my office, exclaiming that her baby had just died. I ran over to her house to find the doctor standing over the baby declaring that she was dead, she had no radial pulse, no carotid pulse, and no pupil response. Having obtained permission from the presiding doctor, I felt the baby's abdomen. When I pressed around the umbilicus, I felt a slight pulsing. I reasoned that this was the moving qi between the kidneys and that the baby might not be dead, even though the pulses were indistinct. I applied shiatsu to this area for about thirty minutes. The baby suddenly started crying, and revived.

This story is of interest not only because of the apparent miraculousness of a simple treatment, but because a seemingly obscure classical Chinese concept, the moving qi between the kidneys, is something we can touch.

Kuzome's diagnosis is supported by the works of other therapists. Denmei Shudo says that to feel a very slight pulsing around or just below the umbilicus is a positive sign, as this is the moving qi between the kidneys, the non-material heart. It is this energy that makes Kuzome's shiatsu therapy so powerful and effective. His work, as follows, shows practically that the abdomen is reflective of both energetic and physical levels of disease and disorder. Treatment based on abdominal indications is indeed root treatment.[3]

General Treatment Procedure

Treatment procedure is similar to diagnosis. Work initially and primarily on the areas that elicit sharp pain or traveling or reflective sensations. Also work on other reactive areas of the abdomen. The most important areas to treat are those that induce sensations that radiate to the areas of the body where the patient's problems manifest. Kuzome calls these places "the origin of the problem." If there are no reactive areas on the abdomen, then the treatment target should become any area of sharp pain sensation.

To treat the reactive areas, use a count of six to apply pressure perpendicularly to the reactive area with the finger tips. The following procedure should be applied continuously for a few minutes.

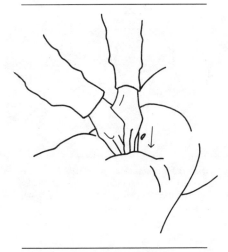

Figure 12.4 Using one hand to support the other, apply pressure perpendicular to the point.

Step	Breath	Practitioner Action
1.	Patient inhales	Poise the fingers over the abdomen
2.	Begin exhale	Begin to apply finger pressure at the count of one.
3.	Exhale continues	Continue pressure, deeper at the count of two.
4.	Exhale continues	The fingers touch at the depth of pressure where reaction is elicited at the count of three.
6.	Exhale continues	The pressure is decreased at the same rate as applied, through counts four and five.
7.	Exhale ends	The pressure is completely lifted by the count of six.

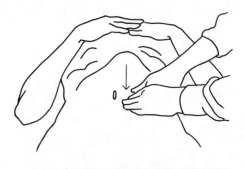

Figure 12.5 The fingers are held at about 60 degrees over the area to be treated with pressure applied straight down.

Repeat the procedure for succeeding breath cycles. If the area is too painful to apply direct perpendicular pressure, apply the pressure less directly by angling the fingers; however, the pressure is still perpendicular to the body.

When treating, as when diagnosing, sudden movement should be avoided. Thumbs as well as fingers may be used, depending on what is most comfortable for the patient. Pressure should not be applied mechanically, as this can be less comfortable; instead, put weight behind the pressure, using the energy from one's hara. When done correctly, this is more comfortable for the patient.

□

These treatment techniques can be applied to virtually all reactive areas on the abdomen. Tense, tight, or painful focii should decrease as the treatment continues; this is a favorable sign. If not, the reactions should decrease as the patient effects home treatment. In most cases the reactions will change in the first few days or weeks of treatment.

This type of treatment can catalyze movement in the body. Should a patient experience nausea or dizziness, the treatment may be broadened to lessen these reactions. Because of such cases, regardless of what areas on the abdomen are reactive, first apply pressure up and under the ribs, along the length of the ribs on both sides. Then treat the reactive areas on the abdomen. Finally, treat the areas beneath the ribs again. This is essential, as it acts to prevent counterflow qi or to treat its occurrence. It also helps keep the rectus abdominus muscles loose during and after treatment. Kuzome talks of this as "emptying the area" below the rib cage. Pressure to the area below the ribs is not applied perpendicularly, but rather at an angle.

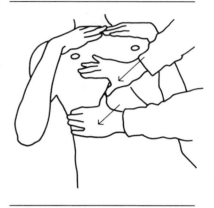

Figure 12.6 Treatment and diagnosis of the subcostal regions should be at about a 45 degrees angle directed up and under the costal border.

The patient should follow this order of treatment at home. Self-treatment should be carried out in a comfortable, supine position, to assure that the abdominal muscles will relax. Such self treatment should last for at least fifteen to twenty minutes a day, more for serious cases. Kuzome gives the example of a seriously ill and hospitalized patient for whom the doctors had given up all hope. She, on the other hand, was determined to heal herself. She would work so intensely on herself while confined to bed that he would have to come to treat her hands and arms, which would get very tired. Of course, this woman improved and was able to leave the hospital.

Special Treatment Techniques

Kuzome sometimes extends his treatment of the reactive areas on the abdomen to cover other points or areas on the body. For example, he has noticed that if there is excessive pain and tightness or tension on the abdomen, such that pressure causes great discomfort, the practitioner should find and treat one or more of the following reactions:

> Pressure pain around SP-10,
> Pressure pain along lines on the upper thigh that are
> continuations of the meridian lines on the abdomen,
> Tension or pain between the third and fourth toes
> (sometimes the second and third toes).
> Pressure pain between ST-36 and ST-38.

Usually these reactions are found on the same side of the body as the most severe reactions on the abdomen. Thus, if you find pressure pain around SP-10, or between ST-36 and ST-38 on one or both sides, treat these painful focii with shiatsu until the tenderness decreases substantially or passes away. You should then find the abdomen less tense and reactive.

Similarly, pressure applied to the lines on the upper thigh will help decrease the tension etc. on the abdomen.

□

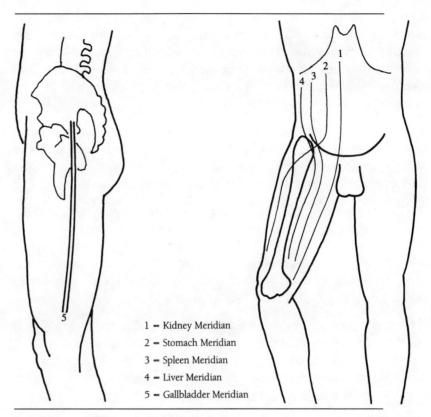

1 — Kidney Meridian
2 — Stomach Meridian
3 — Spleen Meridian
4 — Liver Meridian
5 — Gallbladder Meridian

Figure 12.7

Treating the toes is accomplished in a slightly different fashion. It involves placing the thumbs on the toes, just on the toe side of the metatarsal joint of the third and fourth toes, and below the web of the toes. (See Figure 12.8)

Press the toes apart, comparing left and right sides. Usually there will be more tension or greater pain on the side that was more reactive on the abdomen. As the patient exhales, press the toes apart so as to separate them. After a while, the reactions on the abdomen will lessen, and the toes will become more flexible. As these points and areas can be easily treated throughout the day, with no need to lie down to treat them, they can be included in the patient's self-treatment program.

If a pulsing or palpitation is found on the abdomen, it will usually be accompanied by some tension or tightness. Rather than treat the pulsing directly, which can be quite uncomfortable for the patient, apply pressure to the tense spots next to the pulsing. Try to angle the fingers towards and below the pulsing, as if reaching or pushing below it. Of course, no actual pressure is being applied below the blood vessel. Sometimes, the aorta will be felt; it is situated just in front of and slightly to the left of the spine.

If a lump is found, regardless of its kind and consistency, no direct pressure should be applied. Rather, feel around the edge of the lump. If some spot on the edge elicits a strange reaction with pressure, this is the area to treat. Treat only this area. Kuzome follows this protocol when he treats terminally ill cancer patients. He treats to provide relief from pain and discomfort, journeying to the hospitals near his home to treat these

☐

patients. He finds that he can provide relief of pain and discomfort sufficient to eliminate the need for strong medications like morphine. These treatments are wholly directed at reactive areas on the edge of the tumors. In the case histories that follow there are examples where he has helped patients with cancer; however, he cautions that he does not treat or cure cancer.

If a reactive area around the lump cannot be located, one should work around the entire edge. As we have mentioned, if a lump is found that won't pass with stools or gas, and there is even marginal concern, it is advisable to have a qualified medical doctor examine the patient.

If one finds a noticeably vacant hara, where the fingers easily sink in, look for a tight or tense spot and focus on this area. As one works on it, and as the patient works on it at home, it should become looser. When this occurs, the rest of the abdomen will become firmer and stronger. Such a condition usually takes time to cure. Often, the use of breathing exercises and moxa may help to hasten the healing process.

Infant children who exhibit a vacant (kidney type) hara often inherit it from the mother's identical pre-partum conformation. In treating infants, the prenatal energies residing in the lower hara must be checked. It is also a good idea to have on hand a supply of cloths or diapers, as infants easily and involuntarily pass urine or stool during shiatsu treatment.

Careful reading of the material that follows, before applying it to practice, is strongly recommended. Close attention to the case histories is also advisable. If the diagnostic information seems sparse, remember that the abdominal indications are the only necessary element of the diagnosis. It should be noted that Kuzome's descriptions of his case histories distinguish at what degree of pressure (of the five levels detailed previously) the reactiveness was found. This description provides an indication of the level of pressure at which to be attentive for the reaction discussed.

Substernal Region

Most significant reactions

Board-like with the first degree of pressure.

Swollen with the feeling of a ball inside at second degree of pressure.

A board-like or "corregated board" area with third degree of pressure.

Too soft at the third degree of pressure (like a slug). This is like pressing an octopus, it feels soft on the surface, harder and tighter on the inside.

With less pressure a soft band of muscle, like a thin tongue.

General Comments

Some patients evincing this conformation will feel pain that may travel anywhere, to the head, downward, inward. Usually, if there is pressure pain here, the patient will describe it as "uncomfortable." After pressing this area for a long time the patient may become dizzy, particularly when standing up. In this case, press the patients back at any area found to be tight near the thoracic sixth and seventh vertebrae, on either the *hwa to* points, *shu* points, or outer bladder meridians.

□

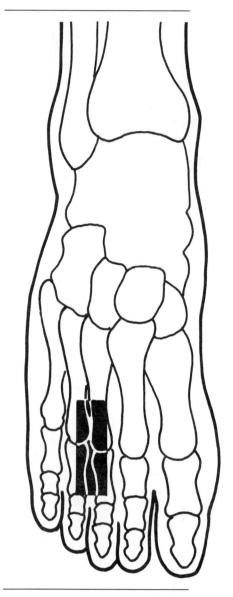

Figure 12.8

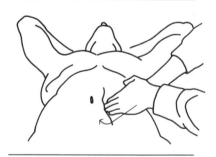

Figure 12.9

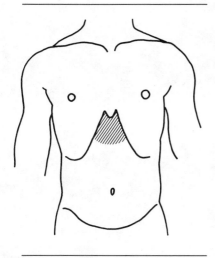

Figure 12.10 Substernal region.

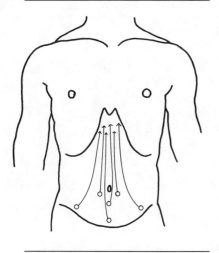

Figure 12.11 Typical areas that commonly accompany substernal reactions.

Associated Symptoms

Headache (usually frontal)
Dizziness
Palpitations
Epilepsy
Feels some suffering inside the chest
Speaking problems
Coughing
Phlegm
Irregular pulse
Neck pain
Insomnia
Overwork of jing and shen (spirit-emotion problems)
No appetite
Epistaxis
Back pain
Easily tired; vacant root qi (basic or source)

If a reaction is found on this area of the abdomen, it is important to palpate the areas shown in Figure 12-11.

Most significant reactions

Positions 1 and 2 are reflex areas for the ovaries and can correspond to emotional problems that are stress-related. If something shows in the substernal region and both of these positions, then the problem reflected at the substernal region is probably emotional, possibly a classical hysteria. Treat areas 1 and 2 with shiatsu.

If one finds the same reaction in areas 3 and 4, which are located halfway between the anterior ridge of the iliac crest and the center of the symphysis pubis, and if there is a lump or knot at the second or third degrees of pressure, treat areas 3 and 4 to correct the problems reflecting at the substernal region and 3 and 4. If the patient has acute stomach pain, gallstone pain, and reaction at position 3 or 4 (particularly on the right side), press here and the pain will decrease.

Position 5 is level with fifth lumbar vertebra; position 6 is just off the pubic symphysis. If, with fifth degree of pressure, a lump or knot is found at areas 5 and 6, and the reaction goes upward to area 4 or towards the lumbar vertebrae, and there is a reaction at the substernal region, then treat areas 5 and 6. The problems reflecting in the substernal region, areas 5 and 6, will be corrected.

Case Histories

Case One: A seventy year old woman suffered from curvature of the spine to the extent that she bowed forward almost 90 degrees. Her body was thin. For the last two months, she had felt stagnation or pressure in the throat with difficulty breathing and bouts of hiccoughs. Following the hiccoughs, she suffered terrible headaches with a pain in the chest that restricted her ability to walk. Subsequently, she became nauseous and vomited frequently. At first, the vomit was clear and watery; then it became darker colored, like coffee. She visited two physicians. The first told her it was a stomach ulcer, the second, after taking X-rays, said she had no stomach problems. The headache, chest pain, and vomiting continued.

Abdominal diagnosis: With deep pressure below the sternum there was the feeling of pressing a board. Between areas 5 and 6 with deep pressure the same board-like structure existed; however, with a very soft sensation just on top. When pressed here, the patient felt a reaction rise to below the sternum and to the inside of the chest. With harder pressure the reaction rose to the head.

Treatment: Shiatsu was administered at areas 5 and 6 until the sensations improved. At this point, the vomiting was eradicated. After several treatments the head and chest pain departed and the spine became much straighter.

Case 2: A seventy year old man had numbness of the lower limbs and inability to move.

Abdominal diagnosis: The area below the sternum was hard and tight; the fingers could not penetrate, and the area felt cold, like a board of ice. The rest of the hara was weak and empty, without elasticity; there was no energy at qihai dantian. Kuzome declined to treat this patient. The man died three days later. The refusal to treat was based on his diagnosis that the man's shen had already departed.

Case 3: A seventy-seven year old woman, of thin build, complained mainly of suffering in the chest (both physical and psychological).

Abdominal diagnosis: On the left side below the rib cage was a lump the size of an egg.

Treatment: Shiatsu was administered at the site of the lump. After treatment the patient felt better. Treatment was repeated several times, and the lump disappeared. She stopped treatment. One year later she discovered a lump in the same place, and administered self treatment, but with no improvement. When she returned to Kuzome for treatment, he found that the lump was back to the same size, but did not move as before. After several treatments the lump got smaller, then returned, got smaller, then returned. The patient died. Her medical doctor reported that she had died of pancreatic cancer. Kuzome was dismayed that he had not administered enough treatment earlier nor followed treatments as perfectly as he should have.

Case 4: A fifty-two year old woman coughed continuously when retiring to bed at night. The problem had endured for two years and nothing had helped. Lethargic, she was flaccidly overweight and her job required constant sitting.

Abdominal diagnosis: With the third degree of pressure below the sternum, there was a soft lump, which when pushed caused a reaction that rose to the throat creating an urge to cough. The rest of the abdomen was unremarkable.

Treatment: She was assigned self treatment to massage the area below the sternum daily. One month later the problem was gone.

These case histories all concern more elderly patients and suggest that with increasing age problems are more likely to occur here, as the shen decreases with age.

☐

Medial Supra-umbilical Region

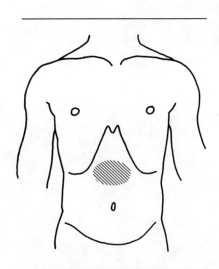

Figure 12.12 Medial Supra-umbilical Region.

Most significant reactions

If you find reaction in this area, pay attention to or look out for the following signs:

With the third degree of pressure, it feels like one is pressing a slug.

The area is swollen.

The area is depressed, tight, and hard.

When palpating, the inside of the abdomen gives the impression of cold.

With the fourth degree of pressure, it feels tight, almost like a lump.

General Comments

When one presses here, the stimulation sometimes rises to the head, to the back, or goes down to the lower abdomen. Sometimes in association there is either hardness, tightness, or weakness in the area below the umbilicus. In the latter case, close attention need be given to treatment progress.

Associated Symptoms

The following are closely associated with this abdominal pattern:

Headache
Insomnia
Dizziness
Stuffed nose
Epistaxis
Stiff shoulder
Shoulder blade pain
Pain around the waist
Tiredness, especially the lower limbs
Feeling of coldness, especially the upper limbs
Knee pain
Cold feeling around the lumbar area
Shortness of breath
Irregular pulse
Extreme thirst
Problems of the eyes (often undiagnosable by allopaths)
Poor eyesight
Acid regurgitation with belching
Constipation
Poor sexual energy
Lumbago
Lumbar pain
Always yawning
No appetite
Hard abdominal mass
Feeling of fullness in the epigastrium
Constant sleepiness
Stomachache

Case Histories

Case 1: A twenty-six year old woman was hospitalized with tuberculosis. She was so profoundly weak that the scheduled operation could not be performed.

Abdominal diagnosis: There was considerable weakness and lack of flexion in this area of the abdomen. The fingers felt cold as they sank in, and there was considerable tightness at the fourth degree of pressure.

Treatment: Shiatsu was administered to this area, and the patient was instructed to treat herself daily. One month later, she became strong enough for the operation she required. After the operation, with nothing else to do, she performed shiatsu on her hara three times a day for 20-30 minutes, recovering from the operation, to the surprise of the doctors, very quickly.

Case 2: A twenty-two year old male suffered with an apparent trachomal infection.

Abdominal diagnosis: The abdomen in this area had a depression that with pressure was very hard.

Treatment: Shiatsu was performed at this area, with instructions to repeat daily at home. The patient reported that the problem completely disappeared.

Case 3: A twenty-four year old woman suffered from constipation, headaches, continual tiredness (leaving her unable to work), and no appetite.

Abdominal diagnosis: There was swelling of the abdominal area. With the third degree of pressure, something like a slug was felt. After self-shiatsu at this area, repeated daily, the problem had completely cleared.

Case 4: A sixty year old woman was told by her doctor that she had stomach cancer. She complained of lack of appetite, though she enjoyed eating two pieces of mochi each day. At 8:00 p.m. every evening, she would experience an upset stomach and would vomit.

Abdominal diagnosis: In this area something like a slug the size of a fist could be palpated. On CV-9, with the second degree of pressure, was a lump that seemed as if floating in water.

Treatment: Self-shiatsu on the sides of the lump, rather than on the lump itself, was recommended. With repeated daily self treatments, and progressive office treatments, the lump decreased until it became the size of a soybean. At this time the woman was able to eat regularly. The doctor who had diagnosed her was very unclear about what had happened to the cancerous growth. She continued to shiatsu the lump until it had gone; her doctor declared that she had been cured of the cancer.[4]

Case 5: a fifty-six year old male suffered from hemiplegia following a stroke. Kuzome had been treating him for the stroke, when his assistant called him to the patient's home. The patient's pulse had become rough and knotted.

Abdominal diagnosis: The area was swollen, reaching almost to the sternum.

Treatment: Shiatsu at the area caused the patient's pulse to become normal and the swelling to diminish. Kuzome comments that following hara

□

shiatsu the patient will often pass gas or belch, which will relieve the symptoms. One should not hastily conclude the existence of a more serious condition.

Substernal Region to Umbilical Region

Most significant reactions

Usually, this area from below the sternum to the umbilicus on the center line feels like a piece of wood. You may also find:

With slight pressure the fingers cannot push into the body. It is very tight, but without pain.

The pressure pain is not too strong or sharp, but the reflex or reactive pain rises to the sternum.

Visible pulsing.

Associated Symptoms

Stomachache
No appetite
Pain in the mouth
Edema
Tiredness of the whole body.

Case Histories

Case 1: a thirty-seven year old woman presented rheumatic symptoms with severe pain. She had been taking heavy doses of cortisone. Her face was very round; she also had soreness and pimples on the gums and soreness at the corners of the mouth. She bruised easily. Her arms and legs were puffy and edematous. She had been taking drugs for three years without much change.

Abdominal diagnosis: There was tightness in the abdominal area.

Treatment: Shiatsu treatment was given several times. When the area became looser, self-shiatsu was recommended. The puffiness of the limbs, soreness of the mouth, gum and bruising problems also improved. But the rheumatism did not improve much.

Case 2: A fifty-two year old male presented with gastritis and swelling of the stomach. He had once had stomach and duodenal ulcers.

Abdominal diagnosis: His abdomen showed tightness in this area.

Treatment: Shiatsu and self-shiatsu were done at this area. After some time, the patient's problems were completely cured.

Supra-umbilical Region

Most significant reactions

The following are commonly found at this area:

Tightness or a knot, round or short and chopstick-shaped, and the size of the pad of the thumb.

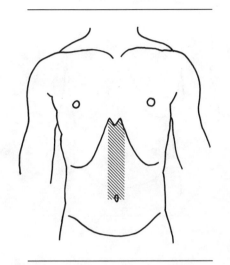

Figure 12.13 Substernal to Umbilical region.

Palpation pressure sends a reaction to the lumbar area, the lower abdomen, or the anus.

This area is one division above the umbilicus (around CV-9) and can be shaped like   or

Associated Symptoms

> Hemorrhoids
> Frigid limbs
> Coldness of the lumbar area and waist
> Pain around the umbilicus
> Problems of urination
> Any symptoms of the stomach
> Alternating constipation and diarrhea.

Case Histories

Case 1: A thirty year old woman would experience three to five days of constipation followed by two days of diarrhea, in continuous alternation.

Abdominal diagnosis: There was tightness in this area.

Treatment: Shiatsu and self-shiatsu were used. After a while the symptoms were completely relieved.

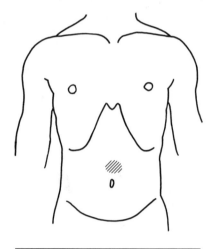

Figure 12.14 Supra-umbilical region.

Supra-umbilical Rectus Abdominus Regions

Most significant reactions

Tension of one or both sides of the rectus abdominus,

The rectus abdominus is hard or tight,

With pressure on the rectus abdominus, the reaction rises to the chest, or travels to the back, usually around the shoulder blade, or to the head or face.

With pressure to the fifth degree, there is tightness, and stimulation goes to the lumbar area, the lower limbs, or to the big toes.

General Comments

The tension or tightness is unilateral or bilateral. If there is tension on the right side of the rectus abdominus, it may often relate to jaundice. Kuzome has good results treating children with jaundice. If there is tightness on the right side of the rectus abdominus, it may often be associated with urinary problems. These patients often need to urinate immediately after the diagnostic palpation or after treatment. The tightness associated with urinary problems occurs in the area just above and to the right of the umbilicus. Tightness at the fifth degree of pressure is often related to a forward curvature of the spine. Treatment may help with this problem, but it is more difficult with age.

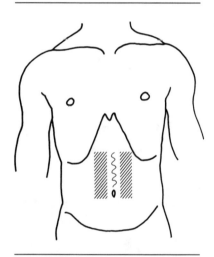

Figure 12.15 Supra-umbilical rectus abdominus regions.

Associated Symptoms

> Stiff shoulder
> Headache
> Back pain
> Insomnia

Lumbar pain
Acid regurgitation
Constant yawning
Stomachache
Hiccoughs
Any symptom of the lower warmer or abdomen (small hara)
Upper or lower limb disease, especially puffiness and edema
(this can also include the face)

Other significant reactions

A supra-umbilical medial palpitation, i.e., a pulsing that can be felt independent of the tension or tightness of the rectus abdominus, may be particularly important when it is coupled with tension of the rectus abdominus. Usually, if there is tension, there is pulsing. Slight pulsing with some tightness or a lump, possibly the size of a soybean, may be felt on the line of the pulse.

Associated Symptoms:

Emotional or psychological problems
Shock
Suffering of the heart
Stomachache
No appetite
Acid regurgitation
Back pain
Vertigo

General Comments

In Kuzome's experience tightness or pulsing in these areas is often associated with surgery performed somewhere on the lower abdomen.

Case Histories

Case 1: A sixty-five year old woman suddenly developed a strong pulsing in this region, and was afraid she was developing a heart problem. This was accompanied by vertigo and night sweats. She went to the hospital and was told that she might be suffering some shock as her husband had died recently.

Abdominal Diagnosis: The pulsing was strongest just below the sternum, with tension of the rectus abdominus.

Treatment: Gentle shiatsu was applied to the pulsing and muscular tension. The patient became relaxed and the pulsing decreased. The patient reported when she returned after three days that this one treatment substantially reduced the sweating the first night. The pulsing had not yet decreased much, but the muscular tension of the rectus abdominus had decreased. Areas of the lower back were treated. After another two days, the pulsing was gone, as was the vertigo and sweating. Kuzome comments that the patient was of a very nervous disposition. She had her right kidney removed at the age of twenty because of kidney tuberculosis. Since then, it was natural that tension and pulsing in these areas would develop and that a nervous upset or excitement would occur.[5]

Fluid Accumulation in the Stomach

Most significant reactions

With pressure in this area, sounds of fluid may be heard, or the patient may report the sensation of fluid moving.

On tapping the area with the tips of the fingers, one hears the sounds of fluid.

With the patient supine, if one were to grasp by the lumbar area and shake lightly, the sounds of fluid may be heard.

A swelling or depression is visible in this area.

Sometimes, the rectus abdominus either side of the area can be tight or tense.

General Comments

The fluid sound is a sign of fluid stagnation; this is often related to tightness or a knot found with deep pressure at the right side of the umbilicus, or a little below the umbilicus. Kuzome feels that the reaction, if found to the right side of the umbilicus, is somehow related to, or causes, the fluid stagnation. The area on the right side of the umbilicus often corresponds to the water dao point, shui dao, ST-28. It can also stretch as far as the spleen meridian. He also feels that these signs are often found in a nervous or emotional and especially an introverted person.

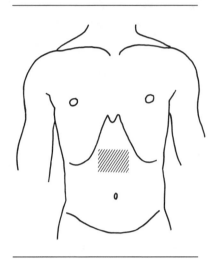

Figure 12.16 Area of fluid accumulation in the stomach.

Associated Symptoms

Palpitations
Difficulty breathing
Hoarse breathing
Coughing
Sneezing
Tightness of the whole body
Constipation
Nausea
Vomiting
Diarrhea
Cold symptoms found anywhere in the body,
   especially the back[6]
Excess saliva production
Tearing eyes
Urination problems
Thirst
Diabetes
Anuria
Dizziness (including travel sickness)
Tinnitus
Headache
Heaviness of the head
Joint pain
Neuralgia
Spasms

Insomnia
Eye diseases
Kidney diseases
Gynecological problems

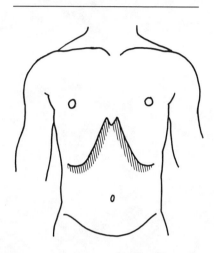

Figure 12.17 Subcostal region - Kyo Kyo Ku man.

Case Histories

Case 1: A fifty-eight year old woman had experienced stomach problems most of her life. Doctors had diagnosed stomach atony and gastroptosis. She had no real relief over the years. She also had headaches, dizziness, cold feet, and no appetite. When she came to Kuzome, she was very thin.

Abdominal Diagnosis: Fluid stagnation was evident, and the right side of the umbilicus was chronically tight.

Treatment: Self-shiatsu was advised. One year later, she had gained weight, the area that was tight had become soft and relaxed, and the fluid stagnation was almost completely gone. In another six months, the tightness and fluid stagnation was completely relieved and she had gained more weight and now looked normal. She told Kuzome that she had been doing shiatsu every day since the first consultation and intended to continue doing it every day so long as she lived.

Case 2: A fourteen year old girl at the age of twelve had developed severe eye problems that her doctors attributed to brain pressure. After surgery, her eyesight improved, only to worsen again six months later. The surgeon who had performed the first operation stated that another operation was necessary, but that it would have only a sixty percent chance of success. Her family refused the second surgery, instead she had spinal taps to relieve the pressure. She reported constant headaches and very bad eyesight. Her facial color was pale.

Abdominal diagnosis: Fluid sounds and swelling were evident; to the right of the umbilicus was a very hard and tight area. L4 and L5 were depressed and exhibited pressure pain.

Treatment: Home shiatsu was done by the girl's mother to the area on the right of the umbilicus. She also massaged the lumbar area and the sides of the spine, especially the sides of lumbar four and five. Every month Kuzome had her return for checkup. After six months of daily home treatment, the spinal taps were unnecessary and the headaches had stopped. Six months later, the eye problems had also disappeared. On last report, after six years, there had been no recurrence of the problem.

Subcostal Region

Reactions in this area correspond to *xiang xie ku man,* Japanese *kyo kyo ku man,* from the *Shang Han Lun.*[7]

Most significant reactions:

When one touches these areas, they are generally tight with one or two small loose areas within them.

The muscle is so tight, that one cannot distinguish between the bone of the ribs, and muscle.

With deep pressure, one feels a lump.

One should compare right and left.

General Comments:

When one presses here, the stimulation can rise to the face, forehead, shoulders, upper limbs, or to the back.

Associated Symptoms:

Headache
Migraine headache
Vertigo
Eye, ear or nose diseases.
Any facial problems
Head tilted to one side
Stiff neck
Tumors that are found around the neck or throat
Diseases of the throat
Stiff shoulders
Diseases of the four limbs, such as dislocation of the joints,
gout, neuralgia, and walking problems.
Any kind of respiratory problems
Shortness of breath
Any symptoms of the heart.
Liver or gallbladder diseases.
Chickenpox
Malaria
Children's digestive disorders
General stomach symptoms
Kidney diseases
Constipation, especially with small rabbit-like stools
Lassitude, easily tired
Tiredness of the whole body
Back pain or lumbar pain
Early stages of fever (as in the *Shang Han Lun*)

Kuzome further comments that if one finds something in these areas, one should be especially attentive to other things found on the hara. If one finds something on the right side, pay special attention to the left side of the umbilicus, or a little below that. If one finds something on the left side, pay special attention to the right side of the umbilicus, or just below that.

Subcostal region - Case Histories:

Case 1: A sixty-eight year old man, in general good health, had felt very tired for the last week.

Abdominal diagnosis: Kuzome found a big lump below the rib cage on the right side, ranging from below the sternum down to the end of the tenth rib, and extending two divisions below the ribs. There was considerable tightness over this area. Kuzome decided to send the patient to a medical doctor instead of treating him, because the patient was quite old, and because of the size and tightness of the lump. He heard that the patient had died ten days later of liver cancer.

Case 2: A fifty-six year old man had undergone an operation for stomach cancer six months prior to his initial visit. Four days before coming to Kuzome, he developed a pain from around the waist to the lumbar area.

□

His medical doctor was unable to relieve this. Kuzome found that the patient was unable to maintain any one position for more than a minute.

Abdominal diagnosis: Even with only slight touching, the palpation areas were very tender, more so than the rest of the abdomen, which was also uniformly tender. From T10 to L3 on the spine and to either side, the muscles were very tense, tight and painful. Kuzome recommended that the patient return to his medical doctor. The patient was then hospitalized and upon further testing was found to have metastasized cancer throughout the body. He died some time later.

Case 3: A sixty-five year old man had experienced nephrosis for the last year, and had been hospitalized. His skin color was blackish, and the face and four limbs were edematous.

Abdominal diagnosis: Perhaps as a result of the patient's medication, the hara was not edematous. On the patient's right side, from under the rib cage and on down to the right side of the umbilicus, the skin was tight like a stone. The skin color was black, and the skin texture thick, soft, and dry.

Starting from under the rib cage and working down to the umbilicus, Kuzome used shiatsu on the tight area. Because the patient's back from the neck down to the lumbar area was tight, he used shiatsu there as well.

He noticed that during and after treatment, the muscles would relax easily, suggesting a favorable prognosis. He taught his assistants and also the patient to use shiatsu on the areas. Several months later, the nephrosis was completely gone.

Case 4: A fifty year old woman had been diagnosed by her medical doctor as suffering from liver cancer.

Abdominal diagnosis: The area from the eighth to the eleventh ribs was visibly swollen. A lump like a short chopstick was found to the left of the umbilicus. He demonstrated his shiatsu techniques to her and instructed her to use the shiatsu at home to treat the lump to the left of the umbilicus.

Over a period of time, as the lump to the left of the umbilicus became less tense and decreased in size, so the lump under the right side of the rib cage became less tense and decreased in size. When the lump to the left side of the umbilicus had gone, so too had the lump under the right side of the rib cage.

As a further comment on this case, Kuzome described another patient suffering with inflammation of the gallbladder, who had refused the requisite surgery. In this case a small slug-like lump was found to the left of the umbilicus. With shiatsu treatment similar to the above case, the lump decreased. The inflammation of the gallbladder subsided correspondingly.[8]

Case 5: A hemiplegic patient who had suffered a stroke complained of constipation, being capable of passing only small rabbit-like stools. A medical doctor also thought that the patient might have liver cancer.

Abdominal diagnosis: Below the right side of the rib cage was a large lump, the size of a fist. As nothing else appeared on the abdomen, Kuzome thought that the patient had a relatively healthy hara, and that the lump might be merely congested stools (as opposed to liver cancer) in the large intestine. So he taught the patient to shiatsu the lump.

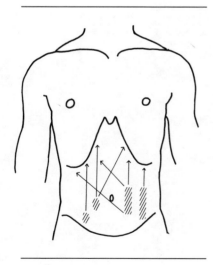

Figure 12.18

The next day the patient called to report that he had passed a large quantity of rabbit-like stools, which were very hard. Kuzome instructed him to continue with the shiatsu on the lump. As the following days passed, the patient continued to pass rabbit-like stools, which became softer and softer. When the lump had completely passed away, the patient's stools had returned to normal.

Case 6: A five year old boy had oozing skin rashes below each ear. They were very itchy and were painful in the evenings. No medication had brought relief of the problem.

Abdominal diagnosis: Kuzome found a chestnut-sized lump below the rib cage (on the side of the more affected ear). He taught the child's mother to shiatsu the lump. When the chestnut-sized lump had completely gone, so too had the skin problems below the ears.

In such cases, reactions that are associated with subcostal reactions are often found to the right or left of the navel, and are commonly seen in the following areas. (See Figure 12.18)

Epigastric Rectus Abdominus Region

Most significant reactions:

One should be careful of these areas becoming tight, especially the muscles of the rectus abdominus.

The skin in these areas is tight, the fingers won't easily sink in, and with deeper pressure the patient might experience reactions such as difficulty breathing, discomfort in the chest, reactions that run from the neck to the shoulder, pain running to and dispersing into the arm, or pain running down from the face dispersing into the neck.

Associated Symptoms:

> Ear diseases
> Diseases of the throat
> Diseases of the front of the neck
> Stiffness of the neck
> Difficulty moving the head
> Pain in the upper limbs
> Suffering or discomfort of the chest
> Shortness of breath
> Stiff shoulders
> Cough
> Intercostal pain

Case History

Case 1: A thirty-one year old man experienced neck pain that made movement of the head difficult. The left upper arm and shoulder area was painful and difficult to move. He had been hospitalized for a while but without much relief of symptoms.

Abdominal diagnosis: The areas of palpation were tense, and with pressure, pain dispersed up into the arms and neck. Kuzome taught the patient to use gentle shiatsu on both areas. After some time of regular self treatment, the tension and the problems were gone.

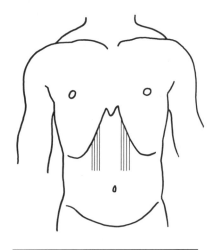

Figure 12.19 Epigastric rectus abdominus region.

Left Umbilical Region

Most significant reactions:

A reaction may be found in an area that extends usually from just above and to the left of the umbilicus to about three centimeters below the level of the umbilicus on the same side.

With the first to second degrees of pressure, it feels tight or hard here, or there is sensitivity or pressure pain, but only in that area.

With the third degree of pressure, it feels tight.

With the fourth to fifth degrees of pressure, it feels tight, and hard like a stone.

General Comments:

With the third, fourth or fifth degrees of pressure, reaction can be caused to rise up to the head, face, or upper limbs, down to the lower limbs, to the lower abdomen or back, along the inside of the right side of the rib cage, or to the same level on the right side of the umbilicus.

If there is an external sexual organ problem and pressure here causes reaction to pass down to the sexual organs or to the urethra, then treating this area with shiatsu can cure the sexual organ problem.

Associated Symptoms:

Headaches
Migraine headaches
Dizziness
Eye pain
Bloodshot eyes
Toothache
Facial spasms
Tendency towards high blood pressure
Tinnitus
Gynecological problems related to blood stasis
Palpitations
Stomach/Intestine problems
Lumbar pain
Vertigo
Skin problems
Numbness or pain of the arms or legs
Symptoms which occur only on the left side
Constipation
Any problems or symptoms of the liver or gallbladder

Case Histories

Case 1: A sixty-five year old woman reported that though she felt usually healthy, she had constipation, and was only able to pass stools twice a month. Now she had been constipated for one month, and had developed a headache.

Abdominal diagnosis: The only symptom found was on this area of the hara, the rest of the hara was in good condition. He treated her with

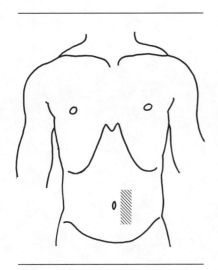

Figure 12.20 Left umbilical region.

shiatsu. She called the next day to report that she had passed stools and that her headache had also passed. On closer examination of the stools, she had also found several black stones in them, and asked Kuzome what they were. She had even tried to shatter them with a hammer to discover what they were, but had been unable to break them. Kuzome said that they were probably "stool stones," stools that had been lodged in the intestines for a great many years.

Case 2: A thirty-eight year old woman had experienced lumbar pain for the last six months. Though she had visited many doctors, she had gained no relief. She had a secondary symptom of headache.

Abdominal diagnosis: She had tension in this area of the abdomen.

Treatment: Kuzome taught her to shiatsu herself on this area, informing her that when this tension had disappeared, she might well be cured. He cautioned her that during the course of treatment, she might pass some very strange stools, but not to worry about them, just continue treating as before.

She came again one month later, having treated herself every day as instructed. She reported that over a period of four days during this month, once or twice a day, she passed strange stools containing blood and pus. After this, the lumbar pain and headache disappeared. Since that time they have not returned.

Case 3: A forty-two year old woman had edema of the left thigh and the right forearm. Other treatment modalities had not helped.

Abdominal diagnosis: There was tightness in this area.

Treatment: Kuzome taught her self-shiatsu for this area. One month later, she called and reported that the edema of the left thigh was almost completely gone, that the edema of the right arm was greatly reduced, but still present, and that she would continue to treat herself.

Case 4: A fifty-four year old man had a constantly high blood pressure, the upper reading being always as high as 250 mm Hg. He also had a stabbing pain from the back of the neck to inside the head, and felt very dizzy and faint with a feeling of wanting to fall down all the time.

Abdominal diagnosis: This area was tense. There was stiffness and tightness from the back of the shoulders to the back of the neck, and from the upper back and down to the lumbar area.

Treatment: Kuzome had the patient come for treatment twice a week. He treated the neck, shoulders, back, and the area on the abdomen each time, and had the patient treat himself on the hara area every day.

After two to three weeks, the patient reported a sudden improvement in his symptoms. He explained that after passing dark, oily, bad-smelling stools twice in one day, his body had become lighter and less tense, and the pain and faintness had passed away.

Case 5: A fifty-five year old man had pain in the external genitals, and difficulty walking and sitting. He had seen many doctors over the last ten years, but without any lasting help.

Abdominal diagnosis: There was tension on both sides of the umbilicus, and pressure caused reaction to go down to the sexual organs and urethra.

Treatment: Kuzome taught the patient to shiatsu himself on both sides of the abdomen.

One week later, the patient reported having a fever for a day. Two to three weeks later, the pain had almost completely gone, and after two months, the pain had completely gone.

Case 6: A fifty-one year old woman had pain in the lower portion of the rib cage on the right side, diagnosed by her medical doctor as gallbladder inflammation requiring surgery. She did not want this surgery, so she had come to Kuzome.

Abdominal diagnosis: He found tightness below the rib cage on the right side, and tension to the left of the umbilicus.

Treatment: He taught her to shiatsu herself on the left side of the umbilicus every day, which she did twice a day. As she did this, she noticed that the pain below the rib cage decreased.

Two to three weeks later, the pain was completely gone, and her doctor advised her that she no longer needed the surgery. One year later, she had a recurrence of the problem. She treated herself again, and the pain left. This occurred again two years later, and she again treated herself, and again the pain disappeared. On last report, five years had passed, and the pain had not returned.

Right Umbilical Region

Most significant reactions:

The right umbilical region is tight, especially with second degree of pressure. Usually with the fourth degree of pressure this area is tight or tense.

General comments:

Kuzome notes that tension here might be connected with fluid stagnation in the stomach, but not in all cases.

Associated symptoms:

> Headaches
> Heaviness of the head
> Stomach problems
> Burping
> Too much phlegm
> Feeling of burning in the chest
> Lower limb problems
> Lumbar pain
> Urination problems
> Spinal cord disease
> Patient always feels cold
> Excess tearing
> Excess salivation
> Dizziness
> Nervousness, oversensitivity

Case histories:

Case 1: A thirty-four year old man had been hospitalized for three years with a spinal cord disease.

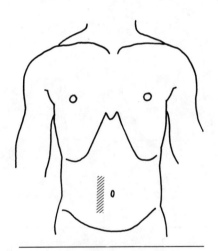

Figure 12.21 Right umbilical region.

Abdominal diagnosis: At the fifth degree of pressure on both sides of the umbilicus, there was a great deal of tightness.

Treatment: Kuzome taught the patient to treat himself on these areas. After two month of treatments, the problem had gone. The patient reported noticing that while treating himself two times a day, the tension would frequently come and go, and that when it disappeared completely, so did his problem.

Case 2: A fifty-two year old man used his right hand continuously while at work, and found that after a while he started developing an empty feeling in his head, with unclarity and difficulty thinking, and also excess salivation. At work, he would frequently have to take rests before he could continue working. He also had tightness and pain of the lumbar area. He had seen many medical doctors, but they were unable to diagnose anything wrong.

Abdominal diagnosis: There was tension in this area on the hara.

Treatment: Kuzome taught the patient to treat himself. Two weeks later, the patient was much improved.

Case 3: A fifty-one year old woman suffered from urinary frequency, having need to relieve this urge every hour. Her lower limbs and lumbar area felt cold.

Abdominal diagnosis: There was tension in this area and fluid stagnation in the stomach.

Treatment: He taught her to treat herself on this area. Two weeks later, her urination had returned to normal and the lower limbs were warmer, but still a little cold.

Lateral Rectus Abdominus Regions

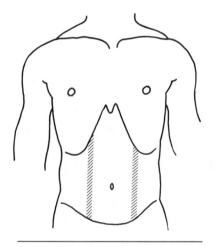

Figure 12.22 Lateral rectus abdominus regions.

Most significant reactions:

A depression may be found on the lateral aspects of the rectus abdominus, sometimes stretching up as far as the level of the nipple.

At the fourth to fifth degree of pressure, there is tightness in an area shaped like a pencil.

At the fourth degree of pressure, a soft lump may be palpated, which may sometimes move along the side of the rectus abdominus muscle.

Between the first and second degrees of pressure, one can feel something like a tense wire along the edges of the area.

At the third degree of pressure, usually level with the umbilicus, a fist-sized lump may be palpated.

Along the same line, but between the rib cage and level with the umbilicus, one can feel tightness at the third degree of pressure.

Associated symptoms:

At the left side, the symptoms are:

Ear diseases
Diseases of the throat
Diseases of the front of the neck
Stiffness of the neck

Difficulty moving the head
Pain in the upper limbs
Suffering or discomfort of the chest
Shortness of breath
Stiff shoulder
Cough
Intercostal pain

Plus:

Joint pain of the lower limbs
Painful left shoulder joint or blade
Abdominal pain
Spinal cord problems
Diabetes

At the right side the symptoms are:

Pleuritis
Cough
Excess salivation
Vertigo, Dizziness
Nausea
Hemiplegia
Lumbar pain
Skin problems especially allergies
Stomach pain
Stomach and intestine diseases
Throat diseases, Eye and ear diseases
Liver disease
Constipation
Urination problems
Abdominal pain, for instance caused by kidney stones

General comments:

Kuzome notes that hemiplegic patients whose right side is affected will have some kind of tightness, etc. on the left side along this line. If the left side is affected, then a similar reaction may be found on the right side along this line.

Case histories:

Case 1: A thirty-five year old man had suffered with a spinal cord problem for the last three years. He had been hospitalized, but was currently convalescing at home. Occasionally he suffered a high fever, and was paralyzed in the lower limbs.

Abdominal diagnosis: On the left side on this line, level with the umbilicus, was a long thin lump.

Treatment: Kuzome taught the patient self-shiatsu. The patient declined to follow Kuzome's regimen, and discontinued treatment.

One year later Kuzome met the patient on the street. The patient began to thank him profusely. He explained that though at the time of his visit, he had not understood the connection between his disease and his hara, he had later, out of desperation and from nothing else to do, started treating himself as Kuzome had instructed.

The fevers started passing, and he started regaining movement in his legs, and now one year later, was able to walk again.

Case 2: A fifty-six year old woman had been diagnosed by her medical doctor as having pneumonia.

Abdominal diagnosis: On the right side, level with the umbilicus, was a lump, almost the size of a fist.

Treatment: Kuzome taught her to shiatsu herself on this area. When the lump had passed, so too had the pneumonia.

Case 3: A sixty year old man had excruciating pain in the abdomen, which a doctor had diagnosed as resulting from a kidney stone.

Abdominal diagnosis: There was tension on the right side from the rib cage down to the pubic bone.

Treatment: He taught the patient to treat himself on this area. The next day the patient passed the kidney stone.

Case 4: A fifty-seven year old man had suffered a stroke, leaving him with hemiplegia and some mental disability.

Abdominal diagnosis: Level with the umbilicus was a fist-sized lump, which moved when touched.

Treatment: He taught the patient to use self-shiatsu on the lump on this area. Sometime later, the lump had completely gone, the patient was able to walk again, and was more clear-minded.

Case 5: A thirty-one year old woman had suffered intermittent allergic skin reactions, on any and all parts of her body. She had suffered from this condition for three years.

Abdominal diagnosis: The area between the rib cage and level with the umbilicus on the right side was tight and knotted.

Treatment: Kuzome taught her self-shiatsu for this area. Over a period of time, the rashes came less frequently, and eventually stopped coming.

Kuzome notes that sometimes following treatments, a rash might flare up terribly. The patient should continue the treatments, as this temporary exacerbation is actually not a bad sign.

Lateral Sub-umbilical Region

Most significant reactions:

A little below the umbilicus, there might be a lump of perhaps indeterminate size. If this lump is deeper, it will be tighter and harder than more superficial lumps. With the second degree of pressure, this same area is very sensitive and painful, even as one removes one's fingers from the area.

General comments:

Pressure pain can radiate to the lumbar area, to below the sternum, to the umbilicus, to the throat, etc. If the lump or tension is one-sided, the stimulation might come to the opposite side, to the rib cage, the breast, or even the upper limb. A lump or pain on the right side can sometimes radiate down to the urethra with pressure. A lump or pain on the left side can sometimes radiate to the same area on the right side with pressure. Kuzome never found that the radiation went from the right to the left.

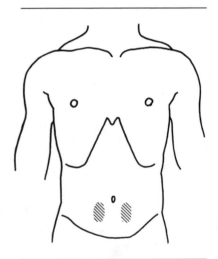

Figure 12.23 Lateral sub-umbilical region.

Associated symptoms:

    Gynecological problems
    Stomach/Intestine problems
    Lumbar pain; Lower hara pain
    Distension of the abdomen
    Diseases of the lower limbs
    Breast diseases
    Diabetes
    Constipation or Diarrhea
    Pain anywhere in the body
    Hernia
    Slight fever
    Vomiting

Case histories:

Case 1: A fifty year old woman had pain on the left side below the rib cage, level with the eighth and ninth ribs.

Abdominal diagnosis: There was a tight knot on the right side, in this area. When the knot was pressed, pressure pain rose up to the area on the painful left side.

Treatment: Kuzome taught the woman to shiatsu herself on this area. When the knot had gone, so had the pain.

Case 2: A fifty-five year old woman was diagnosed by her doctor as having a hernia requiring surgery.

Abdominal diagnosis: She had a scar on the abdomen from a previous operation. There was an egg-size lump on the right side of the abdomen, next to the iliac bone. There was also a tight knot on the right side in this area of the abdomen.

Treatment: Kuzome taught her to shiatsu herself on this area. After some time the lump had gone, and she reported that she no longer needed surgery.

Case 3: A four year old girl had a hernia in the inguinal crease on the right side, for which her medical doctor had advised surgery.

Abdominal diagnosis: On this area on the right side was a tight knot.

Treatment: He taught the girl's mother to shiatsu the knot. One week later the hernia had gone.

Medial Sub-umbilical Region

Most significant reactions:

On this area, at the midline between the umbilicus and the pubic bone, the fingers may encounter a cylindrical lump at the fifth degree of pressure, seeming to start from around the lower lumbar area then to extend forward and downward.

There may be a tight knot, either movable or fixed.

At the fifth degree of pressure, around the level of the fifth lumbar vertebrae, there is a lump which seems to be in front of the vertebrae.

When touching the area, the tip of the fingers sense coldness, as though there were ice in the hara.

There is vacancy and lack of tonus in the area.

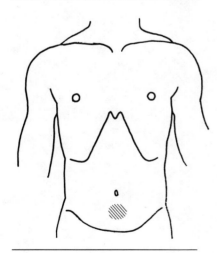

Figure 12.24 Medial sub-umbilical region.

General comments:

The reaction can run to the lumbar area, the back, to below the sternum, up to the throat, to the umbilicus, or to the urethra, anus, or lower limbs, and sometimes to the head and face.

Associated symptoms:

Headache
Facial pain
Toothache
Nervous breakdown
Pain below the sternum
Pain around the umbilicus
Thirst with dry mouth
Decreased sexual energy
Uterine bleeding
Vomiting blood (digestive, not lung related)
Hernia of the uterus
Discharges
Frequent urination
Cold, especially in the lower abdomen
Hemorrhoids
Diseases of the lower limbs
Suffering of the chest
Palpitations

Case histories:

Case 1: A twenty-three year old woman, formerly a prostitute, had experienced constant bleeding from the uterus for the last three years.

Abdominal diagnosis: At the fifth degree of pressure, Kuzome found a tight lump in front of the fifth lumbar vertebrae.

Treatment: He taught her to shiatsu herself. After three days she called to report that the bleeding had stopped. However, she did not return for a follow-up visit.

Case 2: A fifty-four year old woman had a tumor of the uterus requiring surgery. She refused to have surgery, and a while later started bleeding from the uterus, at which point she came to see Kuzome.

Abdominal diagnosis: At the fifth degree of pressure, he found a tight, hard lump in front of the fifth vertebra.

Treatment: He taught her to shiatsu herself in this area. As the tightness of the lump reduced, the bleeding from the uterus reduced, until it stopped.

Kuzome comments that in almost all cases of uterine bleeding, some kind of tightness, hardness, or lump, can be found in front of the fifth lumbar vertebra.

Case 3: A fifty year old woman had sciatica.

Abdominal diagnosis: Kuzome found that the area was tight, and that the areas associated with the sciatic pain were also tight.

Treatment: He taught her to shiatsu all these areas.

After some time of regular treatments, the pain started lessening. On the next visit, she reported that the pain of her previously unreported uterine prolapse was also considerably improved.

□

Case 4: A seventy-three year old woman experienced frequent micturition every morning, approximately every five minutes.

Abdominal diagnosis: The area in front of of the fifth lumbar vertebra was tight and hard.

Treatment: Kuzome taught her self-shiatsu for this area, and the condition gradually improved then disappeared. She also reported that with harder and deeper pressure, she heard peculiar sounds in the abdomen, and it was following these sounds that the urination problem would improve.

Case 5: A seventy year old woman occasionally suffered pain from the lower abdomen up to the chest.

Abdominal diagnosis: The area in front of of the fifth lumbar vertebra was tight and hard.

Treatment: Kuzome taught her self-shiatsu for this area. As the tightness receded, so did the symptoms, until both had gone.

Case 6: A fifty-two year old woman had abdominal pain accompanied by vomiting of blood from the stomach. One doctor had told her it was a stomach ulcer. Another had told her it was not. Confused by these conflicting diagnoses, she went to see Kuzome for treatment.

Abdominal diagnosis: In this area was a scar from a uterine operation performed ten years before. The left side of the scar was particularly tight and hard. He was unable to find anything else on her hara.

Treatment: He taught her self-shiatsu for this area. After two days, the pain and hematemesis had stopped.

Umbilical Region

Most significant reaction:

There is tightness around the umbilicus.

Associated symptoms:

> Poor energy, lethargy
> Anemia
> Weight loss
> No appetite
> Spinal cord diseases
> Constipation
> Lumbar pain
> Low blood pressure
> Inability to maintain one position for any length of time

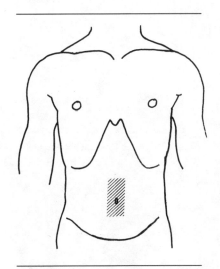

Figure 12.25 Umbilical region.

Case histories:

Case 1: A thirty-two year old woman had suffered from a disease of the spinal cord for many years.

Abdominal diagnosis: The area around the umbilicus was very tight.

Treatment: Kuzome taught her self shiatsu for this area. He also recommended that she see an herbalist, which she did. After treating herself with the shiatsu and taking the herbs, she was completely cured of the disease.

Case 2: A thirty-four year old man had tabes dorsalis, which is a locomotor ataxia from degeneration of the spinal cord. He also had tuberculosis with fever. He had been in hospital for three years. The doctors had given up hope of helping him, suggesting that he spend the rest of his life at home. Kuzome came to see him at home.

Abdominal diagnosis: The area around the umbilicus was very tight.

Treatment: He taught the young man to shiatsu himself in this area. He also taught the patient's mother how to apply shiatsu to the affected areas of the back.

One month later, the patient came by bicycle to see Kuzome at his office. The fever was passing, he had more energy, and was very definitely still doing the shiatsu every day. The patient noticed that the area would alternate from tightness for a few days, to looseness for a few days. Over the course of treatments, this alternation between tightness and looseness decreased in severity and frequency. As the alternations of tightness and looseness decreased in frequency, the pus exudations from the spine also decreased in frequency and amount.

Kuzome treated him over a period of six months, until the tension in the hara had gone. Much improved, the patient was able to return to his farm work again.

Left and Sub-umbilical Region

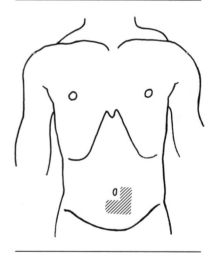

Figure 12.26 Left and sub-umbilical region.

Most significant reactions:

At the third degree of pressure, there is tightness in this area.
At the fourth to fifth degrees of pressure there is tightness in this area.

Associated symptoms:

There is a feeling of something rising from the lower abdomen up to the sternum, causing pain below the sternum.

> The patient fears that their heart is stopping
> Pain in the lower hara
> Bleeding from the uterus
> Discharges
> Rheumatic symptoms
> Neuralgia
> Neuritis
> Ear and eye diseases
> Diseases of the nervous system
> Diseases of the breast
> Diseases of the stomach
> Stiff shoulder

Case histories:

Case 1: A fifty-five year old woman suffered a sudden sensation of something rising from the lower abdomen up to the sternum, with the accompanying feeling that her heart was about to stop. This happened several times.

□

Abdominal diagnosis: Kuzome found tightness of the hara in the left and sub-umbilical area, and with pressure elicited the sensation that rose up to the sternum, upsetting and disturbing the patient.

Treatment: He taught her gentle shiatsu for this area. When the tightness had gone, so too had the symptoms.

Region of the Abdominal Midline

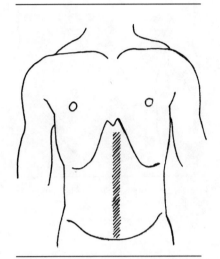

Figure 12.27 Region of the abdominal midline.

Most significant reactions:

From below the sternum, down as far as CV-4, there is: Pressure pain, palpitations or pulsing (strong in some people), and tightness.

Associated symptoms:

> Pain of shifting location
> Weight loss
> Diseases of the head
> Irregular pulse
> Shaking
> Lumbar pain
> Tinnitus
> Diseases of the lower limbs

Case histories:

Case 1: A forty-six year old man suffered from tinnitus (sounding like a drum), which sometimes was strong enough to keep him awake.

Abdominal diagnosis: There was a very big pulsing in the abdominal midline region.

Treatment: Kuzome taught the man shiatsu for this area. After a while, the tinnitus passed away.

Case 2: A sixty year old man had fainted, without regaining consciousness. The family called Kuzome.

Abdominal diagnosis: Without touching the hara, a strong midline pulsing was very obvious.

Treatment: Kuzome refused to treat; the patient died two hours later.

Case 3: While Kuzome was a student, attending lectures, his teacher, Zentaro Koyama, fainted and collapsed. His students found a large pulsing in the abdominal midline area. A doctor was called. He said that Koyama would probably be dead in the morning. Koyama, who was still conscious, refused any treatment from the doctor, and instead instructed the students to take turns in applying shiatsu to the area with the palpitations. The students did this for the rest of the day, and through the night, until the next morning, each taking turns in treating. In the morning the doctor was called again, and to his amazement, found that the palpitations were greatly decreased, and declared that Koyama would probably be allright now. Three days later, Koyama was well enough to travel again.

In describing this case, Kuzome pointed out that a patient who has fainted and is unconscious is in a far more critical condition than a patient who remains conscious. This is why treatment for the unconscious patient was not administered.

□

Lateral to the Medial Line in the Umbilical Region

Most significant reaction:

At the fifth degree of pressure, there is reactiveness lateral to the medial line in the umbilical region.

Associated symptoms:

>   Unusual urination
>   Lower limb problems
>   Lumbar pain
>   Diseases of the spine and buttocks
>   Diseases of the brain
>   Stiff shoulder
>   Ear and eye diseases
>   Testicle diseases
>   Stomach and intestine diseases
>   Pain of the external genital organs
>   Anal diseases

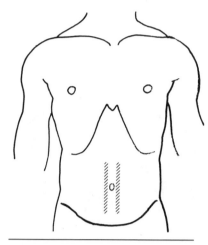

Figure 12.28 Lateral to the medial line in the umbilical region.

Case histories:

Case 1: A sixty year old farmer had discomfort and strange sensations in the head, with occasional headaches, especially when working in the sun, where he would often get dizzy and faint and be unable to continue working. He reported that he had had this problem for thirty years or so. Many doctors had tried helping him, without success.

Abdominal diagnosis: There was almost nothing on the abdomen, except with deep pressure, a very tight feeling in these areas.

Treatment: Kuzome taught the patient to shiatsu himself in these areas. After a while the patient reported that day by day, his head and brain became clearer, he was able to work out in the sun without problems.

Case 2: A fifty-four year old man had pain in the external sexual organs. A medical doctor had diagnosed it as possibly being inflammation of the testicles, and subsequently had surgically removed one of the testicles. This produced no relief, nor did it improve the accompanying lower back pain.

Abdominal diagnosis: At almost the fifth degree of pressure, there was tightness, almost like a stone in the areas lateral to the midline, which caused reaction to run down to the testicle with pressure.

Treatment: He taught the patient self-shiatsu for this area. Some time later, the patient reported that the problem had gone.

Lateral Hypogastric and Iliac Region

Most significant reactions:

Usually this is found on the left side, but it can be found on the right. Lines of tight, cord-like muscles can be seen that pass over the iliac bone. Sometimes these lines can be found with light pressure, sometimes with harder pressure.

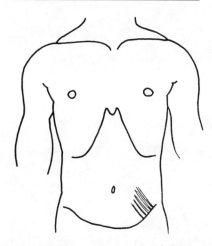

Figure 12.29 Lateral hypogastric and iliac region.

Associated symptoms:

Lumbar pain
Pain or numbness from the buttocks to the lower limbs
Pain around the hip joint
Knee pain
Lower limb pain, especially of the ankle joints.
Headaches

Case histories

Case 1: A fifty-one year old male had very bad pain from the buttocks to the lower limbs. He was unable to stand up properly, having to bend forward at a 90-degree angle all the time. This problem has persisted for about five years.

Abdominal diagnosis: On the left in the lateral hypogastric and iliac region, it was very swollen and tense, and with pressure the reaction went down to the lower limbs.

Treatment: With the first treatment of shiatsu on this area, the patient was able to stand a little straighter, but called up later that day to report that the problem had returned.

The patient continued treating himself daily, and returned to see Kuzome once a week for treatment. After some time, the patient gradually improved to the point where he was able to stand up straight and walk again, and the problem had completely passed.

In relating this case history, Kuzome notes that patients with sciatica will often have this abdominal conformation.

Case 2: A nineteen year old man had arthritis of the hip joint. He had been treated by medical doctors for the last year without success.

Abdominal diagnosis: Pressure in the lateral hypogastric and iliac region caused pain to radiate to the hip joint.

Treatment: Kuzome taught the patient how to treat himself with shiatsu on this area. After some time, the problem was completely relieved.

Abdominal Palpitations

Most significant reactions:

Pulsing of the abdominal arteries; sometimes curving to the left or right of the umbilicus. The artery can be easily felt or seen.

General comments:

Kuzome tells us that if the pulsing of the artery curves to one side or the other, it often signifies or relates to some kind of spinal dislocation, such as a subluxation of the spine.

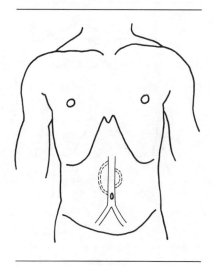

Figure 12.30 Abdominal palpitations.

Associated symptoms:

Lower limb diseases
Lumbar pain
Tension of the rectus abdominus in the epigastric region
   (middle warmer) sometimes emanating from below the sternum
   down almost to the umbilicus

Easily fatigued
Weak energy, no root qi
No tonus on palpation of lower hara
Decreased sexual energy
Tension of lower abdomen/hara
Sweating of the head
Problems of the intestines and susceptibility
   to intestinal problems

Case histories:

Case 1: A sixty-seven year old woman suffered lumbar pain.

Abdominal diagnosis: The abdominal pulsing was felt to curve to the left and deep inside. On the lower abdomen it was very tight.

Treatment: Kuzome taught her to shiatsu both the pulsing and lower hara. After some time, the lumbar pain was completely relieved.

Case 2: A fifty-one year old woman had a disease of the spinal cord, which produced constant backache and fever.

Abdominal diagnosis: The area deep inside and on or around the artery was very tight.

Treatment: Kuzome taught her self-shiatsu for this area. As this tightness decreased, the fever and back pain also decreased until they passed away. In reporting this case history, Kuzome commented that when the pulsing is very clear and stronger on one side, that side of the body or leg develops or has the problem.

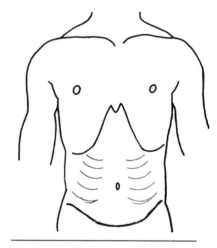

Figure 12.31 Abdominal flaccidity with lines.

Abdominal Flaccidity with Lines

Kuzome reports that one of his teachers, Mr. Iwabe, talked about the kind of hara one comes across when the patient has tapeworms or other worms. Although Kuzome says that he has never come across this kind of problem, he feels it is important to describe it. The hara has the appearance of many depressed lines across it, as though several bands of muscles are clearly outlined, and not as one band.

Supra- and Sub-Umbilical Midline Regions

Most significant reactions:

Tightness is found above the umbilicus on the center line, and looseness and softness below the umbilicus on the center line. The fingers sink in easily. The patient is always tired, either physically or mentally, or both, or has chronic problems.

In this kind of case, shiatsu should be taught for the tight area above the umbilicus. Indirect heat should be applied to the area of the sexual organs (probably with the intention of heating the area around CV-1). Although Kuzome gives no exact description of the preferable method of heating, we can imagine that the heat could be applied by a moxa pole, a hot towel, etc.

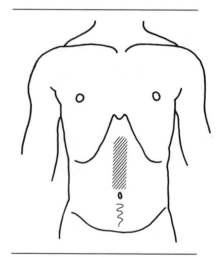

Figure 12.32 Supra and Sub-umbilical regions.

We also recommend in this case to apply moxa directly or indirectly to the most affected points on the ren mai, in the lower hara; e.g., CV-4 or CV-6. Breathing exercises would be helpful as well.

☐

Sub-umbilical Hypogastric Region

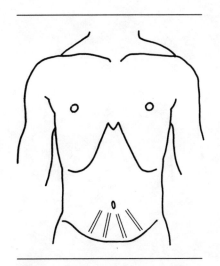

Figure 12.33 Sub-umbilical hypogastric region.

Most significant reactions:

Usually there are three to five lines of muscle tension that can be felt just below the skin or to the fourth degree of pressure. This hara is very commonly seen in patients with vacancy conditions.

General comments:

Kuzome comments that tension of the muscles in this area might be related to fluid stagnation of the stomach.

Associated symptoms:

Frigidity of the lower limbs
Heat of the lower limbs
Pain in the lower limbs
Difficulty stretching or bending the legs
Lumbar pain
No energy
Lower hara is always cold, susceptible to cold
No root qi[9]
Easily tired
Gynecological problems
Urinary problems
Dry throat with thirst

Case histories:

Case 1: A fifty-three year old woman, who easily became fatigued, experienced a perpetual dry throat with thirst, always needing to drink water.

Abdominal diagnosis: The skin of the lower hara was very dry, below the umbilicus were four or five lines of muscle tension, somewhat like chopsticks.

Treatment: Kuzome recommended that she see a medical doctor, who subsequently diagnosed the presence of diabetes. Kuzome also taught her massage to this area. The dry throat and thirst improved.

Case 2: A four year old girl caught cold easily, and had often seen a doctor for this condition. The doctor would prescribe medication. The girl's mother, concerned about the frequent need for medication, brought her to Kuzome. The child's body was thin, she has no energy, and seemed to be overly sensitive.

Abdominal diagnosis: The lower hara had lines of muscle tension. The rest of the abdomen was thin.

Treatment: Kuzome taught her mother to use shiatsu on the problem area. When the tension had gone, the girl started gaining weight, stopped catching cold, and seemed generally healthier.

Lumbar Regions of the Abdomen

Most significant reactions:

The muscles or sides of the abdomen exhibit tension with the second degree of pressure.

The muscles become tense, developing as lines of tension going down and forward.

With the second to third degrees of pressure, the muscles are merely tight.

With finger pressure, the reaction passes to the outside of the thigh.

Associated symptoms:

Weak intestines
No energy below the umbilicus, weakness and lack of tonus.
Lower hara easily becomes cold
Gynecological diseases
Lower limb diseases
Patient feels some problem below the rib cage
Constipation
Lumbar pain

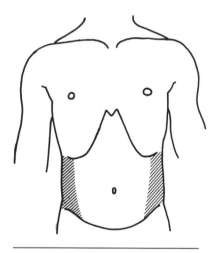

Figure 12.34 Lumbar regions of the abdomen.

General comments:

If a patient has tension along these areas at the sides of the abdomen, the shiatsu can be applied from the side, instead of at the usual vertical angle, so as to be more comfortable for the patient. Also, if the patient is more comfortable drawing the leg of that side up and over, to help relax the area being treated, this is also permissible.

Case histories:

Case 1: A fifty-one year old woman had been having severe pain around the liver for the last five days before consultation. She was also constipated and had pain in the right knee.

Abdominal diagnosis: Below the rib cage and to the right side was a lump or knot, the size of a thumb, which with pressure elicited pain. There was also considerable tension in this area on the right side, extending from the rib cage down to the iliac crest. This tightness was worst at a level with the umbilicus, and at the second degree of pressure. Pressure on this tight area elicited a reaction that rose up to the lump.

Treatment: As Kuzome started applying shiatsu to this area, the tension decreased within minutes, and the pain around the liver decreased. At this point he applied shiatsu to the lump. Very soon after the treatment, the lump disappeared, and the patient passed copious stools. The patient reported that the pain had completely gone.

Lower Left Quadrant Region

Most significant reactions:

On the left side of the abdomen, about level with and in front of the sacro-iliac joint, one finds a lump, ranging from mung bean size to thumb size.

Often at the fourth degree of pressure, one might find a chestnut-sized lump or area of tightness.

General comments:

Kuzome notes that if the patient has ever had peritonitis, something will usually show here.

Associated symptoms:

Stomach diseases
Bleeding of the gums
Bleeding from the anus after passing stools
Vomiting blood (more from the lungs)
Swollen hara
Easily bruised
Anemia

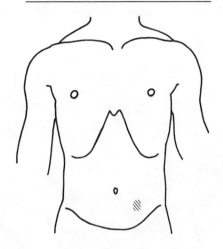

Figure 12.35 Lower left quadrant region.

Case history:

Case 1: A sixty year old woman showed signs of amnesia, being pale of face, skinny, and nervous-looking. She suffered from bleeding from the gums and also bleeding from the anus. If she experienced any kind of shock, she would vomit blood. Her medical doctor thought that she might have tuberculosis, but had not confirmed the diagnosis.

Abdominal diagnosis: Kuzome found a chestnut-sized lump in the lower left quadrant region.

Treatment: He taught her self-shiatsu for this area. Sometime later, the patient reported that the lump had gone and that the bleeding problems had also stopped.

Hypogastric - Iliac Regions

Most significant reactions:

Along the superior edge of the pubic bone, in the abdomen, one might find a lump or knot around the femoral artery, especially on the medial side. One seems to feel a lump that can move, and that traverses the whole area. One feels something like a tendon or cord over the whole area. At the fourth or fifth degree of pressure, one feels a lump which can sometimes be found lying right next to the pubic bone.

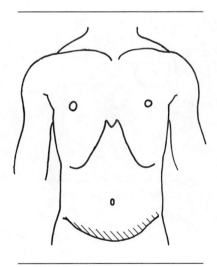

Figure 12.36 Hypogastric - Iliac regions.

General comments:

When one presses here, one can elicit a reaction that goes to the lumbar area, or to below the sternum, or to the urethra or the internal aspects of the thighs of both legs.

Associated symptoms:

> Pain or mass around the stomach or below the sternum
> Gallstone pain
> Hip joint or lower limb diseases
> Lumbar sacral pain
> Discharges
> Abdominal pain

General comments:

If one finds a lump in this area, especially if it is close to the pubic bone, Kuzome tells us that it could be due to some problem or imbalance of the ankle joints, perhaps from improper walking commonly resulting from sprained or fractured ankles years before. In this case one must treat both the lump and the ankles. Either shiatsu or sotai exercise may be used on the ankles and feet.

Also, a lump found here often shows with pressure pain on or around GB-41.[10] Kuzome further comments that if a medical doctor has diagnosed gallstones, a lump will appear around GB-29 on the right side if the patient is overweight. If the patient is not overweight, a lump will not be found around this point.[11] Treatment of what is found should be the same as is usually applied.

Upper Right Quadrant

Most significant reactions:

On the right side, on the outer edge of the rectus abdominus, one can find a knot at the fourth or fifth degree of pressure.

General comments:

Pressure can elicit a reaction that can pass to the left shoulder, to the back or to the right side of the body.

Associated symptoms:

> Pain upper right quadrant
> Urticaria
> Jaundice
> Any stomach problems
> Dizziness
> Pain in the upper limbs
> Lumbar pain
> Vertigo
> Excess salivation

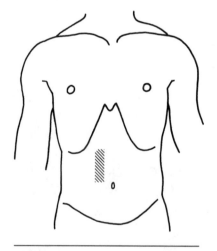

Figure 12.37 Upper right quadrant.

Case histories:

Case 1: A fifty-six year old man, of irritable nature, would feel a sensation of something rising up from the abdomen to inside the chest whenever he became angry. This would cause discomfort of the chest, and confusion of the mind. He also reported having lumbar pain. He had been treating himself by pressing his hara and then pressing his eyes. This was able to give some temporary relief, but the condition always returned. As a visit to a medical doctor produced no diagnosis, he came to see Kuzome.

Abdominal diagnosis: He had a healthy and elastic hara, except in the upper right quadrant area, where Kuzome found a knot and tightness, with strong pressure pain radiating to the lumbar area.

Treatment: He taught the patient to shiatsu the area. So long as the area remained soft, the problems were relieved. But as soon as the symptoms passed away, the patient stopped treatment, so that they would eventually return. The patient did not heal himself because he was too lazy to treat himself.

Case 2: A fifty-seven year old woman suffered from chronic constipation. Four days or so after passing stools, she would begin salivating copiously, get tension in the neck, become muddled of mind, would have frequent urination and vertigo, and develop coldness of the lower limbs. Then she would take medication to pass stools. Each time she passed stools, they were like small stones.

Abdominal diagnosis: This area was very tight, and there was also fluid stagnation of the stomach.

Treatment: Kuzome taught her to shiatsu herself in this area. Over a period of time, the constipation and other problems improved.

Spleen and Kidney Mu Points

The mu points of the spleen and kidney lie at the ends of the twelfth and eleventh ribs.

Most significant reactions:

Palpation of these areas reveals a knot, possibly as large as an egg, on either the left or right sides. The pressure pain may be dull, or strong, or may induce in the patient the urge to defecate. A reaction may go to below the sternum or down to the lower limbs.

Associated symptoms:

> Subjective inability to pass all of one's stools
> Fullness of the epigastrium or stomach
> No appetite
> Stiff shoulders
> Lumbar pain
> Tiredness and weakness around the waist
> Easily tired, especially in the lower limbs

Treatments should be done in the same way as for any other areas found to be reactive.

Scars

Scars on the abdomen from operations can also be problems that require treatment. Single line scars are usually not so hard to treat. If the line is tight with pressure or indented, it can signal a problem or be the cause of problems.

Case history:

A forty-five year old woman had headaches, stiff shoulders, insomnia, dizziness, was easily fatigued, and had no appetite. A doctor had diagnosed her as having low blood pressure, and had prescribed medication, which hadn't helped. She was somewhat overweight, and had a scar on her abdomen from an operation on her uterus. The scar was sunken and deep, and on either side, the muscles were a little swollen, the left side was very tight. Kuzome thought that it was an adhesion problem, so he recommended that she go to see a doctor for another opinion. The doctor thought it might be uterine cancer. She went to see another doctor who thought that it was an adhesion problem, and recommended surgery, to separate the uterus from the abdominal wall. She had this operation. After the surgery, she returned to Kuzome. He found that there was still tightness around the scar, and taught her to shiatsu the area. As the tightness decreased, the symptoms decreased.

Visible Blood Vessels

Veins or blood vessels that are visible on the hara, especially on the lower hara, and that are swollen and clearly defined can be a very serious sign. It would be most advisable to refer the patient to a qualified medical doctor for further testing or treatment.

Final Comments

In his clinical experience with stroke patients, Kuzome found that often something would show on the abdomen on the side opposite to the affected side. He found it particularly useful to pay attention to the unaffected side. For individuals exhibiting problems that might lead to stroke, e.g., high blood pressure, it is preventively important to pay special attention to what one finds on the hara, and to treat what is found there.

Kuzome feels that things found at the first to third degrees of pressure might be related to the intercostal (thoracic) nerves, and things found at a deeper pressure (the fourth and fifth degrees) might be related to the nerves that issue from the lumbar and sacral vertebrae.

Since the surface is yang, it would follow that first and second degrees of pressure could be diagnosing the yang. Since the deeper parts are yin, then the third to fifth degrees of pressure could be understood as diagnosing the yin. It is worth noting that soft lumps or tension are considered to be more yang in nature, while hardness and tight knots are considered to be more yin in nature.

In his experience, patients with vacancy patterns experience pressure pain as comfortable, while patients with repletion patterns experience pressure pain as very uncomfortable.

Finally, Kuzome notes that addressing symptoms found at a deeper depth might be more appropriate for treating root conditions, as such symptoms might be more related to the origin of the disease.

Summary

Treating the hara is in essence doing a root treatment. Drawing on his experience, Kuzome proposes that shiatsu should not be viewed as simply a method of relaxation, but as a method of treating disease. He also stresses the importance of explaining to the patient that even if their symptoms go away, they should not stop treating themselves, until the lump, tightness, or other signs palpated in the hara have completely passed away. Otherwise, the symptoms can easily return.

Naoichi Kuzome is truly a healer in the great tradition of healers. Using abdominal shiatsu almost exclusively, he treats what he finds in the hara, and is famous for remarkable results. The direct simplicity of his work, coupled with his extensive experience, and the empowerment of his patients with their own recovery, stands as a guiding light in our own development as healers.

As a final note, we want to mention some of the research that is being conducted in attempting to grasp and understand the nature of Kuzome's treatments. Already studied in traditional herbal and acupuncture literature, Kuzome is more recently searching in the scientific literature for an explanation of his phenomenal results. In this endeavor, he suggests that perhaps the effects are obtained through stimulation of the greater omentum, lesser omentum, mesenterium, mesocolon, etc. His research has directed him to an examination of some of the body's tissues that we also focus on in this work.

Chapter

- 13 -

Anpuku:

Japanese Anma Massage

Anpuku:
Japanese Anma Massage

Anpuku is another traditional system of therapy that involves massage of the whole body, yet focuses on the same problems as Kuzome's hara shiatsu. These two forms of massage can be easily and effectively combined with needle and moxa treatments and ion-pumping methods, since all are based on hara diagnosis.

Japanese anma massage originated with Shinsai Ota, a contemporary of Waichi Sugiyama in the late 1600's. It is popularly called "anpuku," which translates as "palpating the abdomen." Shinsai Ota was a nearly legendary massage therapist. His work comes to us through Sorei Yanagiya, who translated and explained Shinsai Ota's work. Like Kuzome's hara shiatsu, anpuku is a highly refined and advanced system of massage. Its practical drawback is that skilled teachers are hard to find. Because its focus is on the hara and the application of palpation, its information is applicable to more familiar systems.

Shinsai Ota saw disease as stagnation of basic qi (yuan qi). Once the basic qi becomes stagnant:

> If we do anpuku therapy, it will smooth out the stagnation of the basic qi, producing harmony among the organs, making the flow of blood smooth, the bones and joints more flexible, the muscles less tense, the skin moist, the appetite will be good, urine and stool will come easily, the power of the qi will increase, one's memory will improve. . . .[1]

Since this passage alone mentions most of the basic functions described by Oriental medicine, it is easy to see how central Ota considered the basic qi. He used anpuku to treat all diseases, just as Kuzome does with hara shiatsu. An essential difference of the two systems is Kuzome's involvement of the patient in the treatments. Except in one or two instances, Ota's style requires that the therapist administer the treatment. There are differences in diagnostic style as well. The five significant symptoms that Ota distinguishes are replete hara, vacant hara, pulsing in the hara, tension in the hara, and lump in the hara[2] Replete hara means that the skin of the hara is thick and elastic over the whole hara, with a tiny pulsing, no tension, no lumps, and a slightly moist skin. This is a healthy hara, and by definition, one need perform all therapy as if all diseases were seen as hara vacancy. A vacant hara will have a thin, dry skin. When palpating, there will be a feeling of softness, weakness, or looseness; there will be a stronger or more superficial pulsing without tension or lumps. Pulsing refers to the relative strength of the pulsation usually found. A small, quiet pulsing is acceptable, but an active, strong pulsing is an unhealthy sign. Tension anywhere in the hara is an unfavorable indication, especially if it occurs on the rectus abdominus muscle. Lumps anywhere on the hara require therapeutic attention. There are four kinds of lumps: food lumps, qi lumps, water lumps, and blood lumps.

The therapy performed for any of these signs, tensions, lumps, or pulsings is to treat the back at the same level and on the same side as the indication using the kaisyaku technique of massage. This involves pressure with rotation around a point located in the area. The pressure can be applied firmly or gently according to the patient's relative ease.

Preparatory Work

Have the patient lie down on the stomach in a comfortable position. The practitioner should sit at the left side of the patient level with ming men (GV-4).[3]

Using the right palm, press the two outer bladder lines moving downward from the neck to ming men. The left hand may be used for support and extra pressure by placing it on top of the right hand and using the strength of both arms. Repeat this bladder meridian massage six or seven times on both sides.

Using the pad of the finger or thumb, apply pressure to GV-20, GV-19, the occipital bone near BL-10, and GB-20. Then use the same action to massage the hairline upward to behind the ear. Begin on the right side, then proceed to the left side. Massage the points related to the shoulders — LI-15, TW-14, GB-21. Then massage LI-15 down the upper arm to the elbow on both sides. Be sure to massage both the inside and outside of the lower part of the arm, with both superficial and deep pressure. Next, massage the back of the hand, the heart of the palm, and down each finger to the tips. While doing this, use pressure with the pads of the fingers or thumbs, or use the palm in a squeezing motion. All steps are bilateral.

After completing the first phase, apply pressure between the vertebrae. Begin at GV-14 and massage down to the coccyx, using the thumb. Do the same on both bladder lines, one after the other. Apply pressure to both the left and right side simultaneously. On both sides, massage GB-30, BL-48, BL-49, BL-50, BL-53, GB-32, ST-32, GB-31, and the kneecap. Treat the knot or stiffness at BL-54 and BL-57 until the indication disappears. Then rub along both edges of the tibia and fibula to the ankles, and the ankles and heels. Massage the heart of the sole, KI-1, KI-2, the dorsal, plantar, left, and right sides of the toes.

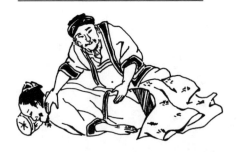

Figure 13.1 Holding pi gen - preparatory work.

With the right hand, stimulate both pi gen points.[4] Using the left palm, massage from GB-30 down to the toes several times. With the left hand stimulate both pi gen points. Then with the right hand massage GV-14 downward to pi gen several times. With the pads of both thumbs, stimulate pi gen for a long time. Release the pressure very slowly and gently.

In this phase, have the patient lie on their back in a comfortable position. Sit to the side of the patient. The treatment technique now is to use the pads of the fingers and thumbs to apply pressure without any sliding

□

motion. Start at GV-20, GV-21, and press across the hairline to the fore-head, coming down both sides to TW-21. Massage above the eyebrows and at the lateral edge of the eyes. Massage below the eyes on the orbital bone, arriving at the zygomatic bone. Massage the sides of the nose, then GV-26, ST-1. Next, massage both sides of the throat and neck down the trapezius muscle (the gallbladder meridian). Massage down the upper arm, elbow, and lower arm, to the hand, then the back of the hand, palm of the hand, and the fingers, to the tips. Be sure to massage both sides and both the upper and lower surfaces. Finally, use a sliding massage down the arms from LI-15 to the ends of the fingers. Do this several times.

Using the simple pressure technique, massage from the iliac bone down the outside of the hip joint, through GB-31 and ST-32 to the knee. Massage the four corners of the knee (around the kneecap). Then massage in a downward direction the internal and external aspects of the tibia from the knee to the ankle. Work around both ankle bones, the heel bone, and between the metatarsals. Finally, treat the heart of the sole and the five toes. Using a sliding technique, massage from the hips to the feet.

Have the patient turn to their right side. Sit behind the patient. With the left hand, apply pressure to both pi gen points. With the right hand, use sliding massage from GV-14 to pi gen. Repeat this step several times. Then use the pads of the fingers to stimulate GV-20, GV-19, the occipital bone (around BL-10 and GB-20), GB-20, and the back of the neck. Next, starting at the left shoulder press downward to the upper arm, to the elbows, to the lower arm, to the wrist, to the back of the hand, and to the heart of the palm and the five fingers.

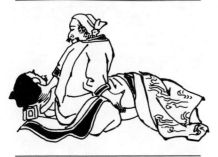

Figure 13.2 Preparatory work continued.

Again use a sliding technique, pressing from LI-15 to the hands several times; then from GV-14 down to the coccyx along the spine. Continue with sliding technique down both bladder meridian lines on the back, several times. Massage the eye of the lumbar points. These points are located 3.7 to 3.8 divisions lateral to the lower border of the fourth lumbar vertebra. To locate the points, Ippo Okamoto suggests having patients lie on the stomach with their hands crossed and beneath the forehead. Stretching the legs, two depressions will be visible around the points. If these depressions are palpated a tight spot or a lump will likely be found. This is the eye of lumbar point.[5]

Then massage GB-30 and the eight liao points, the outside of the hip joint, ST-32, GB-31, the knee cap, and both sides of the gastrocnemius muscle. Press BL-54 and BL-57, moving to around the ankles and the heels; then the pads of the toes. Then press the heart of the sole, KI-1 and KI-2. Stimulate the leg from the hip joint to the toes several times with sliding movements. Now remove the left hand from pi gen. Using the palm of the right hand, move from the shoulders to pi gen several times with a sliding motion. Finally, using the pads of both thumbs, press both pi gen points for a long time. Naturally, one's finger can come over the iliac bone and roll the patient over gently until they are resting on their back.

Basic Techniques of Anpuku

Once the preparatory massage is complete, the patient is ready for the treatment with anpuku techniques.[6]

Techniques for the chest and diaphragm

The patient should be requested to lie comfortably in a supine position. Sitting on the patient's left side, use the left knee to press the patient's left hip, holding the patient still. With the left palm press between each pair of ribs 20 to 30 times bilaterally. Begin at the top of the sternum and work downward to the bottom of the sternum.

Techniques for the right and left sides of the lower edge of the rib cage

With both palms and fingers of the right and left hands, press from the clavicle to the lower edge of the rib cage, applying more pressure with the fingers than the palms. Begin from the sternum and work out, toward the sides of the body. Lead with the finger. Repeat until reaching the bottom of the rib cage. Here, apply pressure to both SP-12 points three times.

Strengthening the rectus abdominus

This technique pulls up any of the large muscles that are sinking. These relate to both the large and small intestine and deep abdomen and are particularly important for weak intestines or a vacant hara. Use the middle three fingers of the right hand to press CV-14, CV-13, CV-12. At the same time, with the fingers of the left hand, press hard with a waving motion on the rectus abdominus muscle on the right side of the hara. Then, with the left thumb, do the same on the left side of the hara. (The third finger of the right hand is still used.) Apply pressure then lift with a light pincer movement.

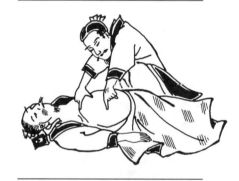

Figure 13.3 The rowing technique

Techniques for drawing down qi

Use the left thumb and forefinger to press ST-25 bilaterally while using the right thumb and forefinger to press the following points at each successive exhalation: ST-19, ST-20, ST-21, ST-22, ST-23, ST-24. Repeat several times.

Rowing technique

To move the rectus abdominus muscles, use the fingers of both hands and "hook" the rectus abdominus muscle on the right side. With the thumbs, hook the rectus abdominus of the left side. Be careful to apply pressure equally with both hands; very regularly, with the exhale, apply pressure with the thumbs in a rowing motion. Repeat for several breath cycles.

Quieting and Relaxing the Palpitation of the Ren Mai

Place the palm of the left hand on the umbilicus, with the thumb on CV-9. Press CV-9. Place the palm of the right hand on the lower part of the sternum and use the right thumb to apply pressure on CV-13, CV-12, CV-11, CV-10, and CV-9 in time with each successive exhalation. Do this several times.

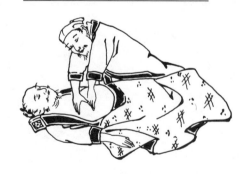

Figure 13.4 Quieting and relaxing the palpitation of the ren mai.

Balancing the stomach

This is good for slight misplacements of the stomach. With the right hand apply pressure below the sternum, between both sides of the rib cage. Repeatedly apply firmer pressure and continue.

Reaching the shen technique

This massage affects the nervous system. The healer should raise slightly onto the knees, facing the patient. With both hands, reach under the body and lift until the top and bottom of the shoulder blade are level. Press down the internal side of the shoulder blade one point at a time with the tips of the finger. Starting at T6 at the edge of the spine, press down to L2. Repeat for the bladder shu and outer bladder lines. If the higher points are out of reach, simply begin lower. If some tension, knot, or stagnation is found on any of these points, apply pressure massage until it is relieved. Then press down from T10 to L2, pi gen. Press the lumbar eye points, GB-30, and the eight liao points. Do the same on the bladder shu and outer bladder lines. Finally, massage the muscles of the lumbar area and the buttocks using the same technique.

Safely relaxing the abdomen

Opening the hands, hook the fingers of both hands over the right side of the body and hook the thumbs at a slight angle across the hara on the left side. Move the hands, applying pressure to both sides of the abdomen in a slow and regular manner. Change the hands so that they angle the opposite way.

Up and down technique

Starting from the collar bone, use the palms of both hands to press down to KI-21 and then back up to the collar bone, down to KI-21. Do this several times. Apply neither too much nor too little pressure. Use either sliding or pressing techniques.

Assisting the metabolism of fluids

This technique is good for fluid stagnation, particularly stagnation of fluid below the sternum. Using both thumbs, repeatedly apply pressure to ST-19 ST-20, ST-21 and then KI-21, KI-20, KI-19, and KI-18. Next, use a sliding pressure technique and stimulate from CV-18 down to CV-10. If this massage produces borborygmus, the fluid will dissipate.

Making jing and shen stable at qihai

Using the fingers of both hands with the palms gently resting on the skin, pull the fingers from the spine to the sternum (between the ribs). It is important to try to use one's own qi while working downward from the first ribs to the last. Below the ribs, pull the fingers from the spine out to qihai. Imagine that all the qi comes to qihai. Work from below the ribs to the sacrum.

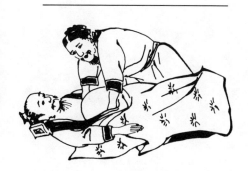

Figure 13.5 Making jing and shen stable at qihai.

Making the shen safe and stabilizing the hun

This technique secures heart and mind at their basic locations. Using the left palm, press the umbilicus and rest the palm there without pressure. Using the right palm, slide and press downward from CV-22 to CV-12. Lift off the body gently at CV-12. Repeat several times.

Using Anpuku for Children

A child's organs child are thin and weak, the flesh is soggy and weak, and the muscles and bones are neither hard nor tight because they are continuously growing. Since children are very susceptible to pathogenic invasion, careful attention must be given when treating them. Generally, if the child is healthy, there is no disease. If anpuku is done regularly the heart, mind, and qi will develop smoothly. The child will be more relaxed and less inclined to oversensitivity or nervous habits. Stagnation of the milk can be avoided, and the urine and stools will pass smoothly. Should skin problems develop (rashes etc.) they will remain light, not serious. Conscientiously applied anpuku will lessen or obviate the need for medications should the child develop some problem such as vomiting milk, diarrhea, acute or chronic cramping or twitching, quick temper or temper tantrums, and skin infections (erysipelas). Without anpuku, these problems are difficult to treat.

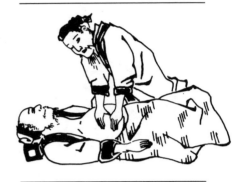

Figure 13.6 Making the shen safe and stabilizing the hun.

To prepare for anpuku massage, have the child lie on the side or have the mother hold the child in position. Begin at GV-14 and GV-12, rubbing down the spine and both bladder lines. Massage the eye of the lumbar points, GB-30, the buttocks, the outside and inside of the hip joints, the outside and inside of the thigh, the gastrocnemius, heel bone, the five fingers and toes, the heart of the sole, and the heart of the palms. Turn the child over and do the same on the other side. Then push both pi gen for a long time, removing the fingers very slowly.

Have the child lie face up. Using the pads of the fingers, apply light pressure stimulation to the chest, the shoulders, the arms, down to the back of the hands, palms, and the end of each finger. Using the left thumb, push left LV-13 placing the forefinger on CV-12, the ring finger on right SP-12, and apply prolonged gentle pressure. Using the forefinger of the right hand, hook under the right side of the abdomen. Then, with the thumb, hook the left side of the abdomen. Apply pressure to both sides with light, pincer-like movements, and pull upward gently. Repeat the whole procedure several times and then apply a rowing motion (see "Rowing technique," above).

Anpuku for Pregnancy

Anpuku is a helpful technique for a woman more than four or five months pregnant.[7] If anpuku is consistently used, a good balance in the abdomen results and the lumbar and leg regions will be warm. It can also correct any malpositioning of the fetus and promote easy labor. Using anpuku should lessen the risk of miscarriage or vomiting before labor. After labor, pain will be eliminated or reduced as will be tissue retention of the amnion and dizziness from blood stasis. Anpuku can stimulate the correct flow of milk. Both the mother and infant will have greater strength and health.

□

To treat, have the woman kneel, sitting on her feet. The practitioner should sit in front of her. Using the pads of both thumbs, press lightly on ST-19 and KI-21. Then, reaching behind the woman, stimulate from T6 down to L2 and L3, down the spine and both bladder lines. Then pull from the spine across the sides to dantian. Move from the upper part of the spine downward to the lower part. This will stimulate the baby, causing it to stir — movement may be felt in the lower part of the abdomen. Apply a very slight rubbing pressure on the ren mai up to the umbilicus. At the upper part of the abdomen, apply a slight rubbing motion from below the breast to above the umbilicus.

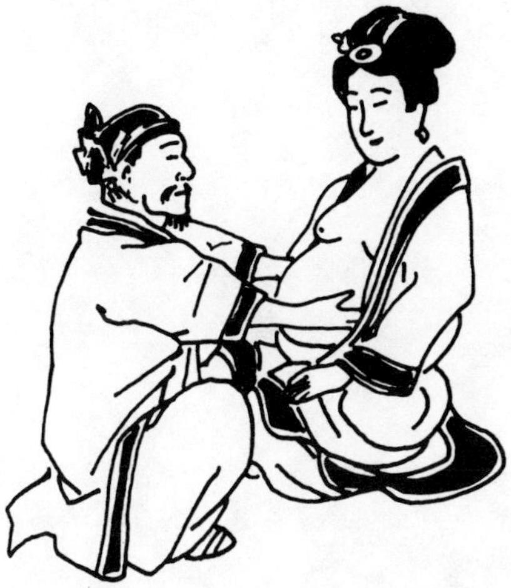

Figure 13.7 Anpuku for pregnancy.

Self-Administered Anpuku

For healthy body management, for long life, and to prevent stagnant or counterflow qi, this massage technique can be performed on oneself. It is best done before going to sleep or first thing in the morning.[8] Repose quietly, swallow any saliva, and do deep hara breathing. With any massage pressure or movement always breathe out. From below the clavicle, massage downward to the umbilicus several times, using the palms of the hands. Rub the face with a motion like washing. Then, using the fingers, massage the bones in front of and behind the ears. Using the thumbs, massage underneath the eyebrow bones. Pinch the nose and move it from side to side. Using the palms, place both hands over the ears, exhaling while pressing. Quickly remove the hands. Using the fingers, lightly press the eyes; pinch the nostrils closed, and breathe out through the mouth.

From the neck down the arm, using the hand of the opposite side, massage with light squeezing motions. End by massaging the back and palm of the hand. Repeat on both sides.

Place the hands at the side with the thumbs stretched behind and beneath the body. Massage the shu points from as high as can be reached to as low as can be reached. Massage down the front of the thighs ending at the knees. With firm pressure massage in order: BL-54, BL-57, ST-36, SP-6, GB-39, the heels. Tuck fingers around the thumb to form a fist. Use the knuckles to massage the soles of the feet. With fist pressure, massage KI-2 and KI-1. With the index finger and thumb, gently roll the toes one at a time. Then, place the fingers between the ribs at the rib cage and gently pull the ribs out toward the side, opening the chest. Then massage LV-13 with pressure; pinch and pull the sides of the abdomen. From ST-19 to ST-25 push with the fingers in a downward direction. Apply slight pressure to the area below the sternum. Finally apply pressure, a little at a time, down from LI-18 on the neck to CV-12 or CV-10.

Chapter

- 14 -

Exercises

to Maintain

a Healthy Hara

Exercises to Strengthen and Maintain a Healthy Hara

Correct deep abdominal breathing is vital to the maintenance of a healthy internal environment. In Japan certain findings on the hara, particularly tension or tightness of the middle warmer, or a stronger middle position of the radial pulse, are commonly ascribed to "stagnation of air." This condition may signal disharmonies of meridian-organ or qi-blood, and should be corrected with exercises to enhance the depth and capacity of the patient's breathing. If proper breathing exercises do not eliminate the signs on the pulse and abdomen then an organ or qi weakness may be suspected. Working with the breath is thus important as therapy and for arriving at clearer diagnostic conclusions.

The following information comes from a variety of sources and is often just common sense in Japan. Much of it may be found in the work of Sorei Yanagiya.

> For any kind of problem, if the breath can be drawn down to below the umbilicus, the patient will have a better chance of living and returning to health. Regardless of whether one has illness now or not, one should be able to draw the breath down to below the umbilicus.[1]

This stresses the importance of drawing the breath down to the hara, as we have discussed previously. This is not meant to imply that literally the air we inhale comes into the abdomen, as this is a physical impossibility; rather it refers to moving the qi down to below the umbilicus, a construct based on an understanding of ideas from many classical sources.

> When inhaling, use the nose, when exhaling use the mouth, but the mouth should be only very slightly open. Send qi to the hara when inhaling.[2]

The *Nan Jing* describes the hara as the source of vital energies, fundamental to the five yin and six yang organs, the root of the twelve meridians, the gate of breathing (*NJ 8:11*). In his commentary on that text, Wang Shu He stated this idea even more explicitly:

> Breath reaches to the inside [of the abdomen]. The qi grows and then becomes solid; this protects against evil injuring the body. Protecting on the inside and defending on the outside, this is qi.[3]

□

In the Western biomedical models, the deep abdominal breathing referred to in the Oriental literature has quite a rational basis. Uses of the abdominal muscles to breathe deeply causes movement of the diaphragm, which increases the volume intake of air into the lungs thus increasing the oxygen levels in the blood. These abdominal muscle and diaphragm movements also compress the abdominal contents, having two basic effects. First, by rhythmically compressing the digestive organs it stimulates the parasympathetic nervous system, increasing parasympathetic activity. Digestive activities and movements are stimulated and the sympathetic activities decreased, thus calmness and emotional balance ensue. Second, the compression and contraction of the abdominal muscles will increase venous return to the heart and increase cardiac output.[4] Though these phenomena are most marked in exercise, they do occur to some extent with abdominal breathing. All these actions serve to decrease excessive mental and emotional activity and generally increase energetic transference and levels of energy in the body.

One simple way of observing the breathing is to ask the patient to breath deeply while supine. Ideally, the abdomen should distend and raise on the inhalation and compress and lower on the exhalation. This draws the diaphragm down on inhalation and up on exhalation. Many patients will distend and raise their *chest* on the inhalation and deflate and lower it on the exhalation, as is commonly the conditioning in the West. This is the first indication of incorrect breathing. A less common indication is simply distention of the chest.

When feeling the abdomen superficially or with slight pressure, if it feels cooler or cold below the umbilicus, and/or warmer or hot above the umbilicus, this could be a sign of weakness of the lower warmer or of improper breathing to this area. Flaccidity of the muscles below the umbilicus (especially if found on or around qihai, CV-6) would corroborate this finding. Another indication would be greater tension, tightness, hardness, or swelling above the umbilicus.

A healthy hara has an even temperature in all three warmers, or a slightly warmer temperature in the lower warmer that may decrease as one moves up the abdomen. Any other temperature variations might be breath-related. Muscular tonus in a healthy abdomen should be slightly greater below the umbilicus, becoming incrementally looser as one palpates further up the abdomen. Variations from this pattern might also be considered as breath-related.

For problems with breathing, we recommend the following four exercises to loosen a tight abdomen and strengthen a weak one, and thereby enhance the patient's capacity for drawing qi down to the hara.

Proper Breathing

Until a patient has learned the appropriate breathing exercises, each treatment should begin with teaching proper breathing. If the patient does not breathe properly, not only is their health affected adversely, but the effectiveness of the treatment itself will not be maximized. The following few exercises have been selected for their simplicity and effectiveness.

□

These exercises should be taught to the patient with the recommendation that they be continued at home. They will help develop the hara and help the patient learn proper breathing. The patient can do Exercises Two, Three, and Four in the office prior to diagnosis and treatment, as well as at home. This will assure proper breathing during the actual treatment.[5]

Exercise One

Instruct the patient to lie flat on their back. They should raise the lower back no more than necessary to be able to fit their fingers underneath. On inhalation, arch the lower back, further, pushing the abdomen up and out. While exhaling very slowly to the count of twenty, lower the back down to the table. At the very end of the exhalation and movement raise the coccyx slightly, then relax completely. The patient should always keep their hand on the lower abdomen during this exercise.

This should be repeated up to ten times, or as many times as feels comfortable to the patient. Instructions to the patient should stress the coordination of the movements with the breath and the cyclical timing of the breath itself. Ideally, this exercise is performed morning and evening.

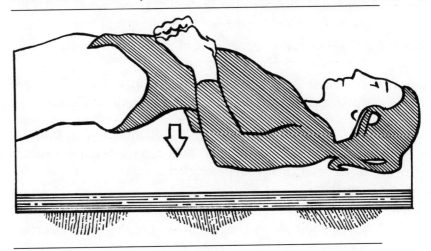

Figure 14.1 Exercise One: Extension of the back.

Step 1: Lie flat and relax, placing the hands beneath the lower back to get the feel of the height to which the back should be arched.

Step 2: Inhalation begins. Raise the back to finger height.

Step 3: Continued inhalation. Raise the back further, arching and pushing the abdomen up and out.

Step 4: Exhalation begins. Begin to slowly lower the abdomen and back.

Step 5: Continued exhalation. During a count of twenty, continue to lower the back, timing the end of the count to coincide with the back returning to a flat position.

Step 6: Exhalation ends. Raise the coccyx slightly, then relax completely. The slight rise of the coccyx is like the "punctuation" of the exercise itself.

Exercise Two

While the patient sits on the table (or on a chair at home) with the legs dangling freely, they should slowly and deeply inhale from the abdomen. The fingers of both hands should be placed along the subcostal border, pointing in towards the ribcage with the palms up. While exhaling slowly, the patient should lean forward slowly from the waist, at the same time pressing the fingers up and under the ribs. At the end of exhalation they should relax completely, letting the body go limp.

This should be repeated as many times as feels comfortable. This exercise is especially good if CV-15 is tight and if CV-6 is very loose, or if the patient is unable to sustain an extended exhalation. In helping the patient to learn this exercise be sure to demonstrate that when leaning forward, the patient's arms come forward too.

Step 1: Take a position on a chair or table sufficiently high to permit the feet to dangle freely, and relax.

Step 2: Inhalation begins. The upturned fingers of both hands rest lightly at the edge of the ribcage.

Step 3: Continued inhalation. Inhalation should continue as deeply as possible, but without any motion or pressure.

Step 4: Exhalation begins. At the peak of inhalation, all motion of the exercise begins as exhalation starts.

Step 5: Continued exhalation. The fingers of both hands exert an upward and inward pressure, sliding beneath the ribs between the ribcage and the internal organs as far as is possible without excessive pressure or pain. Simultaneously, a leaning forward from the waist is performed. Both actions should be coordinated so that maximum extension is achieved at the end of exhalation.

Step 6: Exhalation ends. Remaining in the bent-forward position, relax completely, releasing the pressure of the fingers and resting them at the edge of the ribcage.

Step 7: Inhalation begins. Complete a slow inhalation.

Step 8: Exhalation begins. Lifting the head, return slowly to an upright posture in time with the complete exhalation.

Step 9: Exhalation ends. Completely return to the upright position, with the fingers resting in place lightly but exerting no significant pressure. Relax completely letting the whole body go limp.

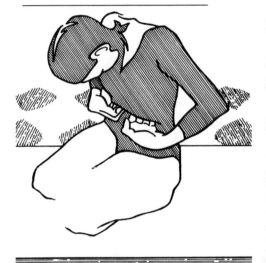

Figure 14.2 Exercise Two: Forward Abdominal Compression

This exercise may also be repeated as many times as is comfortable for the patient. For patients who have difficulty with deep, complete inhalation and extended exhalation, this exercise should be repeatedly performed. While teaching the exercise to your patient, be sure to stress the coordination and fluidity of the pressing inward and leaning forward movements. The exercise should be accomplished smoothly without rapid or violent changes in direction or pressure.

□

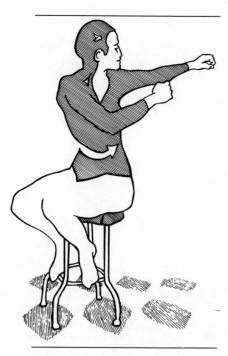

Figure 14.3 Exercise Three: Rotation

Exercise Three

With the patient sitting on the treatment table (or on a chair), legs dangling loosely, the arms are raised straight out in front. Inhaling from the abdomen, the patient should begin to exhale slowly, simultaneously rotating slowly to one side as far as possible. If complete rotation is not possible or is painful, the rotation should go only as far as is comfortable. Then, the patient should relax completely, letting the body go limp. When the rotating motion is done correctly, the turn will be from the waist, and the patient's arms will rise up slightly while twisting. After resting for one breath cycle, the procedure is repeated to the opposite side. Ideally, this exercise may be done a maximum of three or four times in one session, and can be used every day.

Step 1:   Sit on a table or chair with the legs dangling freely. Raise the arms straight ahead, palms down, pointing directly forward.

Step 2:   Complete inhalation. Inhale deeply and completely, without extraneous body movement.

Step 3:   Exhalation begins. Holding the arms in position, turn to one side as far as is possible.

Step 4:   Exhalation ends: Rest in position to the side, then relax completely at the end of exhalation.

Step 5:   Begin and complete inhalation. Continue to rest in position.

Step 6:   Begin and complete exhalation. Return to the starting position, and repeat the procedure on the opposite side.

As with all the exercises, fluidity and grace are to be developed. While teaching this exercise to the patient, it is important to emphasize that the twist be from the waist; if the patient's arms raise slightly during the turn, the movement is correct. If it is particularly painful or difficult for the patient to rotate to one side and not the other, rotation may be performed only to the side that is easier and less painful.

Exercise Four

The patient should sit upright on the table (or on a chair at home) with legs dangling loosely. Inhaling deeply from the abdomen, push the chest up, out, and forward, stretching it. On exhaling slowly rotate the arms backward and upward, stretching the chest even further. This is paced by a slow count of ten. On completion of exhalation, the patient should relax completely, letting the body go limp. This should be done an average of seven times per session, with at least one session per day.

This can be a difficult exercise for some patients, but is very useful for learning deep breathing and correcting the conditions that cause improper breathing. Generally, the greater the difficulty the patient has with the exercise, the greater benefit there is to be derived from its practice.

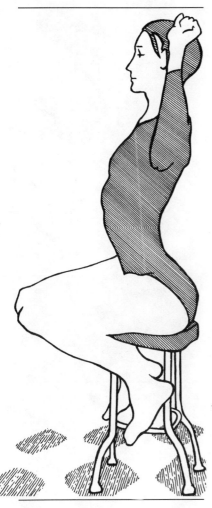

Figure 14.4 Exercise Four: Chest Extension

Step 1: Sit comfortably on a table or chair, with the legs hanging loosely.

Step 2: Inhalation begins. Push the chest upward, outward, and forward, stretching the thoracic area.

Step 3: Continued inhalation. Push the movement of the chest to its greatest extension.

Step 4: Exhalation begins. Slowly rotate the arms back and up, during a slow count of ten. This rotation should be timed with the exhalation such that at the end of the movement the elbows are level with the shoulder and the forearms are facing forward and up.

Step 5: Exhalation ends. Relax completely, letting the body go limp.

Sotai Exercise for Abdominal Tension

One other easy exercise is ideal for simple abdominal tension, specifically tension of the rectus abdominis muscles. It can be done either on one or both sides, depending on the location of the tension. This exercise is from the therapeutic Sotai exercises devised by Keizo Hashimoto.[6]

Have the patient lie supine. Ascertain the side or sides of the abdomen that feel excessively tight. Sitting at the feet of the patient, raise the patient's leg on the side with the tension and rest it on your shoulder, keeping the leg straight. Very gently, holding the leg firmly above the knee, rotate the leg slowly in both directions. Usually the leg will have more restricted or painful motion in one direction. Determine the tighter or more uncomfortable rotational direction of the leg; then perform the following movements three times, slowly, gently, and without strain, on the exhalation.

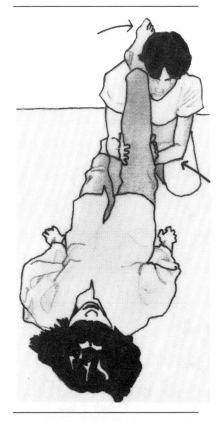

Step 1: Make sure that the leg is turned slightly to the direction with greater tightness.

Step 2: Have the patient inhale deeply.

Step 3: As exhalation begins, the patient should turn the leg slowly in the easier or less painful direction.

Step 4: Continue exhaling, continue the rotation of the leg.

Step 5: Towards the end of exhalation and rotation, begin to apply a gentle pressure to the leg, above the knee, to give a slight resistance to the motion.

Step 6: Once the pressure is applied, count to three, holding the position, then give the patient the verbal request, "Relax."

Step 7: With the word "relax," the patient's breath finishes, movement finishes, and the whole body relaxes.

Figure 14.5 Exercise for tight rectus abdominus muscles.

If necessary, this routine may also be performed on the other leg. When done correctly, the patient should not become tense. If the patient does tense up with the resistance or if the practitioner resists too firmly, the procedure is incorrect. This exercise helps loosen the muscles of the abdomen and improve the flexibility of the hip joints. It can be indicated in any cases of excessive abdominal tension, and has both therapeutic value and diagnostic usefulness.

□

Chapter

- 15 -

Nan Jing

Five Phases

Nan Jing Five Phases

The five phases constitute an important system of theory, diagnosis, and treatment in Oriental medicine. The first text to describe the practice of five-phase acupuncture in detail, and the first text to systematically describe palpation of the hara and explain the importance of this palpation to the source in the hara was the *Nan Jing* (*NJ 8; NJ 16; NJ 56*). From this text, we learn that the five phases have direct relationships to the source or root in the hara, the moving qi between the kidneys. They can directly reflect the condition of this root, and can also directly affect it. Work on the source or root itself can have profound consequences on the patient's health.

In chapter 5, we saw how the Chinese imaged the universe in the abdomen centered around the north pole star, CV-3, ST-25, ST-23, and the umbilicus. The area around the north pole star, which is the center of heaven, was termed the middle palace, ruled by earth. The *Nan Jing*, in partial emulation of this macrocosmic view, placed the earth phase in the center of the abdomen around the umbilicus, mirroring the central location of the middle palace. The other four phases lie around the center. When looking at the abdomen as though one were behind the northern direction, i.e., level with the legs looking up the abdomen towards the chest, this can be seen as follows. The fire phase is above the umbilicus. In the heavens, fire rules the southern palace. The water phase reflects below the umbilicus. In the heavens, water rules the northern palace. The wood phase reflects to the left of the umbilicus. In the heavens, wood rules the eastern palace. The metal phase reflects to the right side of the umbilicus. In the heavens, metal rules the western palace (*NJ 16; NJ 56*). Visually, this description may be represented as in Figure 15.1.

Recapitulation of some basic five-phase diagnostic correspondences will help us comprehend the abdominal findings as viewed within a total pattern of signs that includes the pulses, typical symptoms, areas of the body affected, colors, emotions etc. The following table offers a brief review; readers wishing more detail are encouraged to peruse the first chapters of our earlier work, *Five Elements and Ten Stems*.

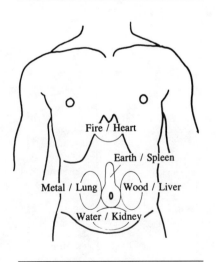

Figure 15.1 While not perfectly matching the heavenly topography, this microcosmic bodily representation works clinically.

Correspondence	wood	fire	earth	metal	water
Season	spring	summer	long summer	fall	winter
Climatic Influence	wind	heat	damp	dryness	cold
Yin organ	liver	heart	spleen	lung	kidney
Yang organ	gallbladder	small intestine	stomach	large intestine	bladder
Opens into	eyes	tongue	lips	nose	ears or two yin
Branches into	nails	face color	lips	skin/body hair	head hair
Colors	blue/green	red	yellow	white	blue/black
Senses	color/sight	smell	taste	voice	body fluids
Emotions	anger	joy	reflection/overthinking	grief	fear/shock/stress
Pulse quality	wiry/tight	flooding/big/scattered	middle/moderate/big	floating/rough/short	soggy/slippery
Odors	greasy/oily	scorched/burnt	sweet	raw flesh	rancid/musty
Tones of voice tastes	strong clear shortened voice acid/sour	drawn out voice bitter	strong throaty voice sweet	loud sobbing voice spicy/hot	weak deep voice salty
Symptoms of each organ	speaking	belching	belching with food	cough	yawning and sneezing
Symptoms of each organ	grief/melancholy	joy	fear(like stress)	grief	fear/worry

The *Nan Jing* made significant contributions to the practice of radial pulse diagnosis. The most easily and commonly used method comes from chapter 18 of the *Nan Jing*, where the meridians are described with reference to the positions of the pulse *(NJ 18:3-4)*.

Left Pulse			
	Inch	Bar	Foot
Superficial	small intestine	gallbladder	bladder
Deep	heart	liver	kidney
Right Pulse			
	Inch	Bar	Foot
Superficial	large intestine	stomach	triple warmer
Deep	lung	spleen	pericardium

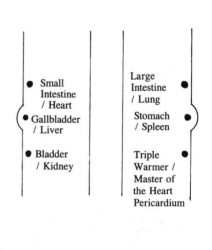

Figure 15.2 *Nan Jing* radial pulse positions.

Qualities of the pulse were assigned more extensive discussions and correspondences. Generally they were correlated to the organs, though no single simple correspondence was given. For instance, in chapter 13 of the *Nan Jing,* the following correspondences were described *(NJ 13:16).*

Wiry or tight pulse	Liver
Flooding, big, or scattered pulse	Heart
Middle, moderate, or big pulse	Spleen
Floating, rough, or short pulse	Lung
Sinking, soggy, or slippery pulse	Kidney

With reference to the seasonal pulse variations, chapter 15 of the *Nan Jing* describes the following qualities. These are particularly interesting when viewed as reflecting the condition of the stomach qi, vital to the thermoregulatory functions of the body:

> In the spring, a wiry pulse: weak, soggy, and long. In the summer, a hooked pulse: arriving quickly, passing slowly. In the fall, a hair pulse: light, empty, and floating. In the winter, a stone pulse; sinking, soggy, and slippery.

Though many of the five-phase correspondences were said to relate to the organs rather than the twelve meridians, the *Nan Jing* clearly states the positional diagnoses of the radial pulse as a means for diagnosing the condition of the twelve meridians. There is a difference between diagnosis of the relative strengths of each of the six pulse positions and diagnosing the qualities of the pulse. This difference is basically the difference between diagnosing the organs and diagnosing the meridians. Because of the strong relationships between the organs and meridians and the interconnectedness of the whole system, this distinction may be·somewhat contrived. Ultimately, the basis for the distinction that the *Nan Jing* emphasizes might be lost to history. Yet there is one possible reason why this distinction may have significance: the importance of accurately and carefully assessing the strengths and weaknesses and relative flow of each of the twelve meridians. As we have described, the source qi comes from the moving qi between the kidneys to the source points of the twelve meridians. We also described the relative flows and cycles of various other qi through the meridians. The pulse diagnosis of each of the twelve meridians would be essential in the assessment of these flows and cycles.

The comments in chapter 8 of the *Nan Jing* concerning the general limitations of pulse diagnosis apply equally to this method of diagnosis. Yet this distinction does provide us food for thought. It may explain why the practice of so-called "five-phase treatments" in Japan, known as *keiraku chiryo* or "meridian treatment style," place strong emphasis on treating and balancing the meridians, and why the positional aspects of the radial pulses are usually seen as the core of five-phase diagnosis and treatments. It may also help explain why, in the practice of herbal medicine, the overall qualities of the pulse are much more significant than the positions of the pulse, since the herbal treatment tends to treat the organs more directly than the meridians, circulating throughout the whole body and thus affecting the overall quality of the pulse. Though this is not always true, it seems to be how the tradition has developed.

□

Most relevant to our current discussion are the two systems of pulse quality correspondences. When pulse qualities are discussed in the *Nan Jing,* the reference may be to organ qualities as described in chapter 13; or to positional qualities, as described in chapter 15. Often the reference is not clear. Examination of eight *Nan Jing* commentaries on chapter 16, for example, gives an even split for either correspondence. Ultimately there is no single interpretation; the reader must be aware of both possibilities. Probably the most commonly used pattern of *Nan Jing* pulse diagnosis is that of the positional differences. Hence it is the method of choice for this and the next few chapters in this text.

Nan Jing Abdominal Palpation Descriptions

Chapter 16 of the *Nan Jing* describes radial pulse findings that correspond to abdominal pulsings and other specific symptoms that may appear with these abdominal signs. The phase diagnosis is determined if the overall picture fits within one phase.

When one finds a liver pulse, and the external symptoms are obsession with cleanliness, blue facial color, easily irritated;

if the internal symptoms are a moving qi [pulsing] at the left side of the umbilicus, and on pressure palpation it feels tight deep inside, or is painful;

if further there are symptoms of swollen or puffy limbs; urination that stops or is difficult to pass; stool that is difficult to pass; calf muscles that cramp;[1]

finding all of these symptoms, we can say with surety that it is a liver problem. But if we don't find all of these, we have to doubt if it is a pure liver problem and need to think more about it.

When one finds a heart pulse, and the external symptoms are red facial color, dry mouth, excessive laughter;

if the internal symptoms are a pulsing above the umbilicus, and on pressure palpation it feels tight deep inside, or painful;

with further symptoms of suffering of the heart, heart pain, fever of the palms, retching [dry vomiting];

on finding all these symptoms, we can say with surety that it is a heart problem. But if we don't find all of these, we have to doubt if it is a pure heart problem and need to think more about it.

When one finds a spleen pulse, and the external symptoms are yellow facial color, profuse belching, thinking too much, thinking about and wanting to eat food too much;

and if internal symptoms are pulsing of the umbilicus, and as one presses harder it feels tight deep inside, or is painful;

if further symptoms are swollen abdomen, inability to digest food well, the body feels heavy and the joints ache; there is constant desire to rest and lie down, the four limbs feel heavy and hard to move;

on finding all these symptoms, one can with surety say that it is a spleen problem. But if we don't find all of these we have to doubt if it is a pure spleen problem and need to think about it more.

When one finds a lung pulse, and the external symptoms are white facial color, profuse sneezing, melancholia, grieving, inability to enjoy oneself;

and if internal symptoms are pulsing to the right side of the umbilicus, and on pressure palpation it feels tight deep inside, or is painful;

if further symptoms are chills, feeling cold, alternating fever and chills, panting;

on finding all these symptoms one can with surety say that it is a lung problem. But if we don't find all of these, we have to doubt if it is a pure lung problem and need to think more about it.

When one finds a kidney pulse, and the external symptoms are black facial color, fear, yawning;[2]

and if the internal symptoms are pulsing below the umbilicus which feels tight deep inside or is painful on palpation;[3]

if further symptoms are counterflow qi, tightness or pain in the small [lower] abdomen, diarrhea followed by spasming of the anus,[4] and if the legs below the knees become cold and then counterflow;[5]

on finding all of these symptoms one can with surety say that it is a kidney problem. But if we don't find all of these, we have to doubt if it is a pure kidney problem and need to think more about it. *(NJ 16:1:26)*.

These external and internal symptoms are interpreted in the *Zhen Jiu Ju Ying* in the Ming dynasty (1529 A.D.) to be symptoms of the coupled yin and yang organs.[6] Though an interesting interpretation, it does not strictly conform to the description in the *Nan Jing*, which does not make the distinction between the external and internal symptoms as referring to the external (yang) and internal (yin) organs.

Nan Jing Lump Descriptions

Chapter 56 of the *Nan Jing* focuses on abdominal palpation and the diagnostic significance of lumps or masses found in the five areas.

A brief comparison of remarks from the *Ling Shu* and *Nan Jing* will help us understand how lumps were seen to develop, and what kinds of lumps there are.

Chapter 55 of the *Nan Jing* distinguishes two basic kinds of lumps, the yin lump, described as the "piling-up lump" 積, and the yang lump, described as the "gathering lump" 聚.

□

Diseases can have accompanying yin lumps or yang lumps. The yin lump is yin qi. The yang lump is yang qi. Therefore yin sinks and is then hidden, yang floats and then moves. The qi that piles up is a yin lump. The qi that gathers is a yang lump. The yin lumps are created (sheng 生) by the five yin organs. The yang lumps are completed (cheng 成) by the six yang organs. The yin lumps are yin qi, they have roots from which they occur. The pain doesn't move from this place, the lumps are clearly defined on all sides. The yang lumps are yang qi, they have no roots and are not clearly defined, the pain is not at this place, they are called yang lumps. This is how one differentiates between yin and yang lumps. *(NJ 55(3):25).*

This discussion is probably in answer or response to an earlier discussion in chapter 46 the *Ling Shu:*

The Yellow Emperor asked, "Some people easily get yin and yang lumps in the intestines; how does one differentiate these?"

Chao Yu answered, "If the skin is thin and dry, the flesh is not hard [elastic] and is muddy [weak and soft] this is a sign of poor intestines and stomach. This means that the evil qi can stay easily. The evil qi will gather and pile up and attack the inside, to the spleen and stomach. [This causes] temperature changes. The evil qi little by little piles up and then a big yang lump will occur" *(LS 46:347).*

Here the yang lumps are seen as resulting from problems of the stomach and intestines, probably cumulative stagnations. The nature and origin of the yin and yang lumps can be seen to be different. The yang lumps are more associated with digestion and the intestines. The yin lumps are more associated with imbalances in the yin organs, transferring through the five-phase cycles, through the changes of the seasons. Chapter 56 of the *Nan Jing* gives fascinating explanations of these differences and processes.

Each yin lump of the five yin organs has a name. By using the months and dates when the lumps occur, we are able to name them *(NJ 56(3):25-27).*

Sosen Hirooka elucidates this for us, expanding on the distinctions between the yin and yang lumps.

The six yang organs carry water and grain. This is the alchemical transformation of one qi, therefore each yang lump has a different form. The five yin organs are different from this [without the alchemical transformations of one qi that the yang organs have]. Also, the form [nature] of each of the five yin lumps is different. Instead, to begin with, the lump comes in the corresponding season of the organ and then becomes lodged. Therefore, in the person's body, the yin organs and yang organs are also dependent on the stems and branches of heaven [i.e., seasonal].[7]

□

The yang lumps have different forms because they represent different manifestations of problems in the digestive system. The yin lumps are different in nature because of the fundamental differences of each of the five yin organs, and also because they have different manifestations in the different seasons.

The *Nan Jing* describes the different types of yin lumps:

> The yin lump of the liver is called "fat qi" 肥氣. The location of the lump is on the left side, below the rib cage. Its shape is like a small upside-down bowl and it has smaller lumps on it. If the lump is not treated for a long time, it will cause coughing, counterflow qi, and nue [hot-cold syndrome], and the patient will suffer from these. It comes in the long summer. A more detailed explanation of this is as follows: lung disease is transmitted to the liver. The liver tries to transmit it to the spleen. But the spleen, which corresponds to long summer, the present season, cannot accept it. The liver tries to return it to the lungs, but the lungs don't accept it. It stays [at the liver] and becomes knotted, creating a lump; this becomes a yin lump. Thus we can understand how the "fat qi" was gotten in long summer, the fifth and sixth of the ten stems.

> The yin lump of the heart is called "hidden beam" 伏梁. It occurs above the umbilicus and reaches to below the sternum. If it isn't treated for a long time, the patient will suffer from more emotional or mental problems. It comes in autumn, at the time of the seventh and eighth of the ten stems. A more detailed explanation of this is as follows: A kidney disease is transmitted to the heart. The heart tries to transmit it to the lungs, but in the autumn, the corresponding season, the lungs don't accept it. The heart tries to return it to the kidneys, but the kidneys won't accept it. It stays and becomes knotted, creating a yin lump. Therefore, we can understand that the "hidden beam" originated in autumn, at the time of the seventh and eighth of the ten stems.

> The yin lump of the spleen is called "stagnant qi" 痞氣. Its location is below the sternum and above the umbilicus. Its shape is like a small shallow saucer. If the problem isn't treated for a long time, the joints cannot contract smoothly or well; jaundice will ensue; the food and fluids will not transform easily. Its origin is in winter, the time of the ninth and tenth stems. A more detailed explanation of this is as follows: A liver disease is transmitted to the spleen. The spleen tries to transmit it to the kidneys, but in winter, the season correspondent to the kidneys, it is not accepted by the kidneys. The spleen tries to return it to the liver, but the liver won't accept it. Therefore, it stays and becomes knotted, creating a yin lump. Therefore we can understand that the stagnant qi was gotten in winter at the time of the ninth and tenth stems.

> The yin lump of the lungs is called *xi pen* 息賁. [8]

The lump is located to the right side of the umbilicus below the ribs. The form of the lump is like a small upside down bowl. If it is not treated for a long time it can cause symptoms of chills, alternating fever and chills, panting and coughing, and stagnation in the lungs.[9] It comes in spring, the time of the first and second stems. A more detailed explanation of this is as follows: A heart disease is transmitted to the lungs. The lungs try to transmit it to the liver, but in spring, the liver's correspondent season, the liver doesn't accept it. The lungs try to return it to the heart, but the heart won't accept it. Therefore, it stays and becomes knotted, creating a yin lump. Thus we can understand that the *xi pen* has its origin in spring at the time of the first and second stems.

The yin lump of the kidneys is called "running piglet" 賁豚. It occurs in the small abdomen [below the umbilicus] and rises up to below the sternum. The condition is like a pig, sometimes ascending, sometimes descending, it is never stationary. If untreated for a long time it can cause symptoms of counterflow panting, weak breathing, and weak bones. It comes in the summer, the time of the third and fourth stems. A more detailed explanation is as follows: A spleen disease is transmitted to the kidney. The kidney tries to transmit it to the heart, but in the summer, the heart's correspondent season, the heart doesn't accept it. The kidney tries to return it to the spleen, but the spleen doesn't accept it. Therefore it stays and becomes knotted creating a yin lump. Thus we can understand that the running piglet was gotten in summer at the time of the third and fourth stems *(NJ 56(3):25-27)*.

Sosen Hirooka explains this last phenomenon:

> Counterflow panting is panting with a sensation of something like a little piglet running up. The weak bones occur because the kidney jing is insufficient, and then the patient can't stand up. The kidneys are the source of each of the qi. If this qi is insufficient, the breath is very weak as both the lungs and kidneys are the qi-yin organs.[10]

Wang Shu He's commentary on this passage from chapter 56 of the *Nan Jing* states that "running piglet" is "movement that starts between the kidneys, and stops at CV-17."

This whole discussion of the nature, causes, and accompanying symptomology of the five yin lumps can help us to understand that lumps are generally more difficult to treat, since they were seen to occur by transmission of disease on the controlling cycle of the five phases, according to seasonal changes. Recall that in the *Nan Jing,* diseases that transmit on the controlling cycle were viewed as more difficult to treat *(NJ 13)*.

In our "modern-day" practice of acupuncture, where energetics and physiology are often seen against the backdrop of Western science and Western medicine, the finding of a lump on a patient's abdomen can be disturbing in light of the fear reactions surrounding lumps, growths, tumors, etc.. It is important to bear in mind that a practitioner need not be overly concerned, nor should the patient be unduly alarmed. Check the signs and symptoms for lumps as described above, and treat accordingly. Where necessary, refer the patient to a medical specialist for corroboration of findings. In this context, a brief case history provides appropriate illustration.

While palpating a friend's abdomen, the author found a clearly defin-able, hard, and immobile fist-sized lump that was sensitive to palpation. The friend nervously stated that the lump had been there for a good while, and that he was very concerned about it. Further diagnosis recommended the use of the ren mai connection, which was applied. Within ten minutes, the "lump" was less than half its original size and substantially less hard and less painful. After a few more minutes of ren mai treatment, hara shi-atsu was applied. By the end of treatment, this terrifying "lump" was a mild muscular tension with pulsing in the area. This example supports the common view that this chapter of the *Nan Jing* is not necessarily referring to abdominal tumors or masses, that areas of tightness or hardness of the muscular wall of the abdomen are the usual signs.

Not all lumps found on palpation require that we refer immediately to a Western medical specialist. If a lump does not respond to appropriate treatment, then it is wise to confer with a medical specialist just to have it checked out. Many clinical cases suggest to us that the lumps referred to by the *Nan Jing* were often areas of tight, swollen muscles, and not "masses" as such. A first step would be to differentiate these, and then in cases where masses are present, to further discern their relative nature and importance.

Modern Extrapolations and Applications of Nan Jing Theory

The preceding descriptions from the *Nan Jing* give us two possible interpretations of the reflex areas of the phases/organs. Pulsings may be found in areas much closer to the umbilicus. Lumps may be found over a larger area of the abdomen, stretching up as far as the ribs on either side. (According to where the pulsings are found, the areas are much closer to the umbilicus. According to where the lumps can be found, the areas are much more extensive, stretching up to the ribs on the right or left sides.) To summarize both ideas, the areas may be visualized as in Figure 15.3.

The experience and study of several eminent Japanese practitioners leads us to suggest that the five areas can be seen in different ways. Though the result is essentially the same, the particular details of what lies where is somewhat different. Kodo Fukushima, an acupuncturist in Japan whose blindness led him to develop unusual sensitivity, described the five areas according to the diagram in Figure 15.4. He offers this explanation for his choices:

> Around the umbilicus from CV-7 to just above CV-12 is the spleen diagnosis area. From just above CV-12 to CV-14 or CV-15 is the heart diagnosis area. Below the right rib cage from GB-24, SP-16 to the side of the umbilicus [probably KI-16, ST-25] is the main lung diagnosis area. To diagnose, compare the equivalent area on the left side. The area to the left also reflects the lungs, but not as commonly as the right side. Below the umbilicus, to the left side from GB-26 to GB-29 is the main liver diagnosis area. To diagnose, compare the equivalent area on the right side, this area to the right also reflects the liver, but

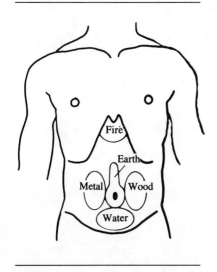

Figure 15.3 Typical interpretation of *Nan Jing* abdominal five-phase areas.

not as commonly as the left side. From CV-7 to just above the pubic bone is the kidney diagnosis area. This area is not just the vertical line or area from CV-7 down to the pubic bone; it can encompass a wider, horizontal area as well. But this varies for each patient.[11]

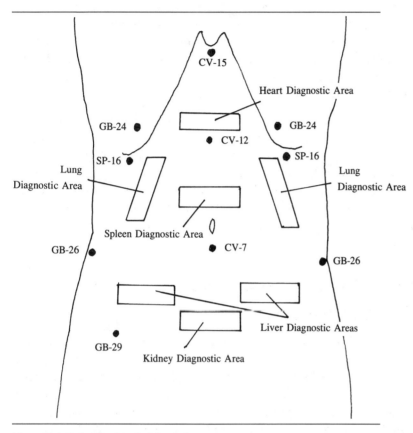

Figure 15.4 Kodo Fukushima's abdominal pattern.

Fukushima uses the abdomen more to confirm the pulse diagnosis. If he finds nothing on the abdomen that confirms the pulse reading, he will check the pulse again. If, for instance, he finds a vacant lung pulse, he will check the lung areas on the abdomen and the spleen area, since in his experience, lung vacancy often comes from a spleen vacancy. When diagnosing the pulse, primarily he checks the relative strength of the six positions of each pulse, as described above.

In his comments on the *Nan Jing* discussion of abdominal pulsing, Denmei Shudo[12] relates that if a slight, gentle, almost imperceptible pulsing is found anywhere on the abdomen and the abdomen is healthy and elastic, then this indicates good health, as this pulsing is the moving qi between the kidneys. If the pulsing is stronger, this is not a good indication. If there is no pulsing, no elasticity, and if the fingers sink in easily, this indicates vacancy.

Shudo also summarizes Ei Maruyama's descriptions of five-phase abdominal diagnosis, whose system concentrates on examination of the area around the umbilicus and exclusive palpation of points that are close to the umbilicus, reminding us of the *Nan Jing* discussion of pulsings in the areas around the umbilicus. Overall, this reflects the significance often accorded the umbilicus and the area around it in abdominal palpation.[13]

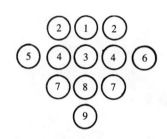

Figure 15.5 Maruyama's reactive points centered around the umbilicus.

1 =   Area just above the umbilicus, between CV-8 and CV-9, for diagnosis of the spleen.

2 =   Area between KI-16 and KI-17, for diagnosis of the kidney.

3 =   The umbilicus, for diagnosis of the spleen.

4 =   KI-16, for diagnosis of the kidney.

5 =   The right side from approximately ST-25 to SP-15, for diagnosis of the lung and large intestine.

6 =   The left side from approximately ST-25 to SP-15, for diagnosis of the liver, gallbladder, and dai mai.

7 =   The areas between KI-16 and KI-15, for diagnosis of the kidney.

8 =   The area just below the umbilicus, between CV-7 and CV-8, for diagnosis of the spleen.

9 =   CV-7, for diagnosis of the kidney.

Shudo comments that in determining a particular problem of a phase, the signs in the radial pulse and abdomen will have corroborative significance. If these signs decrease after treatment, particularly the abdominal indications, the problem will be easier to cure. In clinical cases, when the radial pulse suggested liver vacancy, and abdominal palpation elicited pressure pain on left ST-25, he determined that treating LV-4 would often release the pressure pain on ST-25, thus confirming diagnosis and treatment. Shudo further commented that if the pulse and abdominal indications were substantiated by a pinching diagnosis that elicited pain of the left PC-4, which could be relieved by treating LV-4, this offered definite corroboration of the pulse diagnosis.

In the body of Japanese literature, occasional comments can be found that also discuss distal palpation to diagnose the five phases. The following represent those we have found that are most clearly stated.

Denmei Shudo says that in a lung vacancy, LU-9 can be depressed and/or painful on palpation. In a spleen vacancy, the area from SP-3, SP-4 can be depressed and/or painful upon palpation; also the nail color or shape of the big toe might be changed. In a kidney vacancy, KI-3 can be depressed or swollen, puffy, and painful. In a liver vacancy, LV-8 can be sore and on pressure may have a small, palpable knot.[14]

Kodo Fukushima comments that often points with a relationship to the meridian through the controlling cycle will show some palpable reactions. For instance, LU-10 can become sore in lung problems, and KI-2 in kidney problems.[15] In acute lung problems, such as colds, palpation of LI-11 and LU-10 can elicit soreness. If they are sore, treating these will help treat the cold.[16]

□

Sodo Okabe and Denmei Shudo both discuss the use of pinching techniques along the meridians as further 'diagnostic differentiation or confirmation of the meridians.[17] This technique involves pinching the skin lightly between the thumb and forefinger along the length of the meridian being examined. The nature of the patient response or reaction might be that one or more points feel different from the rest, or feel painful. There might be a difference in the texture of the skin over one or more points. In some areas, the skin might be loose and pinch up easily, and not exhibit normal elasticity; the skin might be loose and pinch up easily, yet exhibit normal elasticity; or the skin might not pinch up easily, and might feel puffy, as if the subcutaneous tissues were being squeezed up with the skin, causing the patient discomfort when pinched. Ideally, the skin should exhibit normal elasticity and be distinct from the underlying tissues. Comparing the palpatory findings of one meridian with another helps identify the most affected meridians and focus treatment.

This pinching technique can also be used on the abdomen within each of the five-phase areas. Sometimes the most reactive, tight, or loose areas are treated directly on the abdomen.[18]

In addition to these basic treatment styles and techniques, there are specific diagnoses and treatments that are extremely useful and in some cases highly effective. Waichi Sugiyama's treatments for various kinds of lumps are perhaps the best known and most developed of classical treatments. Straightforward in nature, they are based on the *Nan Jing* discussions of the types of lumps:

For all kinds of lumps, both yin and yang kinds one can treat, with moxa, ming men, GV-4.

One can also select from and treat CV-13, CV-12, KI-21, KI-20, ST-21, ST-25, LV-14, CV-6, CV-4.[19]

For the lung lump, found on the right side below the ribs, treat LU-5, LV-13, ST-36.

For the heart lump, found below the sternum and above the umbilicus, treat HT-7, SI-3, ST-36, CV-14.

For the spleen lump, found as far as two divisions above the umbilicus and maybe a little to one side, treat BL-20, BL-21, BL-23, BL-66, LV-13, ST-36.

For the liver lump, found on the left side below the ribs, treat LV-13, LV-2.

For the kidney lump, generally found below the umbilicus though it sometimes can move up and down, treat BL-23, CV-3, CV-4, KI-1.

For a qi lump [yang lump] treat BL-20, BL-21, BL-23, ST-21, ST-25[20]

The last and perhaps most intruiging pattern of diagnosis and treatment comes from the Shakuju school of acupuncture in Japan.[21] Here the diagnostic pattern is similar to most classical interpretations:

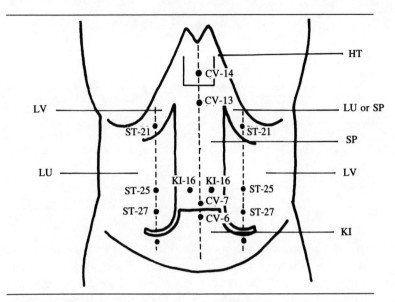

Figure 15.6 Abdominal diagnosis pattern from the Shakuju school.

However, the treatments are quite different, utilizing the back shu points or the bladder points lateral to them. This treatment style uses combinations of the back shu points, according to the area that shows the predominant reaction. Treatments are generally performed using needle or moxa techniques on these points. The abdomen is then reassessed by palpation and compared with the pulse and the general pattern of signs and symptoms to arrive at a firm five-phase diagnosis. In other words, this treatment style can be used as a stepping stone in the process by which one determines the phase that is vacant and the points on the limbs that should be treated for supplementation. Phase diagnosis is often difficult when abdominal signs abound. This treatment will abate or reduce many of the signs, leaving the most significant behind.

This process actually occurs in three steps. The first supplements the relevant back shu points. Supplementation involves application to each point of indirect moxa ten times, or small direct moxa five times, or perpendicular shallow needle insertion for twenty seconds. The abdomen should then be rechecked. If the major signs are still present, one should then proceed to step two. Here the relevant back shu points are dispersed. Dispersion involves application to each point of either direct small moxa, or indirect moxa three times, or perpendicular shallow needle insertion for five seconds. The abdomen should then be rechecked. Any remaining abdominal signs should then be compared with the pulse and any other accompanying signs and symptoms, and a diagnosis determined. Step three involves the supplementation and dispersion of relevant points on the meridians according to the principles described above and in *Five Elements and Ten Stems*.

□

The treatment patterns for steps one and two are as follows. Points are palpated and selected according to reaction:

Reactions:	Step One: Supplementation	Step Two: Dispersion
substernal (heart)	BL-18 + BL-14 or BL-15 or BL-42 + BL-38 or BL-39	BL-13 + BL-23 or BL-37 + BL-47
around or above navel (spleen) + left subcostal	BL-14 or BL-15 + BL-20 or BL-38 or BL-39 + BL-44	BL-23 + BL-18 or BL-47 + BL-42
below navel (kidney)	BL-13 + BL-23 or BL-37 + BL-47	BL-14 or BL-15 + BL-20 or BL-38 or BL-39 + BL-44
left navel (liver)+ right subcostal	BL-20 + BL-13 + right BL-18 or BL-44 + BL-37 + right BL-42	left BL-18 + BL-14 or BL-15 or left BL-42 + BL-38 or BL-39
right navel (lung)+ left subcostal	BL-23 + BL-18 or BL-47 + BL-42	BL-20 + BL-13 or BL-44 + BL-37

Reactions tend to show in the lateral bladder points in the over-30 age group, and closer to the spine in younger patients. It has also been found that pressure pain only, soft lumps, or weak radiation are mild abdominal findings and will clear up after step one. In the order of lesser to greater severity, the following three kinds of abdominal findings generally require steps one and two and often three:

lump (tension, tightness); lump with pressure pain or radiation

pulsing

pulsing with lump and pain.

In the first three treatment patterns, the logic is clear according to five-phase theory: tonify the mother phase and same-phase points; disperse the controlling and controlled phase points. The phasal logic in the fourth and fifth patterns is more convoluted. This is probably because the reactive areas lie on the sides of the navel and are complicated by the crossing spirals of muscle bands that traverse these regions.

Summary

Throughout the history of the use of the five phases as a diagnostic and therapeutic system of acupuncture, there have been many different interpretations and treatment styles. This is essentially due to the complexity and breadth of the *Nan Jing* theories. In our previous works we examined a variety of diagnostic and therapeutic approaches. This chapter summarizes ideas relative to abdominal diagnosis. In the next chapters we will examine five-phase therapeutic principles again with some of Manaka's treatments.

Chapter

- 16 -

Manaka's

Uses of the

Extraordinary Vessels

Manaka's Uses of the Extraordinary Vessels

Dr. Yoshio Manaka, whose ideas we have described throughout this text, is among the most renowned and skillful practitioner-researchers in the field. We have had the good fortune to have studied with him and to have been exposed to many of his treatment ideas and systems in which abdominal diagnosis features as a major component. Some of the many treatment procedures, techniques, and tools that he has investigated and devised are described in the following section. Interested readers may look to a forthcoming study of his work, *Chasing the Dragon's Tail,* for more detail and development of his ideas.

Manaka's theories of diagnosis and treatment of the eight extraordinary vessels are the most coherent available in the medical literature, and his use of the the ion-pumping cords has created a body of clinical results that offer substantial practical justification of his theories. While emphasizing refinement and systematization of diagnosis and treatment to achieve maximum results with minimal stimulation, he takes a slightly different view of his role as a teacher. He feels that autocratic presentation of materials will retard a student's development. It should therefore be noted that while his information is presented procedurally, the exceptions and cautions germane to his ideas are also presented. While rapid mastery of a few techniques is a very comfortable way to learn, a more thorough clinical repertoire is usually the result of comprehending the scope of a theory, i.e., its limitations as well as its possibilities.

Manaka's general premise is that prior to any local or symptomatic treatment, a general or root treatment, *benzhi fa,* should be administered. This general treatment is aimed at clearing abdominal findings, pulse, and general muscular tension, just as was described in the classical literature. Manaka will often use methods or systems such as the extraordinary vessel points, the five-phase points, the daily, ten-day and sixty-day biorhythmic open points, or Tae Woo Yoo's palm points, to achieve these ends. He feels that it is important to have a systematic and demonstrable approach to treatment, and has developed clear palpatory diagnostic patterns that key into specific treatments.

When devising a general or root treatment, Manaka takes many strategies and summarizes them in three diagnostic and therapeutic steps. Observing to the phenomena of yin and yang, we can treat:

1. According to abdominal diagnosis, what Manaka calls the mu areas.

2. According to back diagnosis, which involves the use of moxa, heated needles etc on back shu points related to one's diagnosis.

3. According to the muscular imbalances, with for instance Sotai exercises, often combined with heated needles.

□

Thus, he will treat to rid the abdominal reactions, to rid the back reactions, and to correct muscle imbalances, in a three-step manner. The uses of the ion-pumping cords on the extraordinary vessels described in this chapter represent what is probably the most common application for the first step. Uses of the open points and other specific treatments for patterns of abdominal reaction — like the taikyoku treatment or the palm points treatment described below — represent other common treatments for achieving the goals of the first step, reduction of abdominal reactions. Reduction of back reactions can be achieved in a number of different ways, a simple means being to focus on reducing reactivity of back shu points associated with the diagnosis by direct needle or moxa placement on the associated back shu points — for instance in liver problems, treating BL-18, or for kidney problems, treating BL-23. Two or three pairs of back shu points are commonly treated.

In Manaka's style of treatment, the third step focuses on the importance of correcting exacerbated muscle tension and restricted ranges of motion. He states quite clearly that one step in treatment should be to correct and balance muscle tension. To do this, he utilizes Keizo Hashimoto's therapeutic Sotai exercises, incorporating into the exercises some simple stimulation techniques.

Manaka's Mu Points

From his extensive clinical experience, Manaka has evolved a series of points which he feels are more useful as mu points than many of the classical mu points.[1] We summarize these points here and explain Manaka's reasoning in their selection.

Organ-Meridian	Mu Point
Lung	LU-1 - LU-2
Heart	KI-25, KI-23
Spleen	SP-21
Pericardium	PC-1
Liver	LV-14, LV-13
Kidney	KI-16*
Spleen or Liver and Kidney or Liver and Pericardium	GB-26
Stomach	ST-21
Gallbladder	GB-24, GB-29**
Large Intestine	ST-27
Small Intestine	ST-26
Triple Warmer	ST-25
Bladder	KI-11

Handwritten notes in right margin:

Worsley

IX-1
XIII-14
VIII-13
XIII-15
VIII-14
VII-25

XIII-12
VII-23 & 24
XI-25
XIII-4
XIII-5
XIII-3

* KI-16 also reflects the yin qiao, chong mai, and dai mai.
**GB-29 located at the ASIS also reflects the yang wei mai, yang qiao mai, and yin qiao mai.

Though some are identical to the meridian mu points, many are radical departures from standardized association. These point selections are based on Manaka's practical experience, specifically on the success he had eliminating pressure pain at these points by treating the corresponding meridian, and the source points of that meridian. His selections are based on a thorough knowledge of classical Chinese anatomy and meridian pathways.

Several theories of mu point association are held. Some authors feel that the mu points are related to the organs, some feel they relate to the meridians. Others feel there is no clear distinction between organ and meridian, but that often in a particular disease, reaction will reflect to one side, sometimes to both. For instance, heart disease reflects only to the left side, where liver disease reflects mostly to the right. The meridians are bilateral; how can a blockage of the left or right channel of the meridian be diagnosed by palpating mu points on the midline? Why is the small intestine mu point on the midline, while the large intestine mu point is bilateral? Why are the heart, small intestine, stomach, triple warmer, and bladder mu points, single points on the midline?

Perplexed by these questions, Manaka resolved to find possible solutions. Theoretically, treating the source point of a meridian would eliminate pressure pain on the corresponding mu point, since the source points are able to treat problems of their corresponding organs *(NJ 66)*. Since the distinction between organs and meridians seemed unclear, he felt this was a good place to start researching. He began palpating the mu points and treating the source points. What he found confirmed his suppositions.[2]

When a patient demonstrated a vacant kidney condition, GB-25, the classical mu point, was usually found to be unreactive; instead KI-16 was reactive. Treating KI-3 eliminated the pressure pain on KI-16, confirming KI-16 as a better mu point for the kidneys. As other examples, ST-25, the classical mu point of the large intestine, was not relieved of pressure pain by treatment of LI-4. Instead, treatment of TW-4 relieved ST-25 pressure pain, confirming that ST-25 is a better mu point of the triple warmer. In problems of the large intestine, ST-27 was often found reactive; treating LI-4 relieved the reactivity, confirming ST-27 as a better mu point for the large intestine. This same procedure was used to determine the revised mu points. Manaka further noted that if a meridian on one side is more sensitive than the other, generally the mu point on the same side is more sensitive than the other.[3] These findings led Manaka to conclude that some classical mu points have less therapeutic value than those he found by his own experience, at least when palpated and used in the prone position.

His method of checking the classical mu points involves stretching the correspondent meridian to confirm the mu point indication. This simply means stretching or bending the meridian that corresponds to the mu point being diagnosed. For instance, when palpating CV-4, the small intestine mu point, one should stretch the small intestine meridian by stretching the arm and bending the hand toward the thumb. If stretching the corresponding meridian increases the reaction, this confirms that the mu point is reflecting a condition of the corresponding meridian. In this example, the small intestine would reflect at CV-4.

□

Manaka utilizes this phenomenon as a further means of diagnosing his own mu points. As in all of Manaka's work, this technique progresses in stages and compound configurations. If one finds pressure pain on ST-26, the Manaka small intestine mu point, also check CV-4, the classical mu point. If CV-4 is not reactive, stretch the small intestine meridian, usually on the side where ST-26 is most reactive. Then, palpate both ST-26 and CV-4 again. In confirmed problems of the small intestine, CV-4 will become quite reactive. ST-26 will often become less reactive while the small intestine meridian is stretched.

Pressure pain on ST-25, the Manaka triple warmer mu point, may be indicative of a number of problems. To confirm that ST-25 is reactive because of a triple warmer problem, palpate CV-5, stretch the triple warmer meridian and palpate both ST-25 and CV-5 again. In confirmed triple warmer problems, ST-25 will become less reactive and CV-5 will become more reactive. This technique may be used to differentiate and confirm the other mu points as well. To treat problems found and confirmed in this manner a number of techniques may be used.

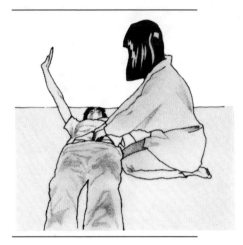

Figure 16.1 While palpating CV-4, stretch the small intestine meridian.

One of Manaka's favorite techniques is simply to treat the source point of the affected meridian. To determine the efficacy of this treatment, place the north pole of a magnet on the skin at the source point of the meridian; leave the magnet in place for a few moments and palpate the mu point again. If the reactivity has decreased, needle the source point after removing the magnet. On occasion, the reaction changes very quickly when one places the magnet on the point, at other times it changes more slowly. Be careful to leave the magnet in place long enough. As an example, when ST-25 is reactive, and stretching the triple warmer creates reactiveness on CV-5, one can test TW-4 on the side most affected. If both sides are equally affected, test both sides with the north pole magnet. If ST-25 becomes less reactive and CV-5 also becomes less reactive with the triple warmer meridian stretched, then needle TW-4.

As further evidence of the usefulness of his mu points, Manaka cites other research utilizing meridian and five-phase relationships. One technique is to treat the phase point corresponding to the mu point of the active meridian at the time of treatment. This development is based on open point theory (described below). Thus, if ST-25 is reactive and confirmed as a problem associated with the triple warmer, and the spleen meridian is active (9-11 am), treat the fire point of the spleen, SP-2. The fire point is chosen since the triple warmer, the problem meridian, belongs to fire, as the supporting fire.

Manaka's Isophasal Concept of the Five Phases

This type of treatment just described is part of Manaka's isophasal concept of the phases. As a further development of this isophasal concept and as a further demonstration of the tai yang, shao yin, shao yang, jue yin, yang ming, tai yin relationships discussed in the classical literature,[4] Manaka describes an inter-meridian relationship.[5]

Within each coupled yin—yang pair, energetic relationships exist between both yin, and yang, and yin—yang pairs. For the shao yin—tai yang relationship, similarly, for jue yin—shao yang, and tai yin—yang ming, this can be seen as follows:

□

yin	yang	yin	yang	yin	yang
shao yin	tai yang	jue yin	shao yang	tai yin	yang ming

heart ⟷ small intestine

kidney ⟷ bladder

liver ⟷ gallbladder

pericardium ⟷ triple warmer

lung ⟷ large intestine

spleen ⟷ stomach

Manaka uses both these interrelationships and the isophasal concept by treating, for instance, the metal point of any of the four meridians of the yin-yang coupled unit in a metal phase imbalance, when the time of treatment corresponds to the active time of any of the four meridians. That is, if it is the time of the bladder and the patient has a metal imbalance (perhaps LU-1 or ST-27 are reactive), treating BL-67, SI-1, KI-7, or HT-4 can treat the metal imbalance. Treatment of these points should elicit a decrease in the reactivity of the diagnostic points or areas. As before, use the north pole of a magnet to select the point that produces the greatest change.

An interesting case history from his practice demonstrates a variation of these ideas. When a patient with a unilateral reaction on ST-27 was tested by placing the north pole of a magnet on LU-9, reactivity of ST-27 on the affected side decreased, but the reactivity on the other side increased. Manaka then placed the north pole on ST-36, reducing the reaction of ST-27 on both sides. He treated ST-36. In this case he was utilizing the large intestine and stomach relationship of yang ming; ST-27 reflects the large intestine, and the yang ming—tai yin relationship.

With similar experiments and a deep knowledge of the classics, Manaka has found other useful treatments for specific reactive points. Needling LV-8 and PC-6 can relieve pressure pain on LV-14. If not, needling GV-20 or palpating and treating reactive points on the ren mai where the liver meridian passes (e.g. CV-3, CV-4, CV-12) will relieve the pain.[6] For pressure pain on BL-23, placing copper on a reactive lower point on the kidney meridian (KI-1 to KI-6, etc.) and placing zinc on a reactive point on the upper portion of the kidney meridian will relieve the pressure pain of BL-23, if good points are chosen.[7] For pressure pain on ST-11, copper may be placed on a reactive point on one of the three leg yin meridians, and zinc placed higher up the meridian on another reactive point. Or, copper may be placed on ST-30 and zinc on KI-1. With one or the other of these two treatments, the pressure pain on ST-11 should be eliminated.[8]

This last case shows that the stream of the extraordinary vessels may well be opposite to the stream of the meridians. Usually, zinc is placed downstream and copper upstream on the meridian. But in this case, with an extraordinary vessel, it is opposite, copper downstream and zinc upstream. This raises some fundamental questions about the nature of the meridians and the extraordinary vessels. In similar experiments using zinc and copper polarity, Manaka has found that if an imbalance exists in a meridian between left and right, as determined using Akabane's diagnostic method of heating the jing points, placing any metal on the tonification or luo point of the weaker side will make that side stronger when tested a few minutes later.[9] This restores the balance and treats the problem.

□

With these kinds of simple clinical tests, Manaka has attempted to demonstrate many classical concepts and theories. Further, recognizing that we live in a quantitatively-minded society, he has clinically investigated the occurrence of pressure pain on relevant diagnostic points, developing a series of diagnostic statistics of the reactivity of some of the more important points. It should be noted that these statistics ought not be taken as absolute figures, merely as starting points in our own quest for knowledge and better practice. The statistics as listed below are based on the palpation of 95 cases, with comparison of the left and right sides of each point. The percentages represent the number of people with pressure pain on that point.[10]

Point	Correspondence	Right	Left
ST-11	chong mai	34.7%	34.7%
ST-12	yin qiao mai	9.5%	12.6%
LU-1	lung	8.4%	18.9%
LV-14	liver	55.8%	10.5%
KI-16	kidney	28.4%	40.0%
ST-25	triple warmer	12.6%	27.4%
GB-26	spleen or liver/kidney or liver/pericardium	10.5%	31.6%
ST 27	large intestine	12.6%	16.9%
GB-29	gallbladder or yin or yang qiao or yang wei	14.7%	44.2%
KI-11	bladder	3.2%	6.3%
LI-4		37.9%	33.7%
CV-22	yin wei mai	12.6%	

Statistics such as these can be useful in the development of a coherent systematic approach to diagnosis, as they can help us discern normal from pathological pressure pain.

History and Development of the Ion Cords

Manaka's invention of the ion-pumping cords came as a result of his medical experience during World War II. During his medical tour of duty, he discovered that applying tin foil to burns not only relieved the pain but also stimulated and seemed to speed the healing process. In his efforts to understand and research this phenomenon, he theorized that possibly the electrical properties of tin, relative to the body's electrical properties, had brought about the effects. He considered that pain was related to a relative imbalance in the sodium and potassium ions inside and outside of the cells, particularly in a burned area where the tissues were actually damaged. Based on these assumptions, he posited that moving electrical currents through the burned area, or "ion pumping," should help. He began by using electroacupuncture to treat burns.

Although this method was partially successful, he found that the needles through which the electricity was passed underwent degeneration, causing local tissue damage. The positive-charged needle would electrolyze into the surrounding tissues, causing local irritation of the tissues and pitting of the needles. Manaka's findings stimulated considerable research in Japan regarding the effects of electroacupuncture, and led to the development and use of much safer and more sophisticated electric machines and techniques. He continued to experiment with tools and techniques that might effect conduction of the electrical current without side effects.

The body works in interesting ways. Manaka's burn treatment theory posited that a repletion of energy in one area of the body, i.e., a burn, would cause a relative depletion or vacancy of energy in another area or areas. The ability to transfer the repletion to the area of vacancy was theoretically inviting. Rather than using an external electrical source, Manaka sought to use the body's inherent relative electrical potentials. He devised the ion-pumping cords, essentially comprised of copper wires attached to clips. One clip contains a diode so that the electric flow can progress in only one direction.

In a 1965 report, he described treatment of thirty-one patients who had second-degree burns. All these patients were in severe pain. Within ten minutes of the initial ion cord attachment, all reported less pain. In twenty minutes, all reported no pain or markedly reduced pain.[11] While studying these clinical results, Manaka noticed that certain points — the extraordinary vessel points — were more effective than others. He was able to develop remarkably effective uses of the ion cords in treatment of the extraordinary vessels. Manaka's later theories about the nature and function of the extraordinary vessels derived in part from this experience.

The treatment for burns is quite simple. Gently press sterilized tin foil onto the burned area, covering the area. Aluminum foil will also work. Then, at the most distal part of the body, select a point by palpation, often an extraordinary vessel point, which has some relationship to the burned area. Insert a needle shallowly into this point. Attach the red clip of the cord to the needle and the black clip of the cord to the foil. In virtually all cases, this will relieve the burn pain, if not immediately, then within a few minutes. It is important to ensure that the patient is comfortable and that the foil maintains good contact with the burned area. The following illustrations, drawn from photographs taken at the Manaka Hospital in Odawara, Japan, demonstrate this procedure. Manaka tapes the foil, cord, and needle firmly in place and leaves it in place for extended periods of time. Sometimes he encourages the patients in his hospital to walk around with the entire assemblage in place. As long as the cord is attached, the pain should be relieved or greatly lessened and the healing process, usually quite slow with burns, will accelerate. In treatment of burns, one burn at a time is treated and the cord should cross over the body. However, it is also possible to treat bilaterally. To do so, do not cross the cords; maintain a bilateral needle—foil connection, remaining on the same sides of the body.

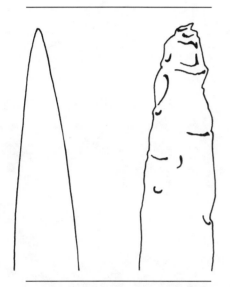

Figure 16.2 An acupuncture needle prior to use in electroacupuncture procedures and the same needle after these procedures.

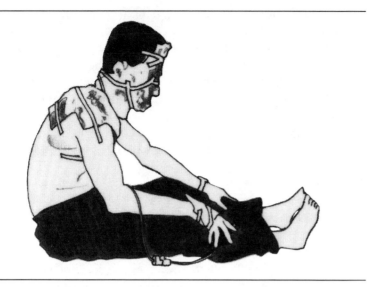

Figure 16.3A From the Manaka Hospital. A patient being treated for burns on the face and right shoulder.

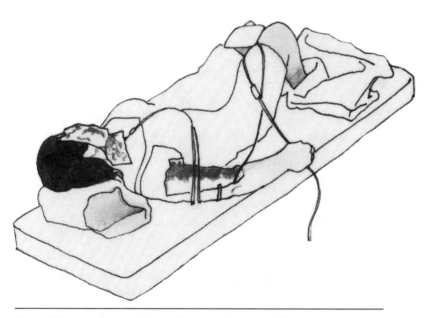

Figure 16.3B From the Manaka hospital. A patient being treated for burns on the face and right arm.

Many have difficulty believing that something seemingly so simple can have such phenomenal effectiveness in treating first and second degree burns. The treatment of burns is an area of medicine that is constantly researched. Hopefully, this procedure can be introduced here in the West.

The selection of points to use for needle treatment in the case of a burn merits further discussion. If, for example, a patient presented with a burn on the right hand, on the small intestine meridian, a number of points could be considered for palpating. Because of the SI-3, BL-62 connection, BL-62 would be an obvious candidate. A point on the liver meridian would be another consideration, as it is chronobiologically opposite to the small intestine meridian by the Chinese clock. According to the five-phase and ten-stem cycles, a point on the kidney meridian might be selected or possibly another point from the liver meridian. Another point might be either SP-6 or GB-35. Manaka speaks of SP-6, three yin crossing, and TW-8, three yang luo, as being able to regulate and control the yin and yang of the body. In conjunction with these points are other points such as GB-35 and Manaka's special point on the pericardium meridian, halfway between PC-7 and PC-3. In all cases, the point selected is determined by palpation. If all the points considered produce no clear choice, palpate GB-35 and SP-6 and select the most reactive.

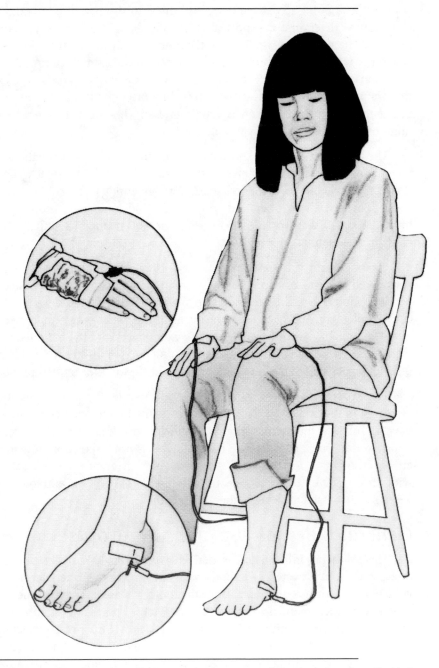

Figure 16.4 Tin foil is taped over the burn. A distal point is needled and taped in place. The black clip of the ion-pumping cord is placed on the foil and red clip on the needle.

During treatment the patient will become noticeably relaxed, sometimes to the point of falling asleep. This is a good indication. When using the ion cords, regardless of treatment goal, the patient should become more relaxed. This crossing over of the cords in the treatment of burns is one of the few cases Manaka describes where the cords cross over the body. In the eight extraordinary vessel treatments using the cords and the other more local treatments, the cords generally do not cross over the body, but are attached unilaterally. One other notable exception to this principle is the treatment of numbness or paralysis.

A paralysis is a vacancy condition; therefore the reverse procedure is used. The red clip is placed on a point in the paralyzed area, the black clip is placed at a point across the body and distal to the paralyzed area. Use palpation to determine the most affected meridian in the paralyzed area, then find the most reactive point on the meridian for needle insertion, and attach the red clip. Numbness may be treated in the same fashion. Makio Maruyama, who has researched Manaka's work on the ion cords, suggests that we palpate and select reactive points then place the black clip on a yin meridian and the red clip on a yang meridian. In effect, this treats the numbness as a condition of yin repletion.[12]

The treatment of burns and paralyzed or numb areas utilizes the supplementing and draining abilities of the cords. Generally, the black clip is draining (dispersing) and the red clip is supplementing. The cords may be utilized specifically to drain and supplement, and have been found to be helpful for treatment of local pain. A series of treatments utilizing the cords in this manner appears later in this text.

Treatment of the extraordinary vessels using ion-pumping cords is not considered in terms of supplementing, or supplementation of the master or coupled points. The classical literature that we have reviewed does not discuss supplementation or drainage of the eight treatment points; one merely treats the points. According to Manaka's experience, and the experience of many others who use the cords, when treating the extraordinary vessels the black clip goes on the master point and the red clip on the coupled point.

The extraordinary vessels represent a different level and manifestation of energy in the body. The *Nan Jing* tells us that when the twelve meridians develop fullness, this fullness drains into the extraordinary vessels, never to return to the twelve meridians. This "fullness" is **not** a repletion. It is more an "overflowing." At this level, the body has different ways of dealing with this relative fullness. The use of ion cords on the extraordinary vessels is discussed in detail in the next section.

General Rules for Use of the Ion Cords

The following information is derived from Manaka's books and lectures, and from private discussions with the authors. Adherence to the guidelines set forth is advisable, since the ion cords are a powerful therapy, thus having the potential to harm as well as cure. Care and attention are required. Experimentation demands a theoretical construct of considerable sophistication. Because of the supplementing and draining properties of the cords, distinguishing between yin and yang symptoms becomes a useful starting point. These distinctions are also helpful in determining the correct application of the cords on the extraordinary vessels.

Yang symptoms include excessive tension or oversensitivity of the muscles, nerves or blood vessels, i.e., *inflammation, pain, or tension*. These are said to result from either excessive accumulation of positive ions or insufficient accumulation of negative ions. Yin symptoms include lack of tonus or slackness of the muscles, nerves, or blood vessels, i.e., *numbness, dullness, or heaviness*. These are said to result from either excessive accumulation of negative ions or insufficient accumulation of positive ions. Except in extraordinary vessel treatments, the black clip should always go where the yang symptoms are evident and the red clip should always go where the yin symptoms are evident.

There are a series of other important rules when using the cords.

1.   When treating the extraordinary vessels, treatment is usually bilateral, connecting one cord from the master point of one side to the coupled point of the same side. Do the same on the other side with the other cord.

2.   When applying treatments that do not involve the extraordinary vessels, it is often the case that only one side is treated. In such cases faithfully follow the procedure recommended.

3.   The cords are generally retained for 10-20 minutes or until the diagnostic signs that indicated their use subside or decrease substantially, provided this remains within the 20-minute period.

4.   Because of the nature of the cords and the sensitivity some people have to them, the practitioner is ill-advised to leave the patient alone during the time the cords are attached. When the cords are correctly attached to the proper points, the patient will relax, sometimes falling asleep. If the cord arrangement is not correct, the patient will develop signs of discomfort, either physical, emotional, or energetic such as flushing, agitation, unease. This can happen immediately after connection, or sometime later, even after the cords have done their job. The practitioner must be present to make a correct assessment of the patient's condition. Misapplication of the cords can exacerbate a patient's condition. No matter how rarely this occurs, we need to be attentive to all patients.

5.   To help the patient relax and stay relaxed, keep a blanket handy to cover the patient from chill. The lights may be turned down, with gentle music played.

6.   Needles used to attach the cords should be inserted shallowly, either in the direction of flow of the meridian or perpendicularly to a depth of no more than 2-4 mm. It is inappropriate and unnecessary to use a deeper insertion or seek a stimulus; the electrical flow is strongest on the surface of the body. Manaka stresses the 2 mm maximum depth very emphatically. Number 2 gauge Japanese needles are ideal for use with the ion-pumping cords. If these are not available, then number 3 gauge will suffice.

7.   The needles and/or clips of the cords may be taped to the body to ensure that the cords do not pull out the needles.

8.   The cords should not be attached to any electroacupuncture machine. They were devised specifically to utilize the body's own electric currents. Thus, each clip of the cords should be attached to a needle on the body.

9.   When using the cords, usually no other points should be needled or treated at the same time. This can disturb the treatment and allay its effectiveness. Extraneous placement of needles may distort the electric fields and flows generated by the ion cords, becoming electrical poles in relation to their negative and positive poles.

10.   All jewelry, ornament, or metal of any kind in contact with the surface of the skin should be removed so as to eliminate the generation of currents or the disturbance of the currents generated by the cords.

11.   When treating the extraordinary vessels, should the patient fail to relax or become uncomfortable, or should the diagnostic signs remain unchanged, remove the clips and reverse the polarities. That is, place the black clips on coupled points and the red clips on the master point. Often, this alone will relax the patient and produce the desired therapeutic effects. This works possibly because it is the coupled vessel connection as a whole that is functioning. At times, no matter how clear the initial diagnosis, the situation is contradictory and it is the opposite connection that works. If the same lack of results continues or discomfort develops, remove the cords and needles and diagnose again; the original diagnosis is likely incorrect.

12.   When using other than an extraordinary vessel treatment, should the patient show the same signs of discomfort, double check that the correct clips are on the correct points. If they are, remove the cord(s) and needles. It is generally inappropriate to reverse the polarity of the cords in non-extraordinary vessel treatments, as this will most certainly increase the possibility of exacerbating the patient's condition. Review and reassess the diagnosis and apply another treatment.

If diagnosis, point selection, and location are correct, the patient will relax immediately and the diagnostic signs, such as pressure pain or tension in certain areas, will decrease almost immediately. Within ten minutes one should be able to assess the treatment. Palpation is obviously important, providing direct evaluation of the effectiveness of therapy. Manaka and other well-known therapists have remarked that if changes on the abdomen can be brought about, immediate disappearance of symptoms is immaterial. The symptoms will naturally improve or disappear. This style of treatment, directed by the reactive areas of the abdomen, is considered a root or general treatment. When the symptoms also vanish, it is, of course, a satisfying experience.

The wearing of jewelry can have repercussions beyond the clinical setting. Since the body has a whole series of electromagnetic fields and currents generated by the various tissues of the body, any kind of metal can interact with the body and affect these fields and currents. In some cases, metal jewelry has been found to be the cause of certain diseases and symptoms. Of course, it is also potentially beneficial if the appropriate piece of jewelry is worn on the appropriate area. Since this is difficult to determine it is probably advisable to wear no metal jewelry. In fact, this recommendation is commonly issued by experienced practitioners.[13] Nylon pantyhose or synthetic clothing can also create noticeable static charges around the body, and should also be avoided.
□

Manaka relates one interesting exception to this recommendation. He has treated a number of patients who have suffered a heart attack and who continue to experience heart problems.[14] Generally he would treat heart problems with cords to the yin wei—chong mai. However, some patients were unable to get into the office regularly for treatment, because their heart problem made travel difficult. He was able to provide a very simple and effective therapy for these patients. He advised these patients to wear a small gold ring on the distal joint of the little finger of the left hand, instructing them to move it up and down around the joint regularly, and further recommending that they not wear any other metal jewelry, to prevent interference from other bioelectrical and ionic currents. Patients reported an easing of their heart problem and greater ease traveling.

The principle of ion-cord treatment, using tiny electric currents to stimulate acupoints, has been extended from the use of ion cords to include the use of all kinds of metals and magnets. Many of these techniques do not even require the insertion of needles, rendering such therapy even easier to use. These non-invasive treatments also produce outstanding results. For example, utilizing all the information and procedures applicable to the use of ion cords, one can tape "Keptone" pellets to the points and attach the cords to the pellets. On very sensitive or needle-phobic patients, this can extend the range of therapy.

Manaka Extraordinary Vessel Treatments

While the development of extraordinary vessel theory is fascinating and complex, we can with fairness simplify its history by considering that modern thought begins with the *Zhen Jiu Da Quan*. The author, Xu Feng, described the eight extraordinary vessels with reference to the temporal sequence of the trigrams and to their eight treatment points. These correspondences are important in the calculation of the sixty-day cycle of open extraordinary vessel points, sometimes called master points or respectable points.[15] Part of Xu Feng's explanation is that the eight vessels are actually four paired sets of vessels: chong mai—yin wei mai; ren mai—yin qiao mai; dai mai—yang wei mai; and du mai—yang qiao mai. He also describes the point/vessel relationships and meeting places.[16]

Extraordinary Vessel Relationships			
Point	**Vessel**	**Relation**	**Meeting Places**
SP-4	chong mai	father	heart, chest and stomach
PC-6	yin wei mai	mother	
SI-3	du mai	husband	lateral edges of the bridge of the nose next to the eyes; the back of the neck; ears; shoulders; arms; small intestine and bladder meridians
BL-62	yang qiao mai	wife	
GB-41	dai mai	male	the lateral aspect of the eyes; behind the ears; cheeks; neck; shoulders
TW-5	yang wei mai	female	
LU-7	ren mai	master	the "supporter of the lungs" (trachea and bronchi); throat and diaphragm
KI-6	yin qiao mai	guest	

As may be seen in Manaka's work, some of these areas where the vessels meet are significant diagnostic sites. The selection of these four pairs of points is probably based on the same pairing found in an earlier text, the *Zhen Jing Zhi Nan (Guide To Acupuncture)* of the Jin dynasty, 1115-1234 A.D.. In this text, SP-4 was paired with PC-6, LU-7 with KI-6, SI-3 with BL-62, and GB-41 with TW-5. However, the *Zhi Nan* made no clear mention of the eight extraordinary vessels in reference to these four pairs of points. The point pairs were described as special points, which when treated singly or together, were able to control and treat a great many disorders.[17]

The *Zhen Jiu Da Cheng* also provides an interesting discussion of the eight vessels, useful diagnostically for selecting treatments and making prognostications.

> The yang qiao, yang wei, du mai, and dai mai can mainly treat diseases of the shoulder, back, lumbar, and thigh that are superficial. The yin qiao, yin wei, ren mai, and chong mai can mainly treat diseases of the heart, abdomen, rib, and side of the body that are in the lining [inside].[18]

Manaka's study of these classics, along with his substantive clinical results, provided the foundation for his general theories of the eight extraordinary vessels. He found that specific target or treatment areas are affected by treating these paired points. In addition to the symptomology of the vessels, there are specific indications for each pair of vessels. These indications help determine the appropriateness of extraordinary vessel treatment and to differentiate which to use. This diagnosis is largely based on palpation. Although it is important to remember that the trajectories of the extraordinary vessels have been described in a variety of ways, and that the pathways and points noted in the basic student texts do not tell the whole story, it is not necessary to palpate too many areas or points. Through skillful and attentive practice, research and study, specific points and areas have been found to be the most significant diagnostically. Manaka has led the field is this research.

Theoretical Perspectives

Looking at the eight extraordinary vessel trajectories we can see a particular symmetry. There is a trajectory passing up the front of the body on the midline, the ren mai, and one passing up the back of the body on the midline, the du mai. A horizontal vessel encircles the body at the waist, the dai mai. Manaka develops this idea of symmetry further, discussing these patterns in relation to the right and left sides of the body, the upper and lower, front and back sections.[19]

This divides the body into eight sections or "octants." The eight extraordinary vessels relate to these eight areas of the body. The ren and du mai divide the left and right sides of the body. The dai mai divides the upper and lower parts of the body. The gallbladder and triple warmer meridians divide the front and back sections of the yang aspect. The pericardium and liver/spleen meridians divide the front and back sections of the yin aspect.[20] Though obvious when presented to us now, these relationships had not been described or stated previously in any form of

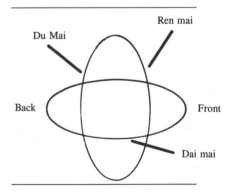

Figure 16.5 The ren mai, du mai and dai mai axes.

therapeutic value. We can see the germinus of these ideas in the *Zhen Jiu Da Quan,* where the eight vessels were discussed in relation to the eight master points.

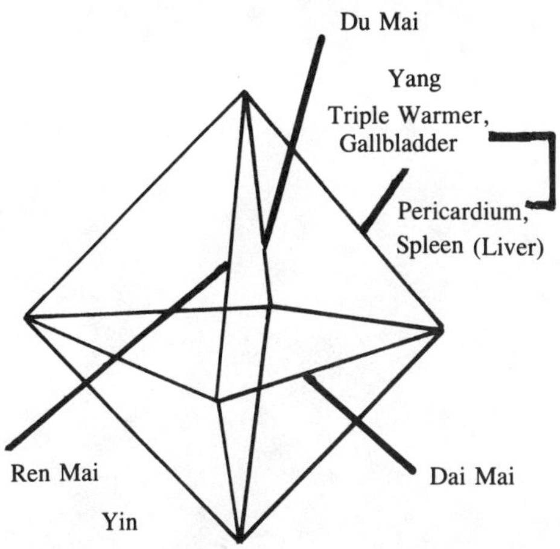

Manaka proposes that these topological dividing lines are related to the selection of these eight points as the master points. The treatment points of the yin wei and yang wei mai, PC-6 and TW-5, lie on the pericardium and triple warmer meridians. The treatment points of the chong mai and the dai mai, SP-4 and GB-41, lie on the spleen and gallbladder meridians. This nearly perfectly fits the pattern of four meridians dividing the front and back portions of the yin and yang aspects of the body. The exception is SP-4 on the spleen meridian, where the liver meridian would be more theoretically satisfying. In noting this variance, Manaka points out that the spleen meridian has a pathway very similar to the liver meridian on the inside of the legs. Even considering the theoretical variance, these four meridians do divide the front and back sides of the body and connect the upper and lower portions. The selection of points on these four meridians as master points relates the extraordinary vessels, which they control, to the same divisions and connections.

The yin qiao and yang qiao mai master points are KI-6 and BL-62. This suggests a relationship of the kidney and bladder meridians because of the close proximity of the kidney meridian to the ren mai and the bladder meridian to the du mai.[21] These too relate to the front and back, upper and lower portions of the body. These distinctions have important consequences in treatment.

Manaka notes that we are best advised to think of the eight extraordinary vessels in relation to the eight corresponding areas of the body, as this supplies a more physical base. We can consider the extraordinary vessel treatments as a means of helping restore body balance and symmetry. From this point of view, there is less emphasis on the nature of the person's disease and more attention to bodily imbalance. When we are thinking about treatment of the twelve meridians and the five yin and six yang organs, we are thinking in terms of each of those meridians and organs and their corresponding functions. This distinction is not absolute. Since we can affect energetics and body balance using both extraordinary vessel and twelve meridian treatments, this distinction is a starting point for our therapeutic problem-solving.[22] Clearly, the extraordinary vessels have direct relationships to the meridians.[23]

Determining a Diagnostic Framework

In utilizing the extraordinary vessels in treatment, our first problem is knowing how to use the theoretical framework of yin and yang. Manaka suggests eight important steps for gathering diagnostic information.

1. When examining the patient determine if the lower part of the body is cold, or if the upper body is easily heated (with sensations of qi rising upward, possibly accompanied by dizziness). Determine if the patient suffers counterflow qi (i.e., vacancy below and repletion above).

2. Ask at what times of the day the symptoms become clearer, worse, or more active.

Figure 16.6 Manaka's octahedral model of the extraordinary vessels.

3. Examine the patient's erect posture. Structural imbalances indicate use of the eight extraordinary vessels.

4. Compare tension between the muscles of the back and the muscles of the abdomen.

5. Palpate on the center line of the abdomen. Apply the same pressure above and below the umbilicus and compare the relative tension of the upper and lower parts.

6. With the same pressure, compare the relative tension of the muscles to the left and right sides of the umbilicus. These areas extend beyond the rectus abdominus muscles (stomach meridians).

7. Check to see if the patient has relative tension, pressure pain, or discomfort below the ribs in the subcostal region (chest distress); compare the left and right sides.

8. Palpate and compare the left and right sides of the following significant points: LI-4, LU-1, SP-21, ST-25, KI-16, ST-40, BL-58, SP-6, GB-29.

It should be noted that Manaka locates GB-29 at the anterior superior iliac spine. This probably follows the alternate location which may be found, for instance, in the *Zhen Jiu Ju Ying:* "GB-29 is below LV-13, the spleen mu point."[24] This location of GB-29 is related to the yang wei and yang qiao mai. Manaka explains that this relationship may be due to a continuous band of muscles originating in this area. The obliquus internus muscles are attached to the anterior superior portions of the iliac spine, extending across the abdomen and continuous with the obliquus externus muscles above the umbilicus. These muscles pass to the sides of the body. They are continuous with the serratus anterior muscles which pass beneath the shoulder blades to attach to the medial border of the scapulae, and with the rhomboideus major and minor muscles which pass to, and attach to, the lower cervical and upper thoracic vertebrae.[25] This would clearly account for the physio-electrical medium of the yang qiao mai relationship and probably the yang wei mai as well. The gallbladder is also said to reflect at this point. This too may be due to the same band of muscles.

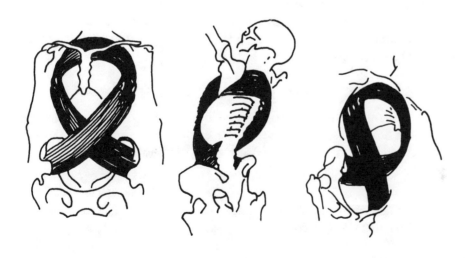

Figure 16.7 Continuous connected muscles serve as a functional muscle group.

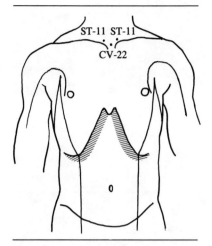

Figure 16.8 The yin wei-chong mai connection.

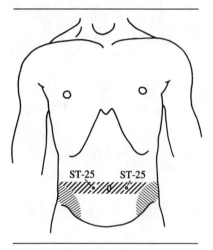

Figure 16.9a The yang wei-dai mai connection.

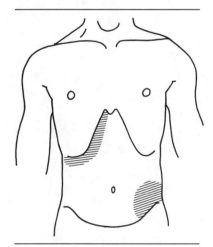

Figure 16.9b Cross-syndrome: yin wei mai— yang wei mai connection.

In following these eight steps, try always to compare the left and right, upper and lower, front and back parts of the body. Check for imbalances or differences. This diagnosis uses the idea of dividing the body into eight parts. If some imbalance of yin and yang is found by this procedure, Manaka recommends a series of ordered steps and treatments. First, examine the yin and yang wei mai connections. If there are imbalances, use the ion cords on the appropriate points for ten minutes. Then, if it is still necessary, check the yin qiao and yang qiao mai connection. If there are imbalances, treat them with the ion cords for another ten minutes. Manaka comments that these imbalances of yin and yang may be caused by many complicated factors. One should pay attention to other imbalances, such as noticeable muscle tension.

It is easy, having arrived at a specific, clear diagnosis, to feel overly secure. The real test comes with treatment. If favorable responses are not obtained from treating these eight points alone, the diagnosis must be reexamined. With a clear diagnosis and treatment at the level of the eight extraordinary vessels, substantial changes often occur without further intervention. But if there are other imbalances from other energetic or physical levels in the body, working with the eight vessels alone will not suffice. Manaka feels that if we are careful and attentive, we will find the most significant paradox in the body. If we find it, treat it. It is generally unnecessary to treat the other, smaller paradoxes. These should naturally resolve themselves. When one has diagnosed the main problem, for instance a problem with the yin qiao mai, the associated problems of headaches, backaches, or digestion will generally disappear, if the yin qiao mai is the true paradox. It may appear that there is a weakness in the kidneys for example, and treatments using the local points offer relief. However, if treatment is directed at the main paradox, it is often unnecessary to treat locally. This is true regardless of the level at which the main paradox resides: organs, meridians, phases, or extraordinary vessels.

Specific Diagnostic Steps

Manaka uses specific steps for diagnosing and confirming each pair of vessels. These reflect not only his cumulative clinical experience, but as well the many classical texts that he has studied. In his explanation of the paired points and their target or diagnostic areas one can see the influence of the *Zhen Jiu Da Quan*.[26]

The yin wei mai connection: Symptoms may be right-sided (yin). There may be symptoms of the yin wei mai or pressure pain or reaction on CV-22; symptoms, pressure pain or reaction of the pericardium meridian; or tension or pressure pain below the ribs in the subcostal region (chest distress).

The chong mai connection: Symptoms of the chong mai are pressure pain or reaction on ST-11. Other indications may be symptoms, pressure pain, or reaction on the spleen meridian.

The yang wei mai connection: Symptoms may be more left sided (yang). There may be pressure pain or other reaction on the yang wei mai or symptoms associated with the yang wei mai. Pressure pain or other reaction on the dai mai, or symptoms associated with the dai mai may also indicate yang wei mai. Pressure pain or other reaction on TW-5 or on the triple warmer meridian and pressure pain or other reaction on GB-41 or on the gallbladder meridian are also indicative. Tension or pressure pain around GB-29 (ASIS) usually on the left points to yang wei mai. Note that right-sided chest distress, a subcostal reaction, associated with the yin wei mai may often be accompanied by reaction around left GB-29. If there is obvious pressure pain or reaction around left GB-29 with right-sided chest distress, this would suggest the use of the yin wei mai connection on the right side and the yang wei mai connection on the left. This is a common abdominal pattern in Manaka's experience which he terms the "cross-syndrome." Treatment for it represents a specialized use of the cords.

The yin qiao mai connection: Most significant indications are pressure pain or reaction on or around the ren mai itself, especially above and below the umbilicus. Compare the relative tension of above and below the umbilicus on the ren mai. Generally tension above with less tension below the umbilicus is an indication of the yin qiao mai. Also look for symptoms associated with the ren mai, which are opposite to the du mai. Compare the relative tension of the back muscles and the rectus abdominus muscles. If the back muscles are overly tense and the rectus abdominus muscles are overly loose, use the yin qiao mai connection. Another indication is pressure pain or reaction on the yin qiao mai or other associated symptoms.

The yang qiao mai connection: Symptoms may include pressure pain or reaction on or just lateral to the du mai (the *hua to* points line), especially on the upper back. Also look for symptoms associated with the du mai, or pressure pain or reaction on the neck or the back of the upper arm. Pressure pain or reaction around the ASIS (Manaka's GB-29) may indicate the yang qiao mai connection. Differentiate a reaction here from the yang wei mai by the presence of pressure pain or reaction on or around KI-11, symptoms or pressure pain or reaction on the cervical vertebrae, and muscle tension or a knot or reaction around SI-10.[27]

The rationale for these symptom-sign indications required a synthesis of a variety of ideas which were randomly presented in the classical texts. For example, we can understand that the yin wei mai connection is made by dividing the front and back portions of the body. PC-6, the "mother point" of yin wei mai, and SP-4, the chong mai "father point," are significant points on the front of the body. They affect a large number of symptoms. Various classical and modern sources tell us that PC-6 is good for symptoms caused by or related to the heart, for instance: palpitations, difficulty or discomfort breathing, dizziness. Some sources say that when a patient overeats or has food poisoning or is suffering in the chest from stomach problems, strong stimulation of PC-6 can cause vomiting and thus treat the symptoms. Stimulating PC-6 can affect the upper part of the abdomen. SP-4 is commonly seen as a major point for digestive problems. By connecting SP-4 and PC-6, one treats the main symptoms of these two points and thus relieves oversensitivity of the middle warmer.

This would explain why a yin wei mai disharmony can be diagnosed by oversensitivity or tension of the muscles in the subcostal region. Overconsumption of alcohol or food (particularly spicy food), or use of medications that cause liver dysfunction, are frequently the cause of this condition. In severe cases, the muscles in the subcostal region will be markedly

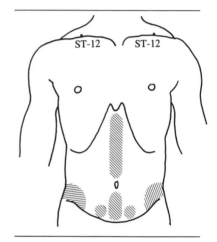

Figure 16.10 The yin qiao-ren mai connection.

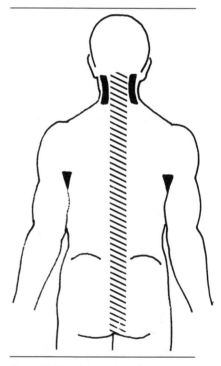

Figure 16.11a The yang qiao-du mai connection.

oversensitive. In milder cases usually the right side alone is involved. There may also be small colored pimples or areas of pigmentation in the Hirata zone on the face.[28] (See Figure 16.12.) Treating the yin wei mai connection for ten minutes will alleviate or remove the symptomatic oversensitivity in the subcostal region, even if only temporarily. The manifested problems will be naturally treated.

The yang wei mai connection is between TW-5, the luo point of the triple warmer, and GB-41, the wood point of the gallbladder. Each is a powerful point, on their respective meridians and in relation to the extraordinary vessels, having many and various effects. The gallbladder and triple warmer meridians divide the front and back of the body, more particularly the yang part. These meridians are able to stimulate or influence the balance of areas on either side of each line. They are like the fulcra of a series of scales. Many of the lines or pathways of the extraordinary vessels pass through these fulcra.

The classic texts tell us that the du mai is the "ocean of the yang meridians," the ren mai the "ocean of the yin meridians." We may conceive of them as the uniting place of all meridians, the oceans into which all rivers and streams flow. The du mai and ren mai are also dividing lines or fulcra. The du mai and ren mai divide the left and right sides of the body, the dai mai the upper and lower parts. The gallbladder and triple warmer are the third dividing lines as they divide the front and back portions of the body.

The classical authors systematized the meridians by attaching their names to the internal organs. The triple warmer and heart-wrapping luo (pericardium) meridians are the only exception. These have rather general energetic correspondences. For instance, the triple warmer represents the relationship of the three warmer functions, a branch of the upper warmer being the meridian circuit. The triple warmer as well can be perceived to function like an ocean of all the meridians. The yin wei mai and yang wei mai function like streams that divide the front and back portions of the body and connect the upper and lower parts. The extraordinary vessels are thus a complete energetic system of oceans that connect and moderate the flow of the twelve meridians. The focus of each is thus expressed in areas, many of which conjoin the related organ meridians.

The yang wei mai connection is indicated by pressure pain or reaction on the dai mai. Since the yang wei mai passes through GB-29, connecting with the gallbladder meridian and the yang qiao mai, pressure pain or reaction around GB-29 indicates the connection. Manaka also notes that while in herbal diagnosis this area is seen as diagnostic of blood stasis, in acupuncture there is generally not a direct parallel.

The focus of the yin qiao and yang qiao mai are the ren mai and the du mai. For the du mai, the focus is on problems or symptoms found on the upper part of the du mai. For the ren mai, focus is on problems or symptoms found on the lower parts of the ren mai.[29] This relationship can be seen as based on the topological relationships of the lower abdomen and upper back.[30]

The classical texts do not explain why SI-3 is considered the respectable point of the du mai or why LU-7 is the respectable point of the ren mai. It may be that the bladder meridian lies at the side of the du mai and

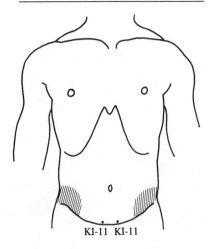

Figure 16.11b The yang qiao-du mai connection.

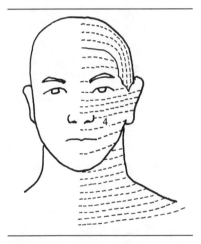

Figure 16.12 The Hirata liver zone.: 4

the kidney meridian at the side of the ren mai. Strong connections and relationships exist between these parallel lines. In the classics, KI-6 and BL-62 were considered lower-limb treatment points for the yin qiao and yang qiao mai. A five-phase relationship is likely the correlation of these two points with the upper limb points, SI-3 and LU-7. Both the yang wei and yin wei mai connect the supporting fire meridians of the arm, triple warmer and pericardium, to the wood and earth meridians of the legs. Both the yang and yin qiao mai connect the water meridians of the leg to important points of the fire and metal meridians of the arm. In part, these relationships maintain a water and supporting fire connection to the other phases, or at least important and powerful points on meridians of the other phases.

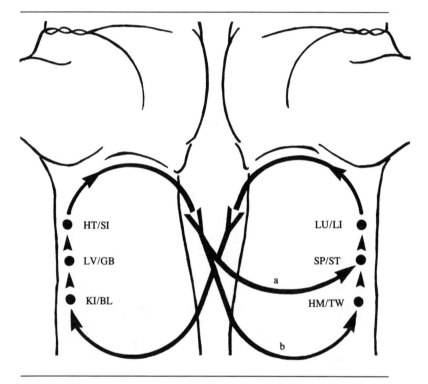

Figure 16.13 *Nan Jing 18* radial pulse diagnosis.
      "a" represents the paths of engenderment.
      "b" represents the possibilities of the continuation of engenderment.

We believe that Manaka's explanations of the five-phase relationships may also be seen in other ways. The following idea is based on our understanding of the creative-cycle process described in the pulse diagnosis system of *Nan Jing* chapter 18. In the right pulse, the fire of triple warmer and master of the heart (pericardium) meridians create the earth of stomach and spleen, which creates the metal of large intestine and lung, which in turn creates the water of kidney and bladder of the left pulse. This, in turn, creates the wood of gallbladder and liver and follows to the fire of small intestine and heart, which feeds back to either the earth of spleen and stomach or the fire of the triple warmer and pericardium. This can be seen in Figure 16.13. If we look at the eight respectable points of the extraordinary vessels and the meridians on which they lie, an interesting relationship appears. One can trace a cycle from yin meridian points, PC-6 to SP-4

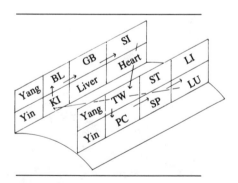

Figure 16.14

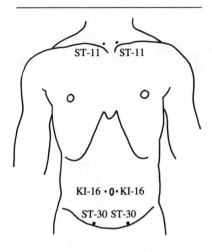

Figure 16.15 Chong mai.

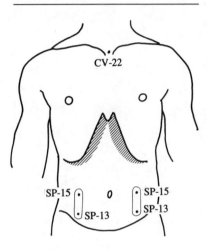

Figure 16.16 Yin wei mai.

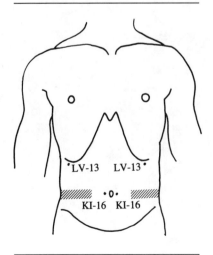

Figure 16.17 Dai mai.

to LU-7 to KI-6, to the yang meridian points, BL-62 to GB-41 to SI-3 to TW-5, then again to the yin meridian points, PC-6 etc. This may be viewed diagrammatically in figure 16.14. Though this may only be a part of the explanation for the connections, at the least it offers a rationale as to why the points of the other four meridians were not selected as respectable points of the extraordinary vessels.

Another connection exists between LU-7 and KI-6 which relates to the pathways of the kidney and lung meridians. The area above the umbilicus is traversed by the lung meridian. It starts at CV-12, passes to CV-10 then CV-13, then to CV-9 and arrives at the large intestine then back to CV-13, and passes upward to the lungs. Part of the area below the umbilicus on the ren mai is traversed by the kidney meridian. It passes through CV-3 and CV-4. This offers reasonable explanation for the emphasis given to palpating the ren mai on the abdomen for the yin qiao and ren mai.

Differential Diagnosis of Extraordinary Vessels

In determining diagnoses of the extraordinary vessels it is important to realize that many of the points corresponding to the eight extraordinary vessels also correspond to one or more of the twelve meridians. One must ensure an accurate differentiation. Each pair of vessels or connections presents further differentiations prior to treatment. For example, with the yin wei mai connection one must carefully determine if the black clip of the ion cords should go on the yin wei mai point, PC-6, or the chong mai point, SP-4. To help in these decisions, Manaka presents a further differentiation for each connection. While these differentiations do help clarify the alignment of the cords, they are not absolute. There are other factors that can overrule these general guidelines.

Diagnosis begins on the abdomen or hara. For each connection and for each of the vessels one begins with the diagnosis of abdominal reactions. The following differential outlines derive variously from Manaka's books, notes, lectures, and private discussions.

Differentiation of Chong Mai and Yin Wei Mai

For the chong mai, pressure pain or reaction will be found on:

KI-16 and around the umbilicus.
ST-11.
The spleen meridian between ST-11 and SP-6.
The spleen meridian, in particular, SP-6 and SP-4.
ST-30.
KI-1.

For the yin wei mai, pressure pain or reaction can be elicited on:

The subcostal regions (chest distress).
CV-22.
The pericardium meridian in general.
PC-6 in particular.
The kidney meridian from CV-22 to KI-9
  (particularly on the abdomen and KI-9).
The areas from SP-13 to SP-15.

Differentiation of Dai Mai and Yang Wei Mai

For the dai mai, pressure pain or reaction may be found on:

KI-16 (or around the umbilicus in general).
The dai mai itself (including LV-13, ST-25 and the area including GB-28, GB-27, GB-26 and GB-29).
The gallbladder meridian.
GB-41 in particular.
BL-23.

For the yang wei mai, pressure pain or reaction may be found on:

The area of the anterior superior iliac spine (Manaka's GB-29).
TW-5.
On the gallbladder meridian between GB-29 and GB-21.
GB-34 and GB-35.

Differentiation of Yin Qiao and Ren Mai

For the ren mai, pressure pain or reaction may be found on:

The whole length of the ren mai from CV-1 to CV-22.
In particular, below the umbilicus and above the umbilicus, with a band of tension on the midline above the umbilicus.
Pressure pain on the lung meridian, in particular LU-1 and LU-7.

For the yin qiao mai, pressure pain or reaction can be found on:

The ren mai (this is particularly important when the area below the umbilicus is weak or has less tension than the area above the umbilicus).
Back muscle and abdominal muscle disparity (the back muscles are tight and the abdominal muscles are relatively weak).
Weakness or flaccidity of the abdomen with areas of tension around the umbilicus, KI-16, GB-29 and KI-11, CV-2.
ST-12.
ST-9.
The kidney meridian between ST-12 and KI-8, especially KI-8.
KI-6 and KI-3.

Differentiation of Yang Qiao and Du Mai

For the du mai, pressure pain or reaction may be found on:

The du mai itself, from GV-1 to GV-20.
In particular, on the du mai on the upper back and often GV-3, GV-4, GV-20.
On the small intestine meridian.
In particular, on SI-3.

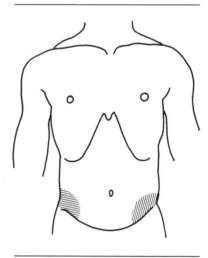

Figure 16.18 Yang wei mai.

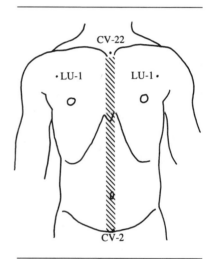

Figure 16.19 Ren mai.

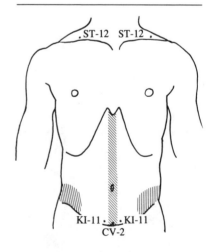

Figure 16.20 Yin qiao mai.

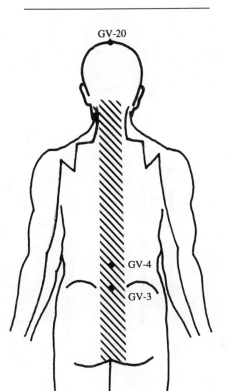

Figure 16.21 Du mai.

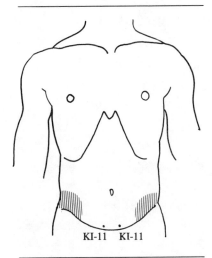

Figure 16.22 Yang qiao mai.

For the yang qiao mai, pressure pain or reaction may be found on:

> The anterior superior iliac spine (Manaka's GB-29).
> On the neck to the sides of the cervical vertebrae.
> On the back of the shoulder, around SI-10, SI-9.
> The KI-11 area.
> The bladder meridian itself, especially between GB-29 and BL-36.
> BL-62.
> GB-21.

It is important to note that KI-16 can indicate the kidney and/or the spleen. Manaka's GB-29 may also indicate the gallbladder, and KI-11 the bladder. Reactions on these points require further differentiation.

A common pattern of abdominal reactions relates to the four quadrants of the abdomen. Manaka suggests we check this pattern carefully. If there is reactivity in the upper right quadrant, especially below the ribs, pay special attention to the lower left quadrant around GB-29. If both of these areas are reactive, yet the other two quadrants are not, this is an indication for using the yang wei mai connection on the left and the yin wei mai connection on the right. This treatment utilizes the extraordinary vessels to helps restore a fundamental balance between yin and yang.

To help us use his overall palpatory system for the eight extraordinary vessels, Manaka presents some interesting and useful statistics regarding the areas and points that he found reactive in 100 of his patients.[31] Utilizing and expanding this information is a task each acupuncturist may perform to enhance clinical understanding and capacity.

The upper right—lower left pattern is the most common; this is part of the reason for its general importance in treatment.

I	II	III	IV	V	VI	Other
35	3	18	15	6	2	21
(F) 14	1	11	2	3	0	7
(M) 21	2	7	13	3	2	14

Manaka's Extraordinary Vessel Symptomology

We can summarize Manaka's extraordinary vessel symptomology in the following table:

Vessel	Symptoms
Ren Mai	gynecological problems; hemorrhoids; asthma; bronchitis; lung problems; neurosis; toothache; ear, nose, and throat problems.
Chong Mai	heart problems; neurosis; stomach problems; gynecological problems; cold feet; liver and gallbladder problems; problems of the anus.
Du Mai	epilepsy; fatigue; problems in the spine and neck; neurosis; insomnia; superficial invasion of cold or external qi; early stages of catching cold (*Shang Han Lun* tai yang disease).
Dai Mai	a feeling of coldness or aching in the lower back; gynecological problems; menstrual problems; problems in the lower abdomen.
Yin Qiao Mai	urination problems; gynecological problems; cold feet; intestinal problems.
Yang Qiao Mai	whiplash; epilepsy; speech disorders; shoulder pain; lumbar pain; unusual sweating; trigeminal neuralgia.
Yin Wei Mai	nervousness; heart problems; palpitations; psychological problems; insomnia; stomach problems.
Yang Wei Mai	dizziness; headache; whiplash; sweating problems; trigeminal neuralgia; tiredness; ear and eye problems.

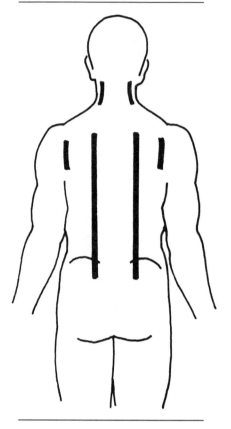

Figure 16.23 Yang qiao mai.

We can see from these lists of symptoms that the range of effects is broad. We can treat a great many problems using just the few points described. In our previous text, *Extraordinary Vessels,* we attempted to delineate this broad range of effects and some of their structural bases using both classical and modern descriptions.[32]

Following Manaka's insight into the topological nature of the extraordinary vessels, we can see the usefulness of combining the symptomology of the vessels, their palpatory diagnosis, and their topological relationships. Another addition to the diagnostic information of the extraordinary vessels are the "meeting" or "correspondence" points of the vessels based on their pathways. The lines connecting these points describe, as Manaka calls them, "dividing lines of the body." These points may be useful both diagnostically and therapeutically. As the *Zhen Jiu Da Cheng* says:

> Examine the right and left, upper and lower [parts of the body]. . . . Feel and palpate the body to find something with your hands, then do some exercises and take the disease away with the [eight] points. This is the rule, according to the rule, one can remove diseases. If the diseases don't pass, one has to ask [palpate] the meeting points [and treat them].[33]

□

The meeting points could be the *he* points, found around the elbows and knees, or they could be the meeting points of the extraordinary vessels. The same character is used in either case. Given the context of the discussion we feel it more likely that this refers to the extraordinary vessel meeting points.

> Make the upper and lower parts connect, make [the patient] comfortable, taking away the suffering or pain.[34]

Manaka's procedures very clearly adopt these recommendations. He uses palpatory diagnosis, as well as therapeutic exercises. He connects the upper and lower parts with cords and emphasizes the importance of the patient's comfort and relaxation during treatment. The meeting points are thus a further step in his treatment style that may be used as required.

Use of the Ion Cords

Using the ion cords requires two diagnoses. The first indicates which connection or pair of vessels to treat (when treating, both master and coupled points are treated). The second differentiates the point that is to be the master point. Place the black clip on the master point of the diagnosed vessel and the red clip on the coupled point of the paired vessel. Thus, if the yin wei mai connection is diagnosed by symptoms of the chong mai, the spleen meridian (tension in the subcostal region; soreness on CV-22 and ST-11), examine all the points and areas of the yin wei and chong mai. Compare the presenting symptomology with the general symptomology of both these meridians. If the most sensitive point is ST-11, and if SP-6, SP-4, and KI-16 are also sensitive, and the patient's symptoms clearly the indicate chong mai, place the black clip on SP-4 and the red on PC-6. However, cases are not always this straightforward; there are other factors that need to be taken into account.

In his lectures Manaka relates that he has found it better to treat the "wei" connections before treating the "qiao" connections. If using the wei connections it is generally better to start treating the wei mai before the chong or dai mai. If using the qiao connections, treat the qiao mai before the du or ren mai. Practically, first place the black clip on PC-6 or TW-5 for the wei connections, or KI-6 or BL-62 in the qiao connections. If clear that treatment of the chong or dai mai is required, it is appropriate to treat these from the outset. However, if it is not a totally clear diagnosis, treat the wei mai first. If the patient does not respond favorably, reverse the connection to treat the chong or dai mai. The same is also true of the qiao mai; unless the diagnosis is clearly of the ren or du mai, treat the qiao mai first.

As has been mentioned, it is important to remain with the patient throughout a treatment using the ion cords. If the patient does not relax and becomes uncomfortable, first reverse the polarity of the cords. If this does not elicit the appropriate reaction, remove the cords and rediagnose. Using magnets to confirm a projected treatment helps reduce the frequency of such diagnostic errors. However, when using ion cords for treatments other than extraordinary vessel treatments, reversing the polarity is not appropriate. If the patient becomes uncomfortable, simply remove the cords and rediagnose.

□

Part of Manaka's reasoning for the precedence of the wei vessels before the qiao vessels and the wei or qiao points before the chong mai, du mai, dai mai, or ren mai points has to do with the names wei and qiao. Generally wei is translated as "linking" or "binding." It is a pictogram of a rope binding or tying things together. More detailed research reveals that the wei character further refers to the action of pulling those things downward. The qiao character is generally translated as heel, as it is a pictogram referring to a heel. As with the wei character, more detailed research reveals that qiao actually refers to the action of the heel kicking upwards; not kicking just a little, but kicking very high. This gives the wei mai the connotation of pulling things down and the qiao mai a connotation of kicking upwards. One of the main indications for the extraordinary vessels is the condition of counterflow qi, repletion above and vacancy below. Since this is a common problem, it is advisable to draw energy downwards first — thus the use of the wei connections first.

In a case where multiple diagnoses seem to occur and deciding priority is difficult, a north-facing magnet of at least 1500 gauss may be placed on the master point of one of the diagnosed vessels, for example, TW-5 for the yang wei mai. After leaving it in place for about twenty seconds (though sometimes up to one or two minutes), check the abdominal reactions. If these have decreased, treat that connection. If there is no change, place the magnet on the master point of the other diagnosed vessel, for instance BL-62. If this decreases the abdominal reactions, even if only mildly, use this point. In this diagnostic testing, the abdominal reactions need to improve only very slightly to be indicative.

This technique is generally not necessary nor is it often used to differentiate treatment. It is more commonly used when biorhythmic variations or the open vessel is used. In some cases, one may have diagnosed the yang wei mai clearly, but the yin qiao mai is the open or active vessel. At times treating the open vessel will provide the most powerful treatment. In these cases use of the magnet to differentiate the treatment is very helpful.

Another factor that needs to be considered is the topographical pattern of the patient's condition. Generally, unless otherwise indicated, treat the extraordinary vessels with ion cords bilaterally, do not cross the body. There are some cases where "crossed" application is employed, for instance in the treatment of burns or in the treatment of certain liver disorders (described in the next chapter). Generally the extraordinary vessels are not mixed or paired except in the common pattern described above, where the abdominal reactions were in the upper right and lower left quadrants. PC-6 (black), SP-4 (red) should be treated on the right and TW-5 (black), GB-41 (red) on the left. In other cases, one may find a right-sided chest distress, which is not related to the liver, but is related to the yin wei mai. This may be treated using right PC-6 (black) and right SP-4 (red). The same might be done if the abdominal reaction were very clearly one-sided and indicative of the yang wei mai. It is more difficult to choose the yang qiao or yin qiao mai as many of the diagnostic signs are on the midline. Remember that these conditions are the exceptions not the rule. Because we attempt to use as few points as possible, it is worth studying these special conditions where the correct orientation and polarity

□

of the cords is sometimes tricky and requires practice and observation. When a clear diagnosis by palpation alone cannot be achieved, the patient's symptoms must be clearly perceived. However, in the more general cases, diagnosing and differentiating the correct extraordinary vessel for treatment is less complex. Very often only palpatory diagnosis is required.

We can summarize very generally the treatment patterns as follows:

Reactions	Indicates	Treatment
subcostal region (usually right) CV-22, ST-11, KI-16, ST-30, SP-6	yin wei-chong connection	usually PC-6 black SP-4 red, right side
ASIS region (usually left) along dai mai, KI-16, along gall bladder meridian	yang wei-dai connection	usually TW-5 black GB-41 red, left side
ASIS region, KI-11, SI-9, SI-10, sides cervical vertebrae, along spine	yang qiao-du connection	usually BL-62 black SI-3 red, bilaterally
ren mai, ST-12, ST-9, LU-1, KI-16, GB-29 KI-11-CV-2 region	yin qiao-ren connection	usually KI-6 black LU-7 red, bilaterally
right subcostal with lower left quadrant regions	"cross syndrome"	right PC-6 black, SP-4 red, left TW-5 black, GB-41 red

As described above polarity reversals of the ion-pumping cords can be chosen based on the total condition.

Summary

The diagnoses and treatments given in this chapter for the use of ion-pumping cords on the extraordinary vessels give a variety of simple, typical approaches to step one in treatment: relief of abdominal reactions. The two chapters that follow will describe a few alternative strategies for step-one treatment. Strategies and procedures for steps two and three and local symptom-control treatments are also described in the next chapter. These include alternative uses of the ion-pumping cords, a simplified use of Sotai exercise therapy, Korean hand acupuncture and dermatome therapy.

Chapter

- 17 -

Secondary

Treatment Strategies

Secondary Treatment Strategies

Palm Diagnosis and Treatment

Although the palm therapy Manaka utilizes was refined and developed in this century by a Korean acupuncturist, Tae Woo Yoo, palm therapy is by no means a twentieth century invention in Oriental medicine. An early reference to examination of the palm comes from the *Ling Shu,* where the finding of a blue vascular spider around LU-10 was seen as an indication of a condition of cold inside the stomach. Red coloration in the same area was interpreted as heat in the stomach and black as bi stagnation *(LS 10:139).* There have been other allusions to palm diagnosis in the classical literature. Publication of the *Zhen Jiu Da Cheng* in 1601 during the Ming dynasty offered one of the first clear and systematic descriptions of this technique.[1]

One interesting concept presented in the *Zhen Jiu Da Cheng* was the assignment of the temporal sequence of the trigrams around the point PC-8 (the center of the palm) and the same assignment around an equivalent point called "external PC-8" on the back of the hand.[2] Although this differs from Yoo's pattern of diagnosis, it parallels his method, where PC-8 is the palmar equivalent of the umbilicus.[3] In Yoo's system, the center line of the palm passing through PC-8 to the center of the middle finger is representative of the ren mai. An opposite line following the back of the middle finger through the center of the back of the hand is representative of the du mai. Starting from this original polar axis, Yoo describes the other extraordinary vessels, meridians, organs, and phases as correspondences on the hand.

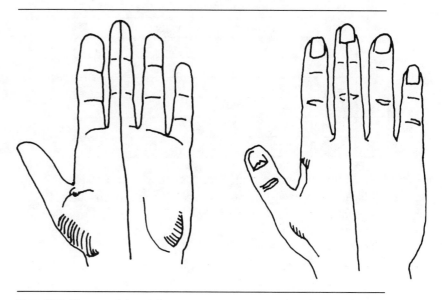

Figure 17.1 The ren and du mai axes.

Combining these correspondences on the palm with the embryologically significant reflex areas derived from Tohaku Ishi's work (described above), Manaka uses these areas in the same way he uses the abdominal reflex areas, considering tension, tenderness, or other signs as diagnostic indicators. Since the area around PC-8 reflects the umbilicus, the line above PC-8 to the middle finger reflects the phasal relationships equivalent to the area above the umbilicus on the abdomen. For example, if he finds tension around CV-12, the earth area, he will treat the earth point of the meridian active at that time according to the Chinese clock (see the next chapter). Alternately, he might needle the earth area on the palm. Either or both techniques will eliminate the tension around CV-12. If the patient has right subcostal tension and tension in the wood area of the abdomen, he might needle the wood area of the palm on the right hand. Manaka will also use an electric point finder to locate reactive points on the palm as a means for determining the exact location of the point to be treated. The point selected is reflective of the patient's problem, such as knee pain. Knowing which meridian the problem lies on will allow us to find the equivalent knee point on the little finger or thumb.[4]

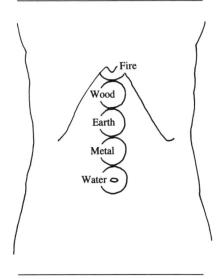

Figure 17.2a Manaka's phasal reflex areas.

Hirata Dermatomes

The Hirata dermatones described by Manaka[5] represent a division of the different areas of the body — back, abdomen, chest, arms, legs, neck, head, and face — into twelve zones. Each zone is numbered and represents one of the twelve systems in the body. (Figure 17.3a,b,c) These correspondences are as follows:

1	Bronchii
2	Lung
3	Heart
4	Liver
5	Gallbladder and exocrine gland of the pancreas
6	Spleen and endocrine gland of the pancreas
7	Stomach
8	Kidney
9	Large Intestine
10	Small Intestine
11	Bladder
12	Sexual organs

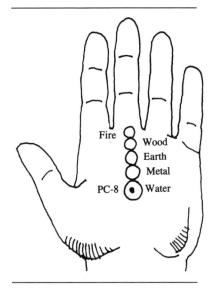

Figure 17.2b The equivalent areas on the palm.

This easily remembered numbering system permits simple reference to these useful diagnostic and treatment zones. One may, for instance, find a pattern of pigmentation of the skin in one of these zones, indicating a problem in that zone. One interesting therapeutic example Manaka cites is his use of LU-6 and SP-7 with ion cords in the treatment of pancreatitis.[6] He selects SP-7 because it lies in the Hirata spleen zone of the leg and LU-6 because it lies in the spleen zone of the arm. In one case he successfully treated right LU-6 (red clip) and left SP-7 (black clip). The right-left polarity here was chosen based on the pattern of abdominal reactions.

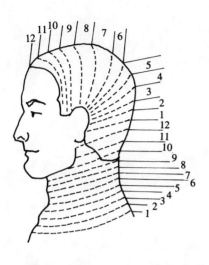

Figure 17.3a The Hirata zones on the head.

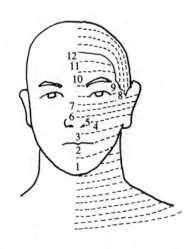

Figure 17.3b The Hirata zones on the face.

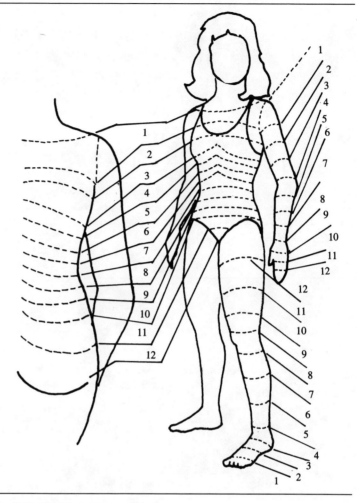

Figure 17.3c The Hirata zones on the body.

Sotai Exercise

When administering treatment, Manaka may frequently employ one or more of the therapeutic Sotai exercises developed by Keizo Hashimoto, an exercise therapist of considerable skill and innovative talent. One exercise that he commonly uses provides relief of abnormal tension of the back muscles.

Have the patient lie on their abdomen; press the heels to the buttocks. If the heels touch without much pressure that is good, but if they don't touch or one leg is tighter than the other, this is a sign of imbalance and too much muscular tension. Usually this tension is accompanied by tension of the muscles of the back. It can often be found with tension or tightness in the subcostal region, specially the right and in the left lower quadrant. This is frequently seen in association with any liver problem, as the liver controls the muscles and muscular membranes *(SW 23; SW 44; LS 1).*

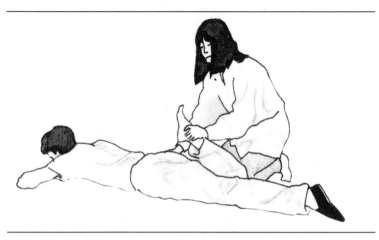

Figure 17.4 Check to see if the heel will touch the buttock.

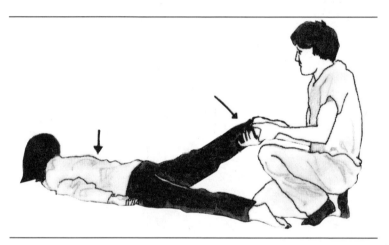

Figure 17.5 As the leg is extended and straightened, resistance is applied with stimulation at BL-18.

In these cases the corrective exercise is to have the patient straighten the leg from a bent position. Once straight, the practitioner resists the motion of the leg slightly, with a gentle pressure. As the patient resists, stimulation is applied to a reactive shu point on the back, usually BL-18, the liver shu. Thus, if the right leg is tighter, (that is, the right leg touches the buttock less easily than the left leg), the exercise is done on the left leg. If there is reaction on the liver shu point, the right BL-18 should be stimulated when exercising the left leg. If there is no reaction on BL-18, check the other shu points below BL-23. If you cannot find reaction by palpation of the back shu points, have the patient bend the legs while palpating, check if there is a point where the back muscles can easily be felt moving as the legs are bent. Apply stimulation to this point. Stimulation may be either the rapid, shallow insertion and withdrawal of a hot needle into the reactive point just at the end of the exercise, as the patient is relaxing, or the application of percussion to the point throughout the exercise movement with a stronger percussive blow at the end of the exercise. This percussion is applied using a small wooden peg and mallet, the Manaka hammer.

☐

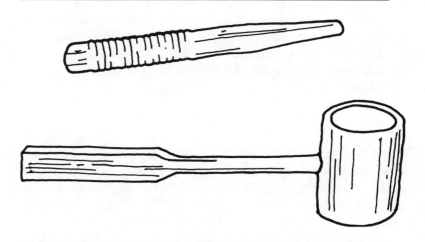

Figure 17.6 The Manaka wooden hammer and peg.

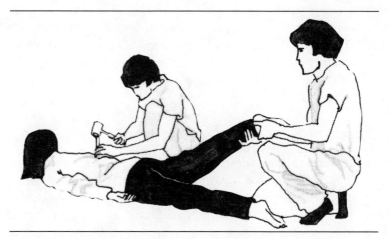

Figure 17.7 Resistance to the leg extension is applied simultaneously with tapping at BL-18.

The exercise should proceed as follows:

Step 1 With the patient lying on the abdomen, pull the leg to be exercised up toward the buttock.

Step 2 Have the patient inhale.

Step 3 Have the patient begin exhaling slowly, at the same time slowly straighten the leg.

Step 4 Continue exhalation and movement.

Step 5 Continue exhaling; when the leg is straight have an assistant apply a slight pressure to resist the motion.

Step 6 Continue exhaling; count slowly "one, two, three" and give the command to relax.

Step 7   At the command "relax" the patient finishes the exhalation and allows the whole body to relax. The practitioner inserts the hot needle into the reactive shu point (e.g. BL-18 on the side opposite from the leg exercised). The insertion of the needle should coincide exactly with the patient's relaxation.

Step 8   Repeat the entire procedure for a total of three turns.

If using the percussion method, the percussion would begin at Step 3 and end with a heavier blow at Step 7. Usually an assistant is required for this exercise. After completing the procedure, test the legs and back muscles again. They should be looser and more flexible. If there is no change, palpate one to two centimeters below the center of the knee on the back of the leg and place an intradermal in the reactive point. Also place an intradermal to the extra point, "back point" on the dorsal aspect of the hand. This will generally help the tension, though Manaka reports an interesting case history where yet more steps were required to achieve good results. His patient suffered from numbness of the left leg. The right leg was tighter. He did the exercise with stimulation on the left leg and this helped a little, but not very much. He then used a hot needle on BL-57, which was very helpful. Manaka is fond of describing exceptions to the rule and not so much the general rule itself.

Some Examples of Local Treatment

In a similar vein, Manaka describes an interesting treatment for ear problems such as deafness. The following is one of his "local treatments" applicable after a root treatment for the extraordinary vessels, phases, or biorhythms. Palpate on a line directly above the top of the ear (affected side); locate and mark the sore point here. Then check the movement of the neck, forward, backward, rotating left then right, and bending (ear to shoulder) to the left and right. Look for the motion that elicits the most reaction or that is the most difficult. Have the patient move from the point of most reaction or resistance in the opposite direction to the looser side as they exhale. At the end of motion, as you apply resistance, ignite a piece of moxa on the reactive point so that it burns to the skin at the point of relaxation. The patient will feel the heat at exactly the point of relaxation. This exercise follows the same principles as the preceding exercise. It should be repeated two additional times. As it is difficult to coordinate the moxa with the resistance and relaxation, one generally needs an assistant. Manaka reports excellent results using this technique.

Further local treatments for relief of symptoms should be applied after applying steps one through three. The first step of treatment is the most important and diverse, thus it is necessary to examine this in more detail.

Selecting Treatment Therapies

In the treatment of liver disorders, which in Manaka's experience are very common, many techniques have been evolved. He uses the treatment of liver conditions to demonstrate his broad-scope approach to treatment. As we will see, Manaka uses a variety of tools and techniques, some of

□

which are considered root treatments and others local treatments. The following information is a slight enlargement from a chart prepared by Manaka.[7]

If the liver is the seat of the patient's condition, how can we think about treating it? There are many approaches that can be used separately or concurrently. Manaka uses most of these at one time or another, depending on what he finds with the patient.

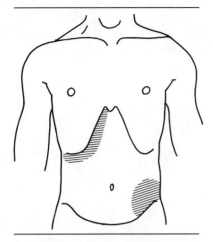

Figure 17.8a "The cross-syndrome". Right yin wei-chong mai. Left yang wei-dai mai.

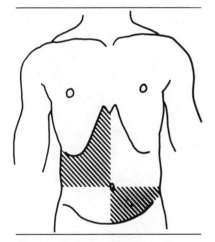

Figure 17.8b Upper right quadrant with lower left quadrant reactions is also part of the "cross-syndrome".

Liver Treatments	
Liver meridian	
Five phases	including: stem—branch cycles, open points and the Chinese clock
Wood points	wood points of other meridians, including: the tai yang, shao yin, shao yang, jue yin, yang ming, tai yin relationships
Muscular meridians	including: combined Sotai exercise and heat therapy
Other therapies	extraordinary vessels herbs medications auricular points palm therapy points liver Hirata zones liver dermatones magnetic fields etc.

In liver problems Manaka has noticed in his practice common diagonal patterns of tension through palpation. He will then treat points on the hand of one side and on the foot of the opposite side. One pattern he focuses on in diagnosis is diagonal tension or reactivity from the right subcostal region to the lower left abdominal quadrant. Tension or pain on the left scapula and the right lower back or vice versa commonly accompanies this.

Manaka uses a variety of means to treat this abdominal pattern: placing the right hand palm-down on a magnetic heater (induction cooker); aligning the patient north (head) to south (feet), needling GV-20, and attaching a small aerial to it pointing west; or treating right SP-4 (red) and right PC-6 (black) and left TW-5 (black) with left GB-41 (red) with the ion cords, to activate yin wei on the right, yang wei on the left.

Based on other factors of the patient's condition and treatment, he will use different patterns. For instance, at the time when PC-6, yin wei mai, is open he might treat right PC-6 (black) and left SP-4 (red). In other cases, for example liver problems, a similar pattern can be utilized. Reactivity in the right subcostal region with particular sensitivity around LV-14, reactivity on left ST-25, left GB-29, and some reactivity on the liver meridian up from SP-10 (around LV-9) on the left leg would be a pattern indicative of liver problems. Manaka comments that one will usually find right LI-4 to be more sore than the left LI-4. Treatment is accomplished by using either the palm on the magnet heater or the right yin wei-left yang wei connection procedures in the list above, or by needling right LI-4 with a silver needle and left LV-3 with a gold needle and attaching the black clip of an ion cord to LI-4 and the red clip to LV-3. This condition usually involves a relative excess of the large intestine, which would explain why LI-4 is so sore. This particular treatment can be useful for hepatitis. This use is indicated when there is not just a simple palpable reaction around the liver, but there is also palpable reaction in the lower left abdominal quadrant and on the left leg.

Manaka has obtained excellent results treating liver conditions such as hepatitis. If the patient has tightness, tenderness, swelling, or tension around the liver, usually centered below the ribs on the right side (which most patients with a liver disease will evidence), and pressure pain and tension to the right of the umbilicus, the following treatment may be applied instead.

Insert a gold needle in right LV-3 and a silver needle in right PC-7. Attach an ion cord to these points, red clip to LV-3 and black to PC-7. This treatment is done only on the right side because the liver is on the right side. Only silver and gold needles should be used. As with other cord treatments, it should be maintained for a maximum period of twenty minutes. The reaction around the liver will decrease. Generally, after several treatments, there will be a marked improvement in the condition. A case history from a Dr. Seki illustrates this treatment.[8]

The patient, a 50-year-old female, had been diagnosed by many other doctors as suffering from chronic hepatitis. She endured severe subcostal pain on the right side and was unable to travel or function well. This condition had lasted for four and a half years. She had been told by one doctor that she would have this condition permanently as nothing could be done for it. Seki applied Manaka's treatment. After ten minutes the patient reported that her pain had completely vanished. As an experiment to ensure the efficacy of treatment, Seki then reversed the polarity of the cords, applying black to LV-3 and red to PC-7. The patient's pain returned. Seki then reversed the cords and the pain disappeared again. Seki reports that the patient did not return for treatment since the pain never came back.

Not all treatments are as instantaneous; often several treatments are required. Manaka offers the following comments about this treatment.[9] Treating right LV-3 and PC-7, the source points of jue yin, will treat not only pressure pain and tension around the liver, but also pressure pain along the liver meridian itself. Applying the treatment will decrease reaction both around the liver and along the liver meridian. Also, placing copper on LV-3 and zinc on PC-7 reduces the same pressure pain and muscular tension. Reversing the polarity, applying zinc to LV-3 and copper to PC-7, will exacerbate the pressure pain and tension. We can thus consider using this treatment for reducing pressure pain along the length of the liver meridian. The treatment utilizes jue yin relationships.

□

Manaka describes another interesting treatment for subcostal reaction that utilizes jue yin—shao yang relationships. Treat TW-4 and LV-3 bilaterally with ion cords for bilateral subcostal reactions. Attaching TW-4 (black) to LV-3 (red) works because the liver to triple warmer meridian connections that exist through the jue yin to shao yang relationships are activated.

Having gained much experience treating patients with liver problems, Manaka has frequently noticed the upper right—lower left abdominal reaction pattern. He has other useful treatments and comments regarding these conditions. In a vacant liver condition, for example, there are often pimples on the face in the Hirata liver zone on the cheekbone. For liver problems in general one frequently finds dark pigmented spots in the triangle on the upper back between the scapulae. In both these cases, when treatment is effective, these pimples or dark spots will slowly decrease.

Many patients with liver problems have reactivity in the right subcostal region and their head is slightly bent to the right. For patients with the upper right—lower left pattern, slowly rotate the head to the left while the patient is lying down. Palpate the areas on the abdomen again; then, have the patient turn their head to the right and palpate again. If the reaction on the abdomen is worse when turning to the left and better when turning to the right, this is a sign that the case will be easier to treat. In serious problems, the rotation will not produce a significant difference in the abdominal reaction.

A series of other general diagnostic and differential signs can be important and useful. Patients who have hepatitis should not go out in the sun frequently, and should particularly avoid sunburning. Manaka has found, contrary to some opinions, that if the patient's hands are red and warm, it is often attributable to poor circulation. If the face is red and the palms swollen, red or hot, this is generally not a good sign. Often one can find warts or dry skin in an area where there is poor circulation. Treat these warts with moxa, focus on treating the worst. Poor circulation is often associated with the liver since the liver stores the blood.

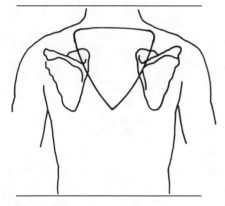

Figure 17.9

The Bidigital O-Ring Test

Sometimes when diagnosing the abdomen and meridians, very little reaction can be found when palpating. This can be due to vacancy or it can be due to medication. Anti-depressants, valium for example, seem to bring about this effect most frequently, though hypertensive medication, insulin, etc., will often bring about the same effects. It is very easy to misdiagnose these cases. Care is required to distinguish no sensitivity from lack of sensitivity. A simple, helpful technique is to pinch as well as palpate the areas and points; often a reaction will show with pinching and not with palpation. A second useful practice is a simple kinesiological technique called the "Omura O-ring" or "bidigital O-ring test." Place the patient's index finger on the area or point to be tested. With the forefinger and thumb of their other hand, have the patient form a circle. Then instruct the patient to hold the finger and thumb together, resisting the practitioner's efforts to pull them apart. If the fingers hold together well, this is a good sign. If they separate easily, the patient not being able to

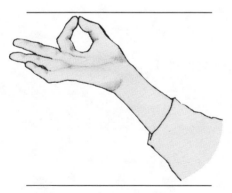

Figure 17.10 The bidigital o-ring.

□

resist, this indicates a problem. Test the reactivity of all the areas and points with which you are concerned. One way Manaka uses this technique is to test just the five-phase areas on the midline above the umbilicus and then treat the appropriate point relative to the affected area and the time of day. Yoshiaki Omura uses this kinesiological technique extensively, more details of which can be found in his literature.[10] This technique enables one to make a clear diagnosis when there are misleading circumstances. Manaka comments that in cases of no reaction, the patient will often develop reactivity in certain areas after a series of treatments. With more treatment this sensitivity will then decline. This is a natural progression that occurs in some patients' course of recovery.

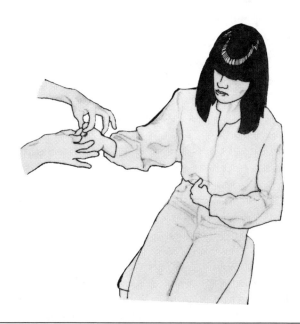

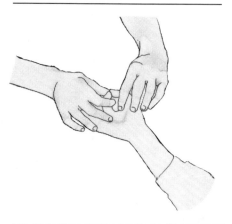

Figure 17.11 The practitioner tries to pull the thumb and index finger apart while the patient tries to keep them touching.

Figure 17.12 The procedure is applied while the subject touches a reflex point with the index finger of the other hand.

The Taikyoku Treatment, or Normal Ion Pumping

Manaka's brilliant taikyoku (Chinese taiji) treatment involves treating four points bilaterally using two sets of ion cords. With this treatment, reactivity on KI-16, LV-13, or SP-15 can be relieved. This means that whatever problems may reflect at these points (kidney, spleen, chong mai, dai mai, yin qiao mai, yin wei mai, liver, gallbladder, etc) can be treated.[11]

Manaka's overall treatment strategy is to treat as much as possible with as few points as possible. He feels that treating meeting points, points on one meridian where other meridians join, potentially treats all the meridians that join there. By joining the points with the ion cords, the whole "Chinese clock," the biorhythmic cycle of the twelve meridians, may be activated. When correctly diagnosed and applied, this type of treatment can have the most amazing results.

□

TW-8 on the arm is three-yang luo, *san yang luo,* the meeting point of the three yang meridians of the arms. SP-6 on the legs is the three-yin crossing point, *san yin jiao,* the meeting point of the three yin meridians of the legs. Manaka theorized that there must be a three-yin crossing of the arms and a three-yang crossing of the legs. Some texts say GB-39 is the meeting point of the three yang meridians of the legs. He tried this point but found that GB-35 (yang crossing, yang jiao), seven divisions superior to the external malleolus, was far more effective. Traditionally there are no descriptions of a three-yin crossing of the arms. Theorizing that it should be on the forearm on one of the yin meridians, Manaka palpated and experimented with a number of points and finally found that an extra point, the Manaka point, halfway between PC-7 and PC-3 on the pericardium meridian, worked best. Needling these four points bilaterally and connecting the ion cords as follows activates the Chinese clock:

Point	Clip		Point	Clip
SP-6	Black	to	Manaka point	Red
TW-8	Black	to	GB-35	Red

Attaching the black clip to SP-6 essentially connects the liver, kidney, and spleen meridians. Attaching a red clip to the Manaka point, the meeting point of the three arm yin meridians, connects the lung, heart, and pericardium meridians:

Ion Cord	Meridian
black	spleen, liver, kidney
red	lung, heart, pericardium

Similarly, attaching a black clip to TW-8 connects the three arm yang meridians — large intestine, small intestine, and triple warmer. Attaching the red clip to GB-35 connects the three leg yang meridians, stomach, gallbladder, and bladder:

Ion Cord	Meridian
black	large intestine, small intestine, triple warmer
red	stomach, gallbladder, bladder

On the Chinese clock, this creates an alternating pattern of red-black connections, half of which are connected with the cords and other half of which are inductively produced (figure 17.13).

This cyclic connection can thus control all the meridians at once and improve the patency of qi flow in the meridians. It increases the patient's natural healing powers. Another name Manaka gives this treatment is "normal ion pumping," which he forshortens to NIP-1. He has found that NIP-1 is able to decrease pressure pain and reaction on KI-16, SP-15, and LV-13. Thus pressure pain on these three points is an indication for this treatment. It is most appropriate to use when the patient has a complex condition that might also be unclear or difficult to diagnose. When a clear diagnosis of some other condition such as liver vacancy or the yin wei mai disturbance can be determined, this treatment is generally unnecessary. However, the treatment gives very good results for restoring physical, energetic, and mental balance; addressing psychological problems, including nervousness; and alleviating tiredness of the whole body. It is also good for knee joint problems, neuritis, high blood pressure, and whiplash, especially when the forward and backward range of motion in the neck is limited.

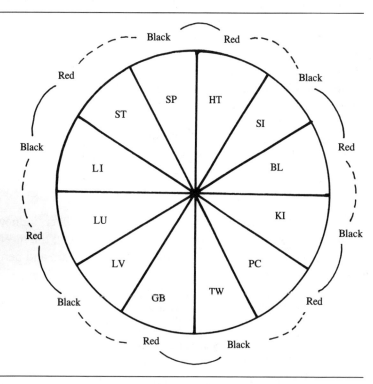

Figure 17.13 The meridian circuit is activated.

Considerable research has been conducted in Japan on Manaka's work. The statistics below come from Yukimichi Seki who researched a number of Manaka's treatments.[12] Using the NIP-1 treatment only, he treated twenty patients with knee problems. For complete recovery, the results were as follows:

Number of treatments	1	2	3	6	8	10
Number of patients	10	3	1	3	2	1

Half the patients recovered from their knee problems with just one treatment. Five patients suffering from generalized joint problems all recovered after one treatment. For eleven patients suffering from neuritis, complete recovery using NIP-1 yielded the following statistics. Again one can see that most patients recovered after only one treatment.

Number of treatments	1	2	3	7	16
Number of patients	7	1	1	1	1

Using the same four points, but with the polarity of the cords reversed, he has found to be useful for treating sprained ankles, neuritis, and numbness of the upper limbs. This he calls "NIP-2."

Point	Clip	Point	Ion Cord
SP-6	red	Manaka point	black
TW-8	red	GB-35	black

Treating Specific Conditions

When using the cords for treatment of specific meridian or extraordinary vessel conditions, as opposed to specific treatments for specific diseases, there are specific points and areas to palpate in order to confirm the diagnosis.

Triple Warmer Problems

Utilizing the techniques of this taikyoku treatment, Manaka has devised a useful treatment for tension and pressure pain at the lateral edge of the abdomen, between the iliac crest and the lower border of the ribs.[13]. The treatment is for reactions that are unilateral. Accompanying this pain and tension there is usually a weak radial foot pulse on the same side of the body, or weakness of both radial foot pulses. Manaka diagnoses this condition as a triple warmer problem. His treatment is to needle TW-8 and SP-6 on the opposite side to the abdominal reaction and apply the black clip of the ion cord to TW-8, the red clip to SP-6. Thus, for tension of the right side of the abdomen, with a weak right foot pulse, he would treat left TW-8 (black clip) and left SP-6 (red clip). This restores the balance and treats the problem.

This treatment utilizes two of the body's major meeting points, TW-8, the three arm yang meeting point, and SP-6, the three leg yin meeting point.

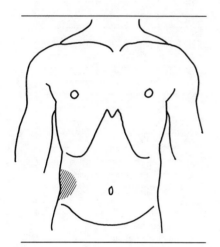

Figure 17.14 Triple warmer problem.

Whiplash

Manaka has also developed a powerfully effective therapy for whiplash. The following treatment is considered so phenomenally effective that it is in part responsible for Manaka's fame. Whiplash tends to affect the cervical vertebrae, making the muscles of the neck overtense and oversensitive. Spasming is easily triggered. This can affect many parts of the body. In Japan it is recognized that in treating problems of the neck where the muscles are oversensitive, it is best not to treat the neck directly. Before applying any direct stimulus, one should use Manaka's ion cord treatment for whiplash. Any stimulus on the neck itself should be very gentle. We usually recommend that treatment of the neck itself should involve the use of intradermal needles or tiny direct moxa, but generally no needling, unless very shallowly and gently done. Manaka's treatment involves treating all the yang extraordinary vessels, specifically the yang qiao mai and yang wei mai connections:

Point	Clip		Point	Clip
BL-62	black	to	SI-3	red
TW-5	black	to	GB-41	red

All points are treated bilaterally so that four cords are used. This treatment alone can be extremely effective, both for acute and chronic whiplash conditions. It is especially good for problems with side-to-side rotation of the head. If treatment of whiplash is started with this therapy, often it will be sufficient on its own. Patients frequently notice immediate improvement. Manaka's taikyoku treatment (NIP-1) is also effective for whiplash, specifically for problems of forward-backward motion of the head. If treating the yang qiao mai and yang wei mai improves the side-to-side motion but forward-backward motion remains a stubborn problem, consider applying the NIP-1 treatment on a future occasion. This should not be done automatically; the applicability of the treatment should be confirmed. When palpating the abdomen, KI-16, SP-15, and LV-13 should be found to be reactive. If two or three of these points are reactive and the patient has other NIP-1 symptoms i.e., problems of a psychological nature, knee problems, etc., the treatment will be appropriate.[14]

In researching Manaka's use of the ion cords, Yukimichi Seki presents statistics confirming that it is possible to obtain extremely good results in the treatment of whiplash.[15] He examined and treated thirty patients with a whiplash condition, assessing the range of motion of the head — side to side, backward and forward — before, during, and after treatment. He applied only the yang qiao and yang wei mai treatment. Here, the number of treatments recorded is the number of treatments required to achieve "perfect recovery," i.e., disappearance of the patient's accompanying symptoms and improvement of the range of motion to an acceptably "normal" range. This is an average of 7.3 treatments for "perfect recovery." Analyzing these numbers, we can see that 30% recovered with only one treatment; a further 27% in two or three treatments. In most cases the treatment was extremely effective, those cases requiring extended treatment were the minority. Seki gives us a case history to illustrate a usual progression of therapy.[16]

The patient, a 62-year-old male, had been unable to move his neck since an auto accident, and was wearing a traction collar. Seki found both side-to-side and forward-backward motion was difficult and restricted. He applied the yang wei mai, yang qiao mai treatment with the cords. After ten minutes he checked the patient's degree of motion. The side-to-side rotation had improved, but the backward-forward range of motion had not improved. After ten more minutes, he found that the forward motion had improved, but that the backward motion was still restricted. On returning three days later, the patient reported that all but the backward motion was better. Seki applied the same therapy. After ten minutes the backward motion had improved. The therapy was discontinued. The patient did not return, claiming that further therapy was unnecessary.

Specific Treatments Using the Ion Cords

The following tables were compiled by Makio Maruyama, M.D., who has done extensive research on the clinical application of the ion cords. These treatments derive from the clinical experience of many practitioners and represent summaries of those that were found to be particularly useful.[17] These treatments are suitable as alternatives to the regular extraordinary vessel ion-pumping cord treatment.

□

Patient	Age	Sex	Treatments
1	47	M	56
2	26	M	10
3	24	F	10
4	23	M	3
5	27	M	13
6	48	M	1 *
7	32	M	19
8	56	F	2
9	28	F	11
10	19	F	10
11	36	M	14
12	26	F	1 **
13	27	M	1
14	14	M	1
15	62	F	2
16	59	F	1
17	37	M	1
18	30	M	10
19	60	M	7
20	68	F	20
21	36	M	10
22	34	F	2
23	59	F	2
24	50	F	2 ***
25	35	M	4
26	55	F	3
27	27	F	1
28	36	M	1
29	38	M	1
30	29	M	2

*   12 years duration.
**   7 years duration.
*** 6 years duration.

Treatment Summaries			
Disease Categories	**Symptoms**	**Black clip**	**Red clip**
Nervous system problems	chest pain	PC-6	GB-34
		(or) PC-6	SP-4
	upper abdomen pain	PC-6	SP-6
		(or) CV-12	SP-9
	lower abdomen pain	CV-4	SP-6
		(or)CV-3	ST-36
Locomotor diseases	rheumatism	TW-5	GB-41
	Whiplash	TW-5	GB-41
	upper limb pain	LI-11	LI-4
		(or) TW-5	SI-3
	lower limb pain	GB-34	GB-30
		(or) ST-36	GB-39
	lower back pain	BL-47	BL-57
		(or) BL-51	BL-60
	lumbar and thigh pain	GB-30	GB-35
		(or) BL-51	GB-34
	lumbar pain	BL-23	SI-3
		(or) BL-47	BL-62
	lateral low back pain	BL-23	GB-29 or GB-34
	numbness	reactive points†	yang meridian
Surgical problems	mastitis	ST-18	SI-3
Gynecological problems		CV-4	ST-36
		(or) CV-4	SP-6
		(or) KI-6	LU-7
Male sexual problems	weak sexual energy	KI-6	LU-7
	(or) impotence		
Urinary problems	night urine	SP-6	CV-4 or SP-9
Eye, Ear, Nose and teeth problems	tired eyes	LI-4	BL-1
	rhinitis	LI-20	LI-4
	tinnitus or deafness	TW-5	GB-2
		(or) TW-3	TW-21
	toothache	ST-6	LI-4
		(or) ST-7	LI-4
Respiratory disease	colds	CV-22	LI-4 or SI-3
	asthma	GV-14	ST-36 or PC-6
	tonsilitis	ST-9	LI-4 or LI-11
Circulatory disease	low blood pressure	BL-62	SI-3
	melancholia	KI-6	LU-7
Digestive problems	stomach atony	BL-62	SI-3
	gastroptosis	ST-36	CV-6 or ST-41
	appendicitis	ST-25	ST-36
		(or) CV-6	ST-40
	stomach pain	PC-6	ST-36
	vomiting, nausea	PC-6	GB-35
		(or) CV-22	ST-36
	diaphragm spasm	CV-22	PC-6
		(or) CV-12	PC-6
	constipation	TW-6	ST-25
		(or) LI-4	ST-36
	diarrhea	ST-36	ST-25
		(or) SP-6	CV-4
Nervous diseases	neurosis	GV-15	PC-6
		(or) PC-6	SP-4
	insomnia	PC-6	ST-36 or SP-6
	facial spasms	LI-4	ST-4
	overtired	BL-62	SI-3
	whole body tired	PC-6	SP-4
	spasm/twitching	GB-20	LI-4
	neuralgia	TW-5	GB-41
	shaking hand	KI-6	LU-7
Headache	front	GV-23	LI-4 or LU-7
	back	GV-15	SI-3 or BL-60
	side	Tai Yang	TW-5 or GB-41
	top	GV-20	LI-4 or LV-3

† Find the points that are reactive on the affected limb; place the black clip on a yin meridian point and the red clip on a yang meridian point.

Manaka offers a few additional pointers relevant to formulating local treatment strategies:

Signs of kidney vacancy may include darkness around the eyelids; ticklishness of the whole body is likewise a sign of kidney problems. One may consider treating the kidney meridian directly; or, if appropriate diagnostic signs are present, treatment of yin qiao-ren mai with the ion-pumping cords may be selected.

Treatment of bladder problems, such as frequent urination, are aided if the patient avoid salty food, curry and hot and spicy foods or condiments.

Patients with skin diseases will show reactions at ST-27, the large intestine mu point. Treatment should eliminate reactiveness on this point.

Patients with stomach problems will manifest a depressed area on the back when they raise up their torso while lying face down. This area should be treated with needle and moxa.

Bursitis patients who manifest pressure pain and puffiness when pinching palpation is administered along the small intestine meridian can gain positive relief when intradermal needles are placed at BL-27 the small intestine back-shu point.

Manaka has described and commented on many different local conditions. His extensive studies and clinical experience are too vast to capture in a single volume. He constantly stresses the importance of undertaking root treatment first, to correct the underlying imbalances, before using local treatments for specific conditions.

Chapter

- 18 -

Manaka's

Biorhythmic

Treatments

Manaka's
Biorhythmic Treatments

The patterns that determine the normal fluctuating activity of the points actually represent biorhythmic changes in the body — the daily, monthly, and yearly fluctuations of external energetic fields and the body's response to them. To apply this information in practice, it is not necessary to understand all the correspondences, nor the complete cycles and where they came from or on what they are based. All that is needed is an accurate timepiece and a Chinese calendar.

The biorhythmic systems described herein are the ten-day cycle of the five phase and source points, the daily biorhythm, the circadian rhythm of the twelve meridians, and the sixty-day cycle of the extraordinary vessel points.

It is useful to note that the stems and branches of Chinese astronomy were correlated to both daily and bihourly periods (one Chinese hour is equivalent to two Western hours). The ten stems describe a ten-day cycle. In conjunction with the twelve-day cycle of the twelve branches, the stems and branches jointly describe a sixty-day cycle. Every day is given a stem and branch correspondence in a continuously repeating cycle of sixty days.

Each bihourly period corresponds to a stem and branch, with twelve bihourly periods in the course of a day forming one complete branch cycle. The stems and branches complete a sixty bihourly period cycle every five days, so that the ten-day cycle of the stems is composed of two complete bihourly cycles. The sixty-day cycle is composed of twelve of these five day, sixty bihourly period cycles.

To read the charts for the ten-day cycle, first determine the stem day, calculated from the tables below, and the time of day. In this cycle there are not always open points available for treatment.

To read the charts for the daily cycle, only the time of day need be determined. To read the charts for the sixty-day cycle, determine the stem-branch-day, calculated from the charts below, and the time of day. For each bihourly period, these charts give a number that relates to the extraordinary vessel master points. The mathematical calculations have already been performed, so that one only need read the tables. There is always an extraordinary vessel point available for treatment.

zi	branch1	B1		jia	stem1	S1
chou	branch2	B2		yi	stem2	S2
yin	branch3	B3		bing	stem3	S3
mao	branch4	B4		ding	stem4	S4
chen	branch5	B5		wu	stem5	S5
si	branch6	B6		ji	stem6	S6
wu	branch7	B7		geng	stem7	S7
wei	branch8	B8		xin	stem8	S8
shen	branch9	B9		ren	stem9	S9
you	branch10	B10		gui	stem10	S10
xu	branch11	B11				
hai	branch12	B12				

Thus a wu-wu, Stem 5—Branch 7 day will be S5-B7.

The Ten-Day Biorhythmic Phasal Treatments

In these treatments, the correspondences of the meridians to the ten stems as the yin-yang aspects of the five phases is important. These correspondences are:

S1	wood yang	gallbladder
S2	wood yin	liver
S3	fire yang	small intestine
S4	fire yin	heart
S5	earth yang	stomach
S6	earth yin	spleen
S7	metal yang	large intestine
S8	metal yin	lungs
S9	water yang	bladder
S10	water yin	kidney

A cycle begins on each day in the ten-day cycle that is associated with the meridian corresponding to the stem assignment for that day; thus each of the meridians, excluding the triple warmer and the pericardium, are described as passing through the same cycle. The yang meridian fluctuations end at the triple warmer. The yin meridian cycle completes at the pericardium. The result of these cycles is a series of points that are "open" at different times of the day and on different days repeating every ten days.

This cycle begins at the jing point of the meridian to which the cycle belongs, jumping through the five-phase points of the other meridians to end on the triple warmer meridian in a yang sequence and the pericardium meridian in a yin sequence. The cycle can be summarized as follows:

□

Comes out	Streams	Passes Through and Streams
jing point	yong point	shu point
Moves	*Enters*	*Is Received*
jing point	he point	TW or PC point.

This gives us a complete cycle as shown below, after the *Zhen Jiu Da Quan*.

	Comes Out	Streams	Passes Through and Streams	Moves	Enters	Is Received
Day	*S1*	*S2*	*S2*	*S2*	*S2*	*S2*
Time	*S1-B11*	*S3-B1*	*S5-B3*	*S7-B5*	*S9-B7*	*S1-B9*
Point	GB-44	SI-2	ST-43 GB-40	LI-5	BL-54	TW-2
Day	*S2*	*S2*	*S3*	*S3*	*S3*	*S3*
Time	*S2-B10*	*S4-B12*	*S6-B2*	*S8-B4*	*S10-B6*	*S2-B8*
Point	LV-1	HT-8	SP-3 LV-3	LU-8	KI-10	PC-8
Day	*S3*	*S3*	*S4*	*S4*	*S4*	*S4*
Time	*S3-B9*	*S5-B11*	*S7-B1*	*S9-B3*	*S1-B5*	*S3-B7*
Point	SI-1	ST-44	LI-3 SI-4	BL-60	GB-34	TW-3
Day	*S4*	*S4*	*S4*	*S5*	*S5*	*S5*
Time	*S4-B8*	*S6-B10*	*S8-B12*	*S10-B2*	*S2-B4*	*S4-B6*
Point	HT-9	SP-2	LU-9 HT-7	KI-7	LV-8	PC-7
Day	*S5*	*S5*	*S5*	*S6*	*S6*	*S6*
Time	*S5-B7*	*S7-B9*	*S9-B11*	*S1-B1*	*S3-B3*	*S5-B5*
Point	ST-45	LI-2	BL-65 ST-42	GB-38	SI-8	TW-6
Day	*S6*	*S6*	*S6*	*S6*	*S7*	*S7*
Time	*S6-B6*	*S8-B8*	*S10-B10*	*S2-B12*	*S4-B2*	*S6-B4*
Point	SP-1	LU-10	KI-3 SP-3	LV-4	HT-3	PC-5
Day	*S7*	*S7*	*S7*	*S7*	*S8*	*S8*
Time	*S7-B5*	*S9-B7*	*S1-B9*	*S3-B11*	*S5-B1*	*S7-B3*
Point	LI-1	BL-66	GB-41 LI-4	SI-5	ST-36	TW-10
Day	*S8*	*S8*	*S8*	*S8*	*S8*	*S9*
Time	*S8-B4*	*S10-B6*	*S2-B8*	*S4-B10*	*S6-B12*	*S8-B2*
Point	LU-11	KI-2	LV-3 LU-9	HT-4	SP-9	PC-3
Day	*S9*	*S9*	*S9*	*S9*	*S9*	*S10*
Time	*S9-B3*	*S1-B5*	*S3-B7*	*S5-B9*	*S7-B11*	*S9-B1*
Point	BL-67	GB-43	SI-3 BL-64 TW-4	ST-41	LI-11	TW-1
Day	*S10*	*S1*	*S1*	*S1*	*S1*	*S1*
Time	*S10-B12*	*S2-B2*	*S4-B4*	*S6-B6*	*S8-B8*	*S10-B10*
Point	KI-1	LV-2	HT-7 KI-3 PC-7	SP-5	LU-5	PC-9

Through the course of the work day, 7 am - 9 pm, this table can be charted as follows:

Open Points on the Ten-Day Cycle							
	7-9am	9-11am	11-1pm	1-3pm	3-5pm	5-7pm	7-9pm
S1		**SP-5**		**LU-5**		**PC-9**	**GB-44**
	TW-6	*SP-1*		*LU-10*		*KI-3*	
S2	**LI-5**		**BL-54**		**TW-2**	**LV-1**	
	LI-1		*BL-66*		*GB-41*		*SI-5*
S3		**KI-10**		**PC-8**	**SI-1**		**ST-44**
		KI-2		*LV-3*		*HT-4*	
S4	**GB-34**		**TW-3**	**HT-9**		**SP-2**	
	GB-43		*SI-3*		*ST-41*		*LI-11*
S5		**PC-7**	**ST-45**		**LI-2**		**BL-65,ST-42**
S6	**TW-6**	**SP-1**		**LU-10**		**KI-3,SP-3**	
		SP-5		*LU-5*		*PC-9*	*GB-44*
S7	**LI-1**		**BL-66**		**GB-41,LI-4**		**SI-5**
	LI-5		*BL-54*		*TW-2*	*LV-1*	
S8		**KI-2**		**LV-3,LU-9**		**HT-4**	
		KI-10		*PC-8*	*SI-1*		*ST-44*
S9	**GB-43**		**SI-3,TW-4,BL-64**		**ST-41**		**LI-11**
	GB-34		*TW-3*	*HT-9*		*SP-2*	
S10		**PC-7**	**ST-45**		**LI-2**		**BL-65**

Points in italics are secondary or auxilliary open points, while those in bold are the primary open points. Primary points tend to be therapeutically more valuable, the secondary open points tend to be more valuable when no primary points are open.

The "secondary" or "auxilliary" points are derived from the close relationship of the opposite stems (e.g. *S1-S6*, *S2-S7*). This is the husband-wife relationship as described in the *Nan Jing*. Thus, on an *S1* day, the points of *S6* are also open as secondary or auxilliary points. Similarly on an *S6* day, the points of *S1* are open as secondary or auxilliary points.

In this context the term "day" on the chart refers to the ten-day cycles of the stems. These can be calculated from the following tables that show the stem and branch for the first day of each month for 1987, 1988, 1989, 1990:

Month	1987	1988	1989	1990
Jan 1	S7-B11	S2-B4	S8-B10	S3-B3
Feb 1	S8-B6	S3-B11	S9-B5	S4-B10
Mar 1	S6-B10	S2-B4	S7-B9	S2-B2
Apr 1	S7-B5	S3-B11	S8-B4	S3-B9
May 1	S7-B11	S3-B5	S8-B10	S3-B3
Jun 1	S8-B6	S4-B12	S9-B5	S4-B10
Jul 1	S8-B12	S4-B6	S9-B11	S4-B4
Aug 1	S9-B7	S5-B1	S10-B6	S5-B11
Sep 1	S10-B2	S6-B8	S1-B1	S6-B6
Oct 1	S10-B8	S6-B2	S1-B7	S6-B12
Nov 1	S1-B3	S7-B9	S2-B2	S7-B7
Dec 1	S1-B9	S7-B3	S2-B8	S7-B1

Knowing the stem and branch for the first of each month enables one to quickly calculate the stem and branch for every day within the month. Thus, August 17, 1987 will be: $S9-B7 + 16 = S5-B11$. December 25, 1987 will be $S1-B9 + 24 = S5-B9$. April 4, 1989 will be $S8-B4 + 3 = S1-B7$. The term "time" on the chart refers to stem-branch cycle through the bihourly sequence of the Chinese clock.

Branch Cycle	
Branch	**Time**
B1	11 pm to 1 am
B2	1 am to 3 am
B3	3 am to 5 am
B4	5 am to 7 am
B5	7 am to 9 am
B6	9 am to 11 am
B7	11 am to 1 pm
B8	1 pm to 3 pm
B9	3 pm to 5 pm
B10	5 pm to 7 pm
B11	7 pm to 9 pm
B12	9 pm to 11 pm

In this sequence, the stems alternate through cycles of ten within the branch hours which cycle in twelves. Thus, on day one, S1, at 11 am to 1 pm, is the time of S7-B7; on day four, S4, at 11 am to 1 pm is the time of S3-B7. For example, for October 28, 1984, the daily stem would have been S2. At 11 am, the branch indicated would have been B7. This was the stem-branch time of S9-B7 and the corresponding open point was BL-54. The auxilliary point was BL-66. On October 26, 1984 at 11 am, an S10 day, the open point was an auxilliary open point, ST-45. It is also possible that there may be no open point at specific times during the stem-branch cycle. On October 22, 1984, the daily stem was *S6* . At 11 am on that day the stem-branch notation was *S7-B7* . At this moment there is no point open. As we will see further, Manaka uses the Chinese clock with the circadian rhythm when there are no open points.

Provided there is an open or auxilliary open point at the time of a patient's visit, treatment can be applied to this point with benefit, regardless of the patient's condition. This kind of biorhythmic treatment is another example of Manaka's taikyoku or tai ji method: by utilizing these points, the condition of whole body can be addressed. Treatment using the open point is able to treat root problems regardless of symptoms or pattern complex. On certain days, at certain times, there may be several open points. In these cases it is advantageous to be able to select the best point for the patient. Manaka has a simple and useful means for testing the applicability of a point, and the general applicability and usefulness of that point for a particular patient.

He places a magnet (1500 gauss or more) with the north pole facing the point. If the reactive points or areas become less reactive after a few moments, sometimes up to five minutes, the point is useful and should be treated. Manaka cites the twelfth century work, *Zi Wu Liu Zhu Zhen Jing,* in explaining how best to treat the point or whether to use needle or moxa. Usually needles can be used to treat the point; however if the patient has yin or cold and vacancy symptoms — wind, cold, damp, numbness, bi obstruction in channels, repletion above and vacancy below, or counterflow qi symptoms, moxa is more appropriate. Overtiredness experienced by men and blood disorders encountered by women also indicate the use of moxa on the open point. For yang symptoms, moxa is not used. From his experience, Manaka feels that shallow needle insertion is sufficient when treating open points. Tonification, dispersion, or other needle techniques are not necessary.

As we have stressed, these treatments are deeply rooted and treat a condition regardless of its symptom picture. Open point treatments may be used on virtually every patient and added to other treatments. Because of the power and effectiveness of this type of treatment, Manaka recommends using open point treatment first. It is often unnecessary to do anything else. For example, a patient with yang qiao symptoms (pressure pain around GB-29, SI-10, and the back of the neck) and a vacant liver (tension below the ribs on the right side, tension to the left of the umbilicus, sensitivity around left LV-8 and LV-9 with a vacant liver pulse) might require both a five-phase and an extraordinary vessel treatment. If the tension below the ribs and to the side of the umbilicus decreases after treating the open point, and if the sensitivity of the left leg decreases and the liver pulse becomes stronger, it would no longer be necessary to tonify the liver. One could simply treat the yang qiao mai with ion cords. Depending on the resulting changes, this could be the complete treatment. Once accustomed to using open point treatments, the practitioner will rapidly discover their broad utility.

□

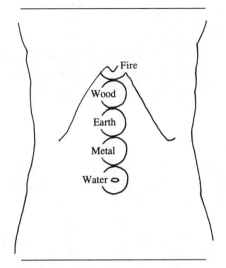

Figure 18.1 The phase correspondences.

Daily or Circadian Treatments

If there are no open points at a certain time, Manaka advises application of the following technique that is in part based on the embryological phase-organ correspondences described by Tohaku Ishi.[1] Begin by palpating the abdomen on the midline, from the sternum to the umbilicus. (See Figure 18.1.) Next, determine the area that is most reactive, for example, the earth area. Then, use the bihourly Chinese clock to determine the active meridian. The clock is as follows:

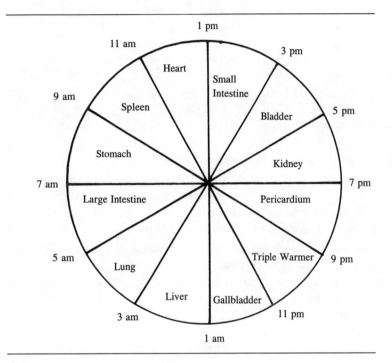

Figure 18.2 Meridian circuit.

For example, 10 am is the time of the spleen meridian. A treatment at that hour would treat the earth point of the active meridian, in this case, SP-3. Following treatment of this point, the earth area would generally be less reactive. This principle is easy to apply. If a patient presents a liver problem and the wood area of the abdomen is reactive and it is the small intestine period (1 pm to 3 pm), we may treat the wood point of the small intestine, SI-3. If the wood area becomes less reactive, then the treatment will succeed in helping the liver problem. Although this type of treatment is useful when there is no point open at the time of treatment, it is also useful any time there is a clearly reactive area on the abdomen above the umbilicus. Manaka reports having a patient come for treatment at midday with acute gallstone pain. Since it was the heart meridian time and the gallbladder corresponds to wood, he treated the wood point of the heart, HT-9. This cured the patient's pain and discomfort.

Manaka has applied and extended the logic of this style of treatment to his isophasal concept of the phases. He posits that whenever a phase is out of balance the areas of the body related to that phase will be reactive. If, for example, the wood phase is out of balance, wood areas and points throughout the body will be active and reflective. The mu points will also reflect phase disharmonies. Thus, if ST-27 (Manaka's large intestine mu point) is reactive, we may remember that the large intestine corresponds to the metal phase, and treat the metal point of the meridian active at that time, thus decreasing the reactivity of ST-27. Similarly, a patient treated between 1 pm and 3 pm (small intestine time) with a lung vacancy pulse and pressure pain on LU-1 (metal), will be benefitted by treating the metal point of the small intestine, SI-1. We will expect a decrease of the reactivity of LU-1 and a strengthened lung pulse.

As with the open point treatments, testing the points with the north pole of a magnet will ensure that they are applicable. Manaka's phasal diagnosis of the ren mai or his phasal diagnosis of the mu points and their appropriate treatments may also be used as specific-phase, bihourly, biorhythmic treatment.

For straightforward cases of vacancy or repletion, there is a relatively simple biorhythmic treatment using the phases and twelve meridians. This treatment method is found in the *Zhen Jiu Zhi Liao Xue,* though even its description is probably based on earlier ideas. It can be used specifically or generally for any vacancy or repletion. If a patient presents a simple lung repletion, one can schedule the patient for treatment at the lung time (3-5 am) and disperse the dispersion point, LU-5. If the condition were simple lung vacancy, treatment might be scheduled for the period after the lung meridian is active, the large intestine time (5-7 am), and the focus of the treatment would be to supplement the tonification point, LU-9. Essentially, the idea is to disperse when at the maximum of energy and to supplement just after the maximum energy, thus slowing the natural energetic decline.

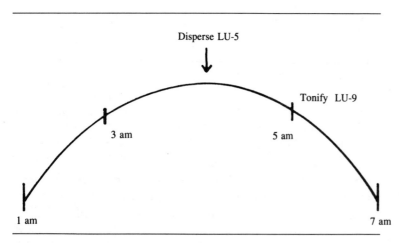

Figure 18.3

These concepts yield the following treatment charts.

Repletion Treatments			Vacancy Treatments		
Meridian	Point	Hour	Meridian	Point	Hour
Lung	LU-5	3-5 am	Lung	LU-9	5-7 am
Large Intestine	LI-2	5-7 am	Large Intestine	LI-11	7-9 am
Stomach	ST-45	7-9 am	Stomach	ST-41	9-11 am
Spleen	SP-5	9-11 am	Spleen	SP-2	11-1 pm
Heart	HT-7	11-1 pm	Heart	HT-9	1-3 pm
Small Intestine	SI-8	1-3 pm	Small Intestine	SI-3	3-5 pm
Bladder	BL-65	3-5 pm	Bladder	BL-67	5-7 pm
Kidney	KI-1	5-7 pm	Kidney	KI-7	7-9 pm
Pericardium	PC-7	7-9 pm	Pericardium	PC-9	9-11 pm
Triple Warmer	TW-10	9-11 pm	Triple Warmer	TW-3	11-1 am
Gallbladder	GB-38	11-1 am	Gallbladder	GB-43	1-3 am
Liver	LV-2	1-3 am	Liver	LV-8	3-5 am

Manaka has found that this simple treatment method works regardless of what is vacant or replete. If a patient presents at 10 am with signs of vacancy, regardless of specific pattern, treating the tonification point for that time (in this case, ST-41), will supplement the vacancy. Similarly if a patient had presented with signs of repletion, treating the dispersion point for that time, SP-5, would disperse the repletion. These treatments seem to have a general or root effect like the open points of the ten-day cycle, and are effective regardless of the specific condition. Thus if a patient presents at 4 pm with weakness in several positions in the pulse, reactions on several areas of the abdomen, and a generally weakened constitution, treating SI-3 can have a general supplementing effect. Manaka further recommends that the needle need only be inserted, and needling techniques of supplementation or dispersion are not necessary.

Manaka adds that it is often difficult to schedule patients late at night and in the early hours of the morning. In cases where one cannot treat at these times, it is possible to treat the phase point related to the vacancy or repletion at the opposite time. Thus, for a vacant or replete liver condition, one can treat the wood point of the small intestine, SI-3, at 1-3 pm. For a vacant or replete lung condition, one can treat the metal point of the bladder meridian, BL-67, at 3-5 pm. (See Figure 18.4.)

In his experience, Manaka has noticed that in a replete condition of an organ and meridian, the patient's symptoms can become worse at the time associated with that organ and meridian. Vacancy condition symptoms can flare at the time opposite the hour when the affected meridian is most active. For a liver vacancy condition, we may expect a worsened incidence from 1-3 pm. For a liver repletion condition, we might see an intensification at 1-3 am. Since for each bihourly time unit an intensification of symptoms may be a repletion of that meridian or a vacancy of the opposite meridian, careful differentiation is necessary before drawing diagnostic conclusions.

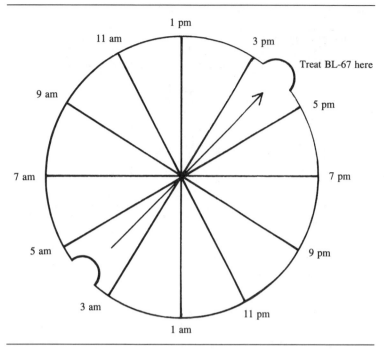

Figure 18.4 For lung problems one can treat at the opposite time of day at that meridian, metal point, BL-67.

There are different ways to use biorhythmic cycles according to the patient's condition. The following examples from Manaka's case histories demonstrate the use of some of these techniques and treatment styles. It is useful to remember that reducing the abdominal reactions with treatment indicates that the patient's condition has also improved. These brief case histories demonstrate how to think about using biorhythmic treatments as well as how effective these treatments may be. Note also that Manaka treats the minimum number of points necessary to produce the desired effect. In the tradition of a great teacher, Manaka places the responsibility for study and understanding on his students' shoulders, encouraging the development of comprehension. A deep understanding of biorhythmic treatments comes after using them and observing their effects.

Case Histories

Case One: A patient suffered from numbness of the whole body. On palpation of the abdomen, Manaka found pressure pain below the sternum and also to the side of the umbilicus on the stomach meridian — i.e., reactiveness in the fire area of the abdomen, along the stomach meridian. As the patient's visit was at 8 am, correlating to the stomach on the Chinese clock, Manaka treated the fire point of the stomach meridian, ST-41. This decreased the abdominal reactions, demonstrating the principle of treating the corresponding phase point of the active meridian. Since the open meridian was also the reactive meridian, its treatment was further indicated.

Case Two: The patient was suffering from lassitude and poor energy. Manaka diagnosed this as a combination of liver and kidney vacancy. Palpation of the abdomen located pressure pain on CV-12 and to the sides of the umbilicus — the area correlating to the water phase. Manaka also reasoned that according to the *Nan Jing*, supplementing the mother will supplement the son; treating the kidney vacancy can thus treat the liver, wood. Since it was the stomach period, 8 am, he treated the water point of the stomach meridian, ST-44. This reduced the abdominal reactions, providing a clear demonstration of the isophasal concept of the phases.

Case Three: A patient with hyperthyroidism who developed palpitations between 12-2 am sought treatment. The pulse showed a liver repletion condition. In this case, Manaka again applied his isophasal concept of the phases. Because of the liver condition, he treated the wood point of the active meridian, ST-43. Since GB-41 was also an extraordinary vessel open point, and coincidentally a wood point, it was also treated. Note also that GB-41 is the treatment point for a liver condition according to chapter 2 of the *Mai Jing*.

Case Four A patient examined at the small intestine time, 1-3 pm, presented severe pressure pain in the fire area — below the sternum — and on left KI-16. Manaka chose SI-5, the fire point of the active meridian. Treatment here eliminated the pressure pain below the sternum. Because KI-16 is his mu point for the kidney, Manaka tested and then treated left KI-3 for the reaction on left KI-16. To do this, he placed a magnet (north pole to the skin) on left KI-3, decreasing the sensitivity of left KI-16. He then placed the magnet (south pole to the skin) on left KI-3, increasing the sensitivity of left KI-16. Because of these reactions he determined that KI-3 was an effective treatment point for the patient. The reactivity of left KI-16 was eliminated. This case history demonstrates the specificity of the points.

Case Five: In a fashion typical of his teaching style, Manaka gives us another case history that demonstrates the exception rather than the rule, leading us to think carefully about what we are doing. Manaka examined a sixty year old who suffered from insomnia and high blood pressure. Examination by palpation located pressure pain along the liver meridian on the feet. The patient had come for treatment in the morning between 9 and 11 am (spleen time). Manaka determined a diagnosis of liver repletion. To treat the patient, he supplemented the spleen. This decreased the pressure pain of the liver meridian. He commented that had he dispersed the spleen, he may well have made the patient's condition worse. While he does not state why this is so, we can suggest that applying the five-phase cycles, wood in repletion will cause vacancy of the spleen. Rather than simply treat a point on the spleen meridian, as could have been indicated by the time of treatment, and run the risk of weakening the spleen by over-controlling earth, he strengthened the spleen, avoiding the potentially harmful controlling-cycle transformation. Since the wood — earth relationship described by the controlling cycle works in both directions, tonifying the spleen further dispersed the liver repletion.

We may note here that the *Nan Jing* describes a great healer as one who treats disease before it manifests or transforms. Supplementing the spleen in a liver repletion condition to prevent the controlling-cycle transformation is an example of the application of this principle *(NJ 77)*.

□

We would like to present two of our own case histories illustrating use of the open points.

Case Six: A twenty-eight year old male with a degenerative disc disease at the fifth lumber vertebra level suffered with low back pain, particularly on the right side. The pain radiated down the right leg. The patient also suffered pain of the left shoulder and a feeling that his back muscles were seizing. Tension and pressure pain below the ribs on the right side, pressure pain on KI-16, CV-7, and CV-9, tension on the stomach meridians to the sides of the umbilicus, and weak liver and kidney pulses, pointed to a diagnosis of liver and kidney vacancy. ST-45 was the open point and was treated on the right side. The patient's back immediately relaxed, literally "sinking into the table." His pain disappeared and the pulses improved. The treatment was completed by placing an intradermal needle in josen, which was sore, to prolong the benefit of the treatment. While not all treatments using only the principle of the open point are so dramatically effective, this treatment does demonstrate how effective they may be. In this case the treatment was one in a series. In the next case only the one treatment was required.

Case Seven: A twenty-three year old female patient presented with a history of cystitis. The current problem marked a seventh recurrence. She had taken medications in the past for the condition, but sought to treat the problem this time without medication. Palpation revealed that the whole abdomen was healthy, except for the detection of some coolness on the area below the umbilicus, and reactive soreness at CV-3, when pressing to the bladder. Her sacrum was also cold. BL-65 was the open point. Right BL-65 was sore, thus right BL-65 was needled. This elicited a sensation up the bladder meridian to the lower abdomen and eliminated the reaction on CV-3. The patient was sent home with instructions to apply dry heat, using a hot stone wrapped in a towel, to both the lower abdomen and sacrum, twenty minutes each, on a daily basis. The patient reported the next week that the cystitis had disappeared the next day and that she would continue the heat therapy until the abdomen and sacrum were no longer cool to the touch.

This case history illustrates how a problem can be cleared with a single open point. It also demonstrates the importance of a healthy abdomen. The therapy may have worked so easily because the patient was actually quite healthy, suffering only from the cystitis, with no major underlying vacancies or imbalances. Though no similar efficacy can be guaranteed in more complex cases, such as illnesses of long standing, multiple problems, or a history of surgery or medication, the open points or biorhythmic meridian treatments prove helpful in most instances.

The dry heat therapy used in this case was employed effectively, using a palm-sized stone roughly the thickness of the palm, having at least one flat surface. To use the stone, it was placed in an oven at 250 degrees for twenty minutes, then wrapped in a towel and settled on the area to be heated. This is an inexpensive and easy therapy for the patient to do at home. In many lower-warmer disorders such as cystitis and gynecologic problems, the lower abdomen and sacrum are cold. Any time coolness is determined here, heated-stone therapy is indicated.

☐

The Sixty-Day Cycle
of the Open Extraordinary Vessels

The last of Manaka's biorhythmic treatment that we present in this work is the "Spiritual Turtle" treatment map as derived from the *Zhen Jiu Da Quan*. Based on information and calculations derived from this text, we may determine the following treatment schedule, abbreviated for regular working hours, 7 am - 9 pm.

Day	7-9am	9-11am	11-1pm	1-3pm	3-5pm	5-7pm	7-9pm
S_1B_1	LU-7	TW-5	SI-3	KI-6	TW-5	BL-62	GB-41
S_2B_2	KI-6	SP-4	GB-41	KI-6	KI-6	TW-5	BL-62
S_3B_3	PC-6	SP-4	SP-4	GB-41	KI-6	LU-7	SI-3
S_4B_4	SP-4	GB-41	KI-6	SP-4	GB-41	BL-62	KI-6
S_5B_5	KI-6	LU-7	GB-41	SI-3	KI-6	TW-5	BL-62
S_6B_6	TW-5	SP-4	GB-41	KI-6	SP-4	GB-41	BL-62
S_7B_7	KI-6	LU-7	GB-41	KI-6	KI-6	TW-5	BL-62
S_8B_8	GB-41	KI-6	KI-6	TW-5	BL-62	KI-6	TW-5
S_9B_9	GB-41	KI-6	SP-4	GB-41	KI-6	KI-6	TW-5
$S_{10}B_{10}$	GB-41	KI-6	SP-4	TW-5	BL-62	KI-6	TW-5

Day	7-9am	9-11am	11-1pm	1-3pm	3-5pm	5-7pm	7-9pm
S_1B_{11}	TW-5	SP-4	BL-62	PC-6	SP-4	GB-41	SI-3
S_2B_{12}	KI-6	TW-5	BL-62	KI-6	KI-6	SP-4	GB-41
S_3B_1	SI-3	KI-6	KI-6	TW-5	BL-62	PC-6	SP-4
S_4B_2	KI-6	SP-4	GB-41	KI-6	SP-4	TW-5	BL-62
S_5B_3	LU-7	SI-3	KI-6	KI-6	TW-5	BL-62	PC-6
S_6B_4	GB-41	BL-62	KI-6	TW-5	BL-62	KI-6	KI-6
S_7B_5	KI-6	TW-5	SI-3	KI-6	PC-6	SP-4	GB-41
S_8B_6	BL-62	KI-6	KI-6	SP-4	GB-41	KI-6	SP-4
S_9B_7	KI-6	LU-7	GB-41	KI-6	LU-7	TW-5	BL-62
$S_{10}B_8$	KI-6	TW-5	BL-62	GB-41	KI-6	SP-4	GB-41

Day	7-9am	9-11am	11-1pm	1-3pm	3-5pm	5-7pm	7-9pm
S_1B_9	KI-6	KI-6	LU-7	SI-3	KI-6	TW-5	SP-4
S_2B_{10}	BL-62	KI-6	TW-5	BL-62	GB-41	KI-6	SP-4
S_3B_{11}	BL-62	PC-6	PC-6	SP-4	GB-41	KI-6	LU-7
S_4B_{12}	KI-6	TW-5	BL-62	KI-6	TW-5	SP-4	GB-41
S_5B_1	PC-6	SP-4	BL-62	GB-41	KI-6	LU-7	SI-3
S_6B_2	SP-4	TW-5	BL-62	KI-6	TW-5	BL-62	GB-41
S_7B_3	TW-5	BL-62	KI-6	TW-5	SP-4	GB-41	KI-6
S_8B_4	KI-6	SP-4	TW-5	BL-62	KI-6	TW-5	BL-62
S_9B_5	KI-6	TW-5	SI-3	KI-6	TW-5	SP-4	GB-41
$S_{10}B_6$	KI-6	SP-4	GB-41	BL-62	KI-6	TW-5	BL-62

Day	7-9am	9-11am	11-1pm	1-3pm	3-5pm	5-7pm	7-9pm
S1B7	LU-7	TW-5	SI-3	KI-6	TW-5	BL-62	GB-41
S2B8	KI-6	SP-4	GB-41	KI-6	KI-6	TW-5	BL-62
S3B9	LU-7	SI-3	SI-3	KI-6	TW-5	BL-62	PC-6
S4B10	BL-62	KI-6	TW-5	BL-62	KI-6	KI-6	SP-4
S5B11	KI-6	LU-7	GB-41	SI-3	KI-6	TW-5	BL-62
S6B12	TW-5	SP-4	GB-41	KI-6	SP-4	GB-41	BL-62
S7B1	KI-6	LU-7	GB-41	KI-6	KI-6	TW-5	BL-62
S8B2	GB-41	KI-6	KI-6	TW-5	BL-62	KI-6	TW-5
S9B3	TW-5	BL-62	KI-6	TW-5	BL-62	GB-41	KI-6
S10B4	TW-5	BL-62	KI-6	KI-6	SP-4	GB-41	KI-6

Day	7-9am	9-11am	11-1pm	1-3pm	3-5pm	5-7pm	7-9pm
S1B5	TW-5	SP-4	BL-62	PC-6	SP-4	GB-41	SI-3
S2B6	KI-6	TW-5	BL-62	KI-6	KI-6	SP-4	GB-41
S3B7	SI-3	KI-6	KI-6	TW-5	BL-62	PC-6	SP-4
S4B8	KI-6	SP-4	GB-41	KI-6	SP-4	TW-5	BL-62
S5B9	BL-62	PC-6	TW-5	SP-4	GB-41	KI-6	LU-7
S6B10	KI-6	KI-6	SP-4	GB-41	KI-6	SP-4	TW-5
S7B11	KI-6	TW-5	SI-3	KI-6	PC-6	SP-4	GB-41
S8B12	BL-62	KI-6	KI-6	SP-4	GB-41	KI-6	SP-4
S9B1	KI-6	LU-7	GB-41	KI-6	LU-7	TW-5	BL-62
S10B2	KI-6	TW-5	BL-62	GB-41	KI-6	SP-4	GB-41

Day	7-9am	9-11am	11-1pm	1-3pm	3-5pm	5-7pm	7-9pm
S1B3	BL-62	GB-41	PC-6	SP-4	GB-41	KI-6	KI-6
S2B4	SP-4	GB-41	KI-6	SP-4	TW-5	BL-62	KI-6
S3B5	BL-62	PC-6	PC-6	SP-4	GB-41	KI-6	LU-7
S4B6	KI-6	TW-5	BL-62	KI-6	TW-5	SP-4	GB-41
S5B7	PC-6	SP-4	BL-62	GB-41	KI-6	LU-7	SI-3
S6B8	SP-4	TW-5	BL-62	KI-6	TW-5	BL-62	GB-41
S7B9	GB-41	KI-6	SP-4	GB-41	SI-3	KI-6	TW-5
S8B10	TW-5	BL-62	GB-41	KI-6	SP-4	GB-41	KI-6
S9B11	KI-6	TW-5	SI-3	KI-6	TW-5	SP-4	GB-41
S10B12	KI-6	SP-4	GB-41	BL-62	KI-6	TW-5	BL-62

The allocation of these points is derived through the sum of the numerical values of the daily and bihourly stems and branches at any time divided by six or nine and then interpreted through the temporal sequence of the trigrams and its relation to the magic square.

Magic Square		
4	9	2
3	5	7
8	1	6

Each number corresponds to an extraordinary vessel point as follows:

Number	
1	BL-62
2, 5	KI-6
3	TW-5
4	GB-41
6	SP-4
7	SI-3
8	PC-6
9	LU-7

Thus, for November 2, 1987 an *S2-B4* day, at 2:30 pm, the active extraordinary vessel is KI-6, the yin qiao mai. Since Manaka uses these tables when using the ion cords, we recommend following these calculations when using the open points or active vessels.

Manaka uses these tables as part of the theory behind his application of the extraordinary vessels. He has found that when an extraordinary vessel point is active, for instance KI-6, its coupled point, LU-7, is also active. Thus, when using the cords on the yin qiao connection we can orient the polarity of the cords based on palpation. For example, if there were tension on the ren mai above the umbilicus, looseness below the umbilicus, looseness of the rectus abdominus muscles relative to the back muscles of the lumbar region, and pressure pain on ST-12, the yin qiao mai would be indicated. We would then orient the ion cords by placing the black clip on KI-6 and the red clip on LU-7. However, if the symptoms were more obviously of the ren mai, an opposite orientation on LU-7 would be indicated (black clip on LU-7, red on KI-6). If the symptoms clearly indicated another extraordinary vessel connection it would be necessary to determine whether the active vessel or the vessel indicated by the symptom-sign picture were most applicable for the patient. Treatment of the active extraordinary vessel, like the open point treatments, is a deep, root treatment. Despite the capacity of these methods to treat deeply, it is sometimes necessary to determine the treatment most important for the patient. One can use the north pole of a magnet on the master point of the open vessel and then the indicated vessel. The point that reduces the reactions the most is the vessel that should be treated.

Case Histories from Dr. Manaka

We may see from the following case histories how to begin thinking about matching the open points with the diagnostic signs.

Case One: A patient came for treatment complaining of problems of the left leg. Abdominal palpation located tension on the upper right quadrant of the abdomen below the ribs and in the left lower quadrant of the abdomen. At the time of his visit, KI-6 was the open point. To treat this problem, Manaka needled left KI-6 and LU-7 bilaterally. He attached ion cords with the red clips bilaterally on LU-7. Both black clips were attached to KI-6 on the left. This eliminated the palpable tension.

□

Case Two: A patient with the same abdominal pattern described above came for treatment when PC-6 was the open point. Manaka treated right PC-6 with the black clip and left SP-4 with the red clip. This eliminated the palpable tension.

In these two cases Manaka was utilizing the open vessel and orienting the cords according to the patient's abdominal pattern, regardless of symptomology. We have described several other treatments for the common syndrome where the upper right and lower left abdominal quadrant are reactive. These case histories show that the open extraordinary vessels are also a means by which this pattern may be approached. As discussed above, Manaka's purpose is not to demonstrate hard and fast rules and treatments, rather to illustrate ways of thinking about treatment and how to utilize what is presented at each moment.

We would like to conclude with another of our own case histories. This case also stresses the importance of focusing on key symptoms and parts of the pattern and applying the logic of different systems to the biorhythmic treatments.

Case Three: A twenty-four year old female came to the clinic for relief of her coughing spells. Every evening from 5-7 pm she would cough for one to two hours. This coughing was usually accompanied by tightness in the chest and occasional difficulty breathing. The condition had persisted for several years. Medical doctors had been unable to help her. The medications she had taken in the past caused stomach problems, so she had discontinued them on her own initiative.

At the time of her visit, KI-6, the yin qiao mai, was open. Her abdomen was generally quite healthy except for slight tightness and soreness on right ST-24, ST-25, and ST-26. Pressure on both right and left KI-23 prompted the urge to cough. Bilaterally, KI-27 was uncomfortable with pressure and LU-1 was tight and sore. Placing a north-facing magnet on right KI-6 decreased the reactivity of all the points. The ion cords were applied to KI-6 (black), LU-7 (red). Within minutes the patient reported an improvement in her breathing and relief of the tightness in her chest. After treatment all points evidenced decreased reactions, but KI-23 and KI-27 were still a little reactive. North-facing magnets of 500 gauss were placed bilaterally on KI-23 and south-facing magnets bilaterally on KI-27. The patient was sent home with these magnets taped in place. The patient called two weeks later. She had not coughed since the treatment. Since KI-23 and KI-27 were no longer sore, she was instructed to remove the magnets.[2]

The logic in this case was that the cough was related to the kidney meridian. This conclusion was reached due to the time of occurrence and the reaction of the kidney points. Since KI-6 is both on the kidney meridian and related to the yin qiao mai, then treating KI-6 when it is the open point should treat both the yin qiao mai and the kidney simultaneously. Again, the importance of a healthy abdomen is clear. The patient may have responded so well to treatment because she was basically healthy. Treating the main paradox, as Manaka terms it, at the right time in a basically healthy person can be powerful and effective.

☐

The treatment procedures described in this chapter represent both a facet of Manaka's treatment style and a generally useful set of procedures for any style of treatment. As we have stressed throughout, the biorhythmic treatments represent a very fascinating and brilliant aspect of treatment by acupuncture. They are essentially practical and reach to deep levels of the patient's energetics.

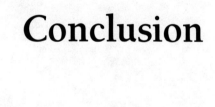

Conclusion

"All of this will not be finished in the first one hundred days,
nor will it be finished in the first one thousand days,
nor even perhaps in our lifetime on this planet;
but let us begin."

————————————————— John F. Kennedy, Jr.

Reflections on the Sea

One of the most interesting qualities of Oriental Medicine is its extremely broad patterning of ideas and the grand scope of treatment that follows such a remarkable conception. In the literature we find descriptions that range from the broadest levels of action — the movements of the stars and planets and the cycles of the seasons — to the finest and most detailed observations of microcirculation and microscopic function. Because of the unified nature of these concepts, the concept of qi for example, this range of observation is really a continuum. Detailed examination of any classical theory always reveals a continuous thread of ideas that links layers of action and response. We find descriptions of how the circulation and fluctuations of qi in the body are affected by the rhythms of the seasons and descriptions of how these rhythms result in and are affected by the movement of qi. At the most profound levels of human function we find parallels of universal motion.

The consequence of researching such a philosophical view is that we gradually lose our native Western conception of linear, single-cause diseases and begin to conceive of our being as affected both constructively and adversely by external and internal events that are cosmological, astronomical, environmental, macroscopic, and microscopic. As we become aware of how we each manifest cyclic adaptations to those influences we perceive in our own lives, we acquire a functional sense of our own sensitivity to environment. Our concept of environment expands and our ideas of health become increasingly relative.

This experience is a challenge to our thought process. While the intuitive sense of this grand vision appeals to our sense of consensual reality and our personal experiences, and is logically justified by many of the discoveries of our own culture's sciences, our logical training nonetheless sounds an alarm. Continually, we halt and incline toward the process of reducing our investigations to the clearly stated, clearly quantified, and practically measurable hypotheses that offer us greater comfort.

This dissonance is most poignantly felt as we approach therapy. From all these observations there flows a vast range of diagnostic and therapeutic ideas. Throughout the history of Oriental medicine we find literally hundreds of different patterns of diagnosis and treatment. Indeed, it might be suggested that in sheer numbers Oriental medicine has forgotten more protocols than Western medicine has as yet described. Multiplicity, however, is only the first challenge. Some of these therapies are hard, perhaps even impossible, to use today, because of the peculiar manner of their recording. Others concern diseases that no longer exist, a sobering experience as our

☐

relatively youthful medical science has only just begun to experience this phenomena. Some treatments were designed for conditions we will never see, some even for conditions we now consider normal and healthy. Yet, within this vast array of patterns, we find brilliant descriptions based in the clinical experience of practitioners whose insight is captivating. Chinese observation, being precise and lengthy, provides us with much that remains in common use today, crossing barriers of time and culture to become part of our therapeutic repertoire.

It is our persistent insight that the dissonance between Oriental and Western patterns of thought is both less dramatic than it seems and more a matter of translation than substance. As in a conversation where both parties are speaking a non-native language with which they are only nominally expert, similarities are blurred and differences of word choice induce unintended misunderstanding. Just as the use of the appropriate dictionary might resolve the problems of a second-language conversation, the application of the appropriate logical process can resolve the conceptual problems of understanding Oriental medicine.

In modern Western terminology the Chinese continuum of concepts and models would be described as a "systems theory." As our concept of reality becomes increasingly complex, and as our awareness of the need to express precisely the interaction and interdependence of all events expands, we have begun to recognize the need to use logical devices that are able to organize and predict the results of hypotheses that simply cannot be clearly stated, precisely quantified, and tested within known controls. As with the Oriental models, our explanations for observable phenomena have become more functional, more philosophical, more relative, and less absolute.

The logical models that we use to coordinate a complexity of interaction are formulations of interlocking systems. Each level of function is seen as a system; all systems are seen to interact with all other systems. For example, a person may be seen as one arbitrarily described level of complexity within the universe:

Galaxy
Solar system
Planetary body
Biosphere
Mankind
Society, Nation
Culture
Subculture
Community
Family
Levels of conduct, experience: "person"
Systems
Organs
Tissues
Cells
Organelles
Molecules
Atoms
Subatomic particles

□

None of these levels can be absolutely separate from any other level. The distinctions we make are consensual, the commonsense separations described by our natural and created methods of observation. We tend not to see that our observations through telescopes relate to our observations through microscopes.

Increasingly, however, we are learning of relationships we have not perceived. In any given medical situation, some influence from all these systems is always manifest. Some influences are dominant, others dormant, and others are exerting tertiary effects through the behavior of some aspect of the system that is not directly related. The job of the healer is to examine and assess the potential for influence of all these interrelating systems over the patient's current medical condition and general life. In particular, this is what many Oriental medical systems suggest that we do.

In the context of systems theory we are provided the logical tools by which we may order our perception of similarity and difference. Oriental theoreticians placed less stress on systems of interpersonal relationship than we do. These were not ignored or forgotten, but perceived as relative to social and environmental systems. As well, they attend to the macrocosmic environment, the upper three levels of this model, with greater diligence. They were also particularly interested in other, less personalized systems: local environmental phenomena such as weather, seasonal influence, variations of temperature and humidity. Indeed, their awareness of the consequences of these phenomena on human health was so acute that these events provided the names of many pathogenic concepts.

The Oriental scientists were also intrigued by cycles and patterns at all levels of their universe views, and consequently formulated descriptions of many rhythmic systems. Because they focused more on universal changes and cycles, we can adapt the preceding diagram to their viewpoint very simply:

> Universe
> Galaxy
> Star systems
> Solar system
> Atmosphere
> Climate
> Local environment
> Person
> Tissues
> Organs
> Cells
> Biochemistry
> Quantum

If we focus on the uses of the various systems of diagnosis and treatment, even without delving into many of their implications, we can generalize system elements as follows:

● Yin and yang may be perceived as ranging from the top to the bottom. In the medical models, yin and yang are described in their numerous interactions, permutations, and cycles by both the five-phase theory and the language of complementary antagonism. In modern language, we may achieve the ability to describe yin—yang interactions by reference to nonlinear oscillators and self-replicating systems.

□

● In their simplest correspondences, five-phase dynamics cover phenomena from the solar system to the level of biological organs. This theory was used to describe the numerous cyclic phenomena with which we interact. In more advanced form, the five-phase theory describes events through the entire continuum. The stem and branch system, as a further development and refinement of these cycles, is equally inclusive. Here again, modern Western concepts such as open systems, information theory, and non-linear, fractal geometries may serve as useful models.

● Xu Wen Bai's "open point" theories and treatments fit the macro-cosmic to human interactions of the continuum. If these theories are accurate interpretations of the *Nan Jing*, the *Nan Jing* theories also fit at these levels. As these are particularized concepts of relationships, they are subsets of the larger systems.

● The largest cycles — the precession of the equinox, the sixty-year, ten-year, and annual cycles, the seasonal, bimonthly, monthly, biweekly, twelve-day, ten-day and daily cycles, the bihourly and pentadecanary daily cycles are all aspects of the five-phase model, ranging from the cosmic to the organ and cellular levels.

● The extraordinary vessels, in general, range from the local environment and the individual to the organ level, but extend to the upper levels via concepts of biorhythmic fluctuation.

● The triple burner and master of the heart theories begin somewhere at the level of the individual and extend downward through the quantum level. The anatomical basis of the triple burner, master of the heart, and meridian systems cover the individual to the cellular (and possibly deeper) levels.

There are a number of more specialized techniques that focus on particular areas of this continuum. For instance, the methodology of the eight parameters considers data derived from the atmospheric to the organ levels. Logically and historically, it has developed to organize and coordinate the class of information that is most readily available from these areas of phenomena, with a particular emphasis on data considered most consequential to the health practitioner. In this sense, it is a subset of yin—yang theory in the same way that bridge-building formulae are a subset of geometry.

Models in the Oriental medical framework each fit this picture and each are a single element of the whole system of interacting systems. Each model has a particular focus and goal. All models can be clearly defined according to their intention and nature. It is obvious that they overlap to a considerable degree. Practically, we can focus on treating via the five-phase theory and still correct a problem that could have been described as belonging to the extraordinary vessel model. All models are by nature limiting; we create them to reduce the observations with which we must contend. This is why, following the tradition of Oriental medicine, we recommend learning many models and approaches. A completely mature practitioner is rarely limited to one approach.

In this attempt we are aided by the use of principles, such as the concept of qi, that serve as unifying ideas. We are simultaneously impaired by our tendency to feel comfortable only with quantifiable concepts. However, if we are careful to distinguish that we are using conceptual tools and not positing mystical substances or fuzzy concepts of relationship, we are able to recognize logical parallels and analogies that serve us well. The qualitative approach is consistent in Chinese thought; we must not rush to quantify concepts such as qi prior to having acquired a sufficiently qualitative understanding. Western thought can contribute to this effort as well.

The philosopher John Ratcliffe describes how there have been a number of approaches to the understanding of reality in the West. He feels that we have evolved through five distinct inquiry systems, all of which are still in use in various fields and disciplines. These approaches are: the deductive approach of Liebniz, the inductive logic of Locke, the synthetic logic of Kant, the dialectical system of Hegel, and the relative approach to inquiry developed by Singer. The more recent and most sophisticated approach is relativistic. This method recognizes that what we take to be correct is conditioned by our assumptions and the method we adopt. What we consider truth is only correct relative to the goals and objectives of the method chosen and the assumptions of the inquirer.

Ratcliffe further argues that the distinction between qualitative and quantitative approaches is false, since all inquiry systems are essentially qualitative. The assumptions that must be made in all systems of inquiry are essentially judgments about what is and what is not "real."

We feel that Oriental medicine and Oriental thought is, in general (not in every feature and detail), an excellent example of a relative and qualitative approach to inquiry. Given the recognition that all things interact at all times, that all systems interact continuously, it is very good sense to attempt, as does Oriental medicine, to analyze as many of these levels as is possible at once. While it is not always overtly stated that methods of analysis in Oriental medicine are limited and yield conditioned information, the existence of broad patterns, the prevalence of unifying concepts, and the very existence of multiple systems implies that Oriental thinkers have wrestled with a relative universe. A culture that honored an absolutist, or theoretically quantitative "reality," would have been unlikely to develop as many interlocking models.

If our analysis is correct, then the Chinese of two or more thousand years ago acquired an understanding of reality that we in the West are only now beginning to recognize (or perhaps allow to surface). The implications of this premise are profound. Some scientists in the West, conditioned by the now-suspect quantitative presumptions of Western science, criticize Oriental medicine for its supposed unscientific nature, its lack of rigor, its lack of a quantitative approach, and for the extremely broad ideas it proposes. Yet the assumption that scientific inquiry concerns only problems that can be well-structured, and reduced to quantifiable hypotheses, can no longer be praised as wisdom and must be recognized as limitation. As the relativistic mode of inquiry becomes ever more necessary, as the problems presented to science become more complex, as the implicit qualitative nature of our methodology becomes clear, all science and all medicine will share an increasing need for the logical power of systems theories.

□

While it is probable, very probable, that concepts within Oriental medicine will not survive the scrutiny of even the most sophisticated analysis, it is just as probable that methods and results that have come to us from its inquiries will prove to be continually useful. It is our hope that this text, in its attempt to approach a single precept from the vast accumulations of Oriental medicine with the broadest possible conception, will contribute not only to practitioners' repertoire of effective tools, but also to the statement of Oriental medical principles in such manner as will permit a grasp of their elegance and logical beauty. To the extent that we have succeeded, we must praise the brilliance of the original formulators of the ideas we have attempted to explain. To the extent that we have failed, we offer the hope that our colleagues will remedy our deficits.

To allow the full benefit of Oriental medicine to participate in the enhancement of the quality of life on this planet, an enormous amount of research, scholarship, and practice is necessary. We envision a new medicine, a truly energetic medicine, that is comprehensible and accessible to all. Let us begin.

□

Notes

Chapter Notes

Notes to Chapter 1

[1] For an interesting conceptual and social analysis of the hara, see Karlfried Durkheim, *Hara, the Vital Centre in Man.*

[2] The group was founded by A.J. Ayers and based upon interpretations and readings of Ludwig Wittgenstein's *Logico-philosophico-tractatus.*

[3] Quotations from the *Su Wen* are cited in the text using first letter abbreviation, followed by the chapter number and page reference. For example, *Su Wen* chapter 39 would be cited as follows: *(SW 39).*

[4] See: K. Hashimoto M.D., and Y. Kawakami M.D., *Sotai, Balance and Health Through Natural Movement.*

[5] *Dao De Jing,* from *Lao Zi, Zhuang Zi* p. 82. See also K. Matsumoto and S. Birch, *Five Elements and Ten Stems* p. 195. p.195.

[6] The basic theories of the *Nan Jing* are described in *Five Elements and Ten Stems* (op.cit.).

[7] Quotations from the *Nan Jing* are cited in the text using first letter abbreviation, followed by the chapter number and page reference. For example, reference to *Nan Jing* chapter 8, vol.1, p.11, would be cited as: *(NJ 8(1):11).*

Notes to Chapter 2

[1] Quotations from the *Ling Shu* are cited in the text following the style of the *Su Wen* and *Nan Jing,* using first-letter abbreviation, followed by the chapter number and page reference. For example, *Ling Shu* chapter 4, would be cited as follows: *(LS 4).* See also *Five Elements and Ten Stems* p. 110.

[2] Wang Shu He, commentary on *Nan Jing* 1(1):1.

[3] Manaka, *Hukubusyoken to Hukusyo,* p.16 passim.

[4] Quotations from the Morohashi Encyclopedic Dictionary may be found cited in the text as follows: *(Mor).*

[5] For instance: The *Han Shu* and the *Shi Jing,* from the *Morohashi Encyclopedic Dictionary.*

[6] For a good, brief discussion of this school and some of their beliefs, see Joseph Needham, *Science and Civilization in China* 2:359-363.

[7] Needham, *Celestial Lancets* p.85.

[8] This passage is also interesting as it explicitly describes a moving "landscape." See also *Five Elements and Ten Stems* p.153.

[9] Often interpreted as ST-25, this is more likely KI-16.

[10] For a translation of the complete quote, see *Five Elements and Ten Stems* pp.160-161.

[11] Respect for the ideas in this passage are among the reasons why the insertion tube was invented and is ubiquitous in Japan. While the left hand finds the acupoint and prepares it with various rubbing techniques, the right hand is used to insert the needle, handle first, into the tube. The tube is then rotated, inverting it so that the needle is ready to be used. By placing the tube between the fingers of the left hand, the needle may be tapped into the point without losing contact with the insertion area. This takes practice, but allows the left hand to find and prepare the acupoint, feeling the qi.

[12] Quoted from *Zhong Yi Zhen Duan Xue* p.129.

[13] From the *Shang Han Lun*, quoted from Nagahama, *Toyo Igaku Gaisetsu* p.130-131. See also page 52 of the *Shang Han Lun Yi Shi*, where further differentiation of this sign with appropriate herbal formularies may be found.

[14] See *Shang Han Lun Yi Shi* p.87-88.

[15] Nagahama, *Toyo Igaku Gaisetsu* p.132. See also *Shang Han Lun Yi Shi* p.52.

[16] Yanagiya, *Kanmei Humon Shinsatsu Ho* p.293.

[17] Ibid. p.288.

[18] Li Shi Zhen, *Qi Jing Ba Mai Kao* 1:18.

[19] *Zhen Jiu Jia Yi Jing Yu Xue Zhong Ji* p.298 passim.

[20] Ibid. p.308 passim.

[21] Ibid. pp.309,313,315 passim.

[22] Ibid. p.316 passim.

[23] Sun Si-Mo, *Qian Jin Yao Fang* 12:141.

[24] Gao Wu, *Zhèn Jiu Ju Ying* p.152-153 passim. See also *Five Elements and Ten Stems* p.167-168.

[25] Manaka, *Hukubusyoken to Hukusyo* p.11 passim. For a review of the history of abdominal palpation systems, including the Mubunryu style, see also Manaka and Itaya, *American Journal of Acupuncture* 13, no.3 (1985):223-234.

[26] Sugiyama, *Sugiyama Ryu Sanbusho* p.113 passim.

Notes to Chapter 3

[1] Rene Descartes, *Discourse on Method* p.53.

[2] Quotations from *Fujido's Etymological Dictionary* are cited in the text using an abbreviation, followed by chapter number and page reference where pertinent. Thus, *Fujido's Etymological Dictionary* would be found cited in the text as *(Fuj)*.

[3] In modern times, "diaphragm block" or "diaphragmatic armoring" have become commonplace terminology for various systems of healing. Modern observation thus confirms the ancient observations of Chinese medicine. See for instance: W.E. Mann, *Orgone, Reich, and Eros* p.66-67.

[4] Quotations from the *Huang Di Nei Jing Tai Su* are cited in text using the following abbreviation: *(TS)*.

[5] Xie Lin, *Nan Jing Zheng Yi* p.61-62.

[6] *Lie Zi* 5:240-241 passim.

[7] *Zhen Jiu Da Cheng* p.120.

□

Notes to Chapter 4

[1] Quotations from the *Shisi Jing Fa Hui* are cited in text with the following abbreviation: *(Shisi)*. This entire text deals with the meridians.

[2] Quotations from the *Nei Jing Jie Po Sheng Li Xue* are cited in text with the following abbreviation: *(Li Xue)*.

[3] Shinji Imamura, "Zofu Keiraku Oyobi Chukankeiraku no Ruchi ni Tsuite (Pathways of the Internal Meridians)," *Ido No Nippon Magazine* (June 1983):6-14 (July 1983):45-54. Quotations from Dr. Imamura's article are cited in text with the following abbreviation: *(Ima)*.

[4] Yoshio Manaka, *Ika no Tameno Shinjutsu Nyumon Kuoza* p.185.

[5] *Lao Zi and Zhuang Zi* 17:378.

[6] Sosen Hirooka, *Nangyo Tekkan* p.27-28 passim.

[7] Ibid.

[8] Ibid.

[9] Liu Wan Su, *Su Wen Xuan Ji Yuan Bing Shi* p.165.

Notes to Chapter 5

[1] For some of the following discussions of astronomy and relative star movements, we have used H.A. Rey, *The Stars, A New Way to see Them,* which very simply and clearly explains some of the basic principles and terms of astronomy. See also the excellent discussions of the Chinese astronomies, in Joseph Needham, *Science and Civilization in China* vol. 3; and *Daikanwa Jiten (Morohashi Encyclopedic Dictionary)*.

[2] Quotations from Needham's *Science and Civilization in China* are cited in the text using the following abbreviation: *S&C*.

[3] Both the *Morohashi Enclyclopedic Dictionary* and *Fujido Etymological Dictionary* attest to this, as does the *Kakusareta Kamigami* (1975) p.45.

[4] Quotations from the *Huai Nan Zi*, with commentary by H. Kusuyama, are cited in the text using the abbreviation *(HNZ)*, followed by chapter and page reference.

[5] *Zhou Yi*, quoted from *Ki no Shiso* p.238.

[6] Honda, *Yi Jing* 2:296.

[7] *Tong Ren Shu Xue Zhen Jiu Tu Jing* p.116.

[8] Liu Wan Su, *Su Wen Xuan Ji Yuan Bing Shi* p.169.

[9] Henri Maspero, *Taoism and Chinese Religion* p.369. He is quoting the *Jin Que Di Jun San Yuan Zhen Yi Jing*.

[10] Ibid. p.370.

[11] Ibid. p.351. Here Maspero quotes from the *Tai Shang Dao Jun Shou Yuan Dan Shang Jing*.

[12] See Hiroko Yoshino, *Kakusareta Kamigami Kodai Shinko to Yinyo Gogyo* p.145.

[13] Sango Kobayashi, *Toyo Igaku Koza* 15:16 passim.

[14] "Experimental studies have led to the conclusion that the geomagnetic field is a very important space-time coordinate for living organisms." A.P. Dubrov, *The Geomagnetic Field and Life: Geomagnetobiology* p.210. This text is a very useful and stimulating survey of the modern literature.

[15] It should be noted that Needham prefixes the first four stars with the term "tian," (heaven), where the *Morohashi Encyclopedic Dictionary* does not.

[16] The *Zhou Bi Suan Jing* talks of this. See *Science and Civilization in China* 3:261.

[17] From the *Nung Cheng Chuan Shu,* circa 1600. See *Morohashi Encyclopedic Dictionary* 7:783 for a picture.

[18] *Five Elements and Ten Stems* p.75.

[19] The *Shi Ji* says it means beginning. See the *Morohashi Encyclopedic Dictionary.*

[20] The *Lei Jing* writer feels that this is both upper and lower qihai (CV-17 and CV-6), though several other commentaries suggest only CV-6.

[21] See *Five Elements and Ten Stems* pp.65-75 for further elaboration of this.

[22] The *Huang Ting Jing* makes reference to these.

[23] Henri Maspero in *Taoism and Chinese Religion* discusses extensively the dantian and the various related breathing techniques.

[24] Different authors describe it differently. Needham and others refer to cinnabar as Mercuric sulphide. Maspero sees it as Mercuric sulphate, $HgSO4$. See *Taoism and Chinese Religion* p.271.

[25] Cf. *Su Wen* 4 for color correspondences. See Shohaku Honma's poetic description of the nature of the fire phase, which can be found on pages 77-78 of our previous publication, *Five Elements and Ten Stems.*

[26] See for instance the *Huang Ting Wai Jing Jing.* This reference can be found in the *Morohashi Encyclopedic Dictionary.*

[27] Shohaku Honma, *Shinkyu Byosho Gaku* p.80.

[28] See for instance Henry Maspero, *Taoism and Chinese Religion* p.459.

[29] See Mr. Yang's commentary on the *Nan Jing* in Wang Jiu Si, *Nan Jing Ji Zhu* 5:4.

[30] Henri Maspero, *Taoism and Chinese Religion* p.268.

[31] For brief discussions of this, see Matsumoto & Birch, *Five Elements and Ten Stems* pp.170,176.

[32] Bunshi Shiroda, *Shinkyu Chiryo Kiso Gaku* 295, quoting *Su Wen* 58:292.

[33] Ibid.

[34] *Zhou Yi,* quoted from the *Ki No Shiso* p.238 passim.

[35] *Shuo Wen Jie Zi,* quoted from *Ki No Shiso* p.27.

[36] *Han Shu Lu Li Zhi,* from the *Dao Jiao Da Zi Dian* p.93.

[37] *Huang Ting Jing,* from *Ki No Shiso* p.146.

[38] *Tai Bing Yu Lan,* supposedly quoting from the *Huai Nan Zi* from *Ki No Shiso* p.138. The foregoing discussions were all taken from the excellent Japanese study of qi, *Ki No Shiso,* quoting various sources, mostly classical in origin.

[39] *Hou Han Shu,* from *Ki No Shiso* p.7.

[40] *Chun Qiu,* from *Ki No Shiso* p.177.

[41] Waichi Sugiyama, *Sugiyama Ryu Sanbusho* p.103.

[42] *Ki No Shiso,* p.177.

□

[43] Shinsai Ota, *Zukai Anma Jutsu* p.91.

[44] Quotations from the *Kadokawa Etymological Dictionary* are cited in the text using the following abbreviation: *(Kad)*.

[45] Needham has a particularly good discussion of these concepts; see *Science and Civilization in China* 2:554-556.

[46] *Lie Zi* p.28. See also Zhuang Zhou, from *Lao Zi, Zhuang Zi* p.408.

[47] See for instance: Louis Kervran, *Biological Transformations;* Louis Kervran and G. Ohsawa, *Biological Transformations* See also, Peter Tompkins and C. Bird, *The Secret Life of Plants.*

[48] Louis Kervran, *Biological Transmutations* p.10.

[49] Ibid.

[50] Ibid. pp.156-157.

[51] Lao Zi, chapter 78 of the *Dao De Jing*, from *Lao Zi, Zhuang Zi* p.145.

[52] T. Sawada, *Kaitai Hatsu Mou* p.32.

[53] Louis Kervran, *Biological Transmutations* p.156 passim.

[54] Zhuang Zhou, from *Lao Zi, Zhuang Zi* p.378.

[55] Ibid.

[56] *Lie Zi* p.31-33.

[57] Zhuang Zhou, from *Lao Zi, Zhuang Zi* p.404.

[58] This passage mirrors the *Yi Jing* and was probably added into the *Su Wen* by Wang Bing in the eighth century.

[59] *Lei Jing* p.15.

[60] Quoted from *Huang Di Nei Jing Su Wen Jiao Zhu Yu Yi* p.29.

[61] *Lu Shi Chun Qiu; Zhou Yi*, quoted from *Ki no Shiso* p.238, and from *Morohashi Encyclopedic Dictionary*.

[62] David Bohm, *Wholeness and the Implicate Order* p.191-192.

Notes to Chapter 6

[1] See the commentary on *Ling Shu* p.198.

[2] From the *Shuo Wen Jie Zi*, and from Ma Shi; see *Nei Jing Jie Po Sheng Li Xue* p.228.

[3] *Jing Luo Shi Jiang*, pp.64-65.

[4] *Ji Yun* and *Zheng Zi Tong* from the *Morohashi encyclopedic dictionary*. The *Ji Yun* defines po ang as the umbilicus.

[5] For instance, in the *Lei Jing* p. 249, and the modern text, the *Jing Luo Shi Jiang* pp.64-65.

[6] The content of this entire quote clearly implies that the author must have performed some anatomical surgery or have been familiar with anatomical studies. The midterm months are particularly indicative of actual observation. Later in the text we will deal with embryology and anatomy in more detail. The organ — sense organ correspondences are also provocative as they contradict other correspondences given in the *Su Wen* and *Ling Shu*.

[7] It cannot for instance be found in the *Zhen Jiu Jia Yi Jing (Systematic Classic of Acupuncture and Moxibustion)* of 282 A.D., which was the first text to systematically describe the acupoints.

□

[8] *Zhen Jiu Jia Yi Jing Yu Xue Zhong Ji* p.304.

[9] *Zhen Jiu Juying* p.248 and *Zhen Jiu Da Cheng* p.160. See also *Five Elements and Ten Stems* p.69 for the complete reference.

[10] Kikuo Chishima, *Revolution of Biology and Medicine* 9 (Gifu: Neo-Haemotology Society of Japan, 1972).

[11] Nigel Wiseman et al., *Fundamentals of Chinese Medicine* Brookline: Paradigm Publications, 1987) p.i.

[12] Bunshi Shiroda, *Shinkyu Shinzui* p.258.

[13] Bunshi Shiroda, *Shinkyu Chiryo Kisogaku* p.185 passim.

[14] Waichi Sugiyama, *Sugiyama Ryu Sanbusho* p.103 passim.

[15] *Lie Zi* p.33.

[16] Sosen Hirooka, *Nangyo Tekkan* 1:26

[17] Henry Maspero, *Taoism & Chinese Religion* p. 465 passim.

[18] Wang Shu He, in his commentary on the *Nan Jing* 38(3):3.

[19] See for instance Waichi Sugiyama, *Sugiyama Ryu Sanbusho* p.60 passim, where these relationships are described.

[20] In the *Su Wen*, the water — fire duality is seen as a fundamental yin—yang duality. See *Su Wen* 5:32.

[21] Wang Shu He's commentary on *Nan Jing* 8(1):12.

[22] Sosen Hirooka, *Nangyo Tekkan* 4:31.

[23] Zhang Jie Bin, *Lei Jing Fu Yi*, quoted from the *Zhong Guo Yi Xue Shi Lue* p.211.

[24] *Lun Heng* 20:5.

[25] Waichi Sugiyama, *Sugiyama Ryu Sanbusho* p.104. See also *Five Elements and Ten Stems* pp.80-82.

[26] Li Shi Zhen, *Qi Jing Ba Mai Kao* 1:14.

[27] For a more complete discussion of qi jie see Matsumoto & Birch, *Extraordinary Vessels* pp.31-34.

[28] Sun Si-Mo, *Qian Jin Yao Fang* 20:362. Here it is interesting to note that the circling of the "way of shen" is the same name as GV-11.

[29] *Kaitai Hatsumou* p. 29.

[30] *Tong Su Shang Han Lun,* from the *Zhong Guo Yi Xue Shi Lue* p.211.

[31] *Kaitai Hatsumou* p.32-34.

[32] *Yixue Rumen,* quoted from the *Nei Jing Jie Po Sheng Li Xue* p.296.

[33] Ryoan Terashima, *Wakan Sansai Zue* 11:27.

[34] Waichi Sugiyama, *Sugiyama Ryu Sanbusho* p.103.

[35] Ibid. p.103 passim.

[36] Ibid. p.107.

[37] Ibid. p.116-117.

□

[38] Sosen Hirooka, *Nangyo Tekkan* 1:28.

[39] Ibid., concerning *Nan Jing* 25:27-28.

[40] Yang, from Wang Jiu Si, *Nan Jing Ji Zhu,* 5:4.

[41] Ibid.

[42] Hua Shou, *Nan Jing Benyi* p.32.

[43] Ding, from Wang Jiu Si, *Nan Jing Ji Zhu* 1:22-23.

[44] Yang, quoted from Wang Jiu Si, *Nan Jing Ji Zhu* 4:32.

[45] He Ruo Yu, *Zi Wu Liu Zhu Zhen Jing* p.122.

[46] Wang Shu He's commentary on the *Nan Jing* 25:20.

[47] *Nan Jing Ji Zhu* 5:4-5.

[48] See Matsumoto and Birch, *Extraordinary Vessels* p.6 passim.

[49] *Nan Jing Ji Zhu* 5:4-5.

[50] See *Extraordinary Vessels* p.36 for a more complete quotation.

[51] Ibid. p.13-18.

[52] Wang Bing's commentary on the *Su Wen,* quoted from the *Nei Jing Jie Po Sheng Li Xue* p.120.

[53] Li Shi Zhen, *Qi Jing Ba Mai Kao* 1:14.

[54] Xie Lin, *Nan Jing Zheng Yi* p.67.

[55] Ibid. p.14.

[56] Ibid. p.65.

[57] Ibid. p.48.

[58] Liu Wan Su, *Su Wen Xuan Ji Yuan Bing Shi* p.231.

Notes to Chapter 7

[1] For a good example of a text that consistently notes and details these parallells, see Yves Requena, *Terrains and Pathology in Acupuncture.*

[2] See, "Translators Foreword," *Fundamentals of Chinese Medicine* p. vi.

[3] It continues to be a major effort to accurately identify all the elements of the fascial system as referenced by each author. Hopefully, later work will clearly delineate the various energetic pathways and trajectories within this vast system of fascial tissues.

[4] *Han Shu,* the "Wang Mang" chapter.

[5] Akira Ishihara, *Kanpo* p.50.

[6] This could be the four directions with the upper (heaven) and lower parts (earth) or the upper, lower, left, right, front, and back portions.

[7] Ippo Okamoto, *Shinkyu Azeyoketsu,* quoted from Bunshi Shiroda, *Shinkyu Chiryo Kisogaku* p.185.

[8] Ryoan Terashima, *Wakan Sansai Zue* 11:19. This same passage from Chen Yan is also cited by Xie Lin in his Qing dynasty commentary on the *Nan Jing,* the *Nan Jing Zheng Yi* p.67.

□

9 *Wakan Sansai Zue* 11:9.

10 Ibid.

11 Ibid. p.17 passim.

12 Hua Shou, *Nan Jing Ben Yi* p.38.

13 Quoted from the *Nei Jing Jie Po Sheng Li Xue* p.308.

14 Yu Bo, *Dan Xi Yi Xue Zheng Bo* 1:8-9. Our special thanks to the Harvard University Yenching Library for allowing us to access this volume.

15 Xie Lin, *Nan Jing Zheng Yi* p.116.

16 Ibid. p.45.

17 Ibid. p.67.

18 *Nei Jing Jie Po Sheng Li Xue* p.297.

19 We are grateful to Mikhail Santaro for allowing us to see part of the working translation of this unpublished text.

20 Tang Zong Hai, *Xue Zheng Lun*. The *Guang Ya* and the *Ji Yun* from the *Morohashi Encyclopedic Dictionary*.

21 *Kang Xi*, a dictionary of the seventeenth to eighteenth centuries, from the *Morohashi Encyclopedic Dictionary*.

22 See Henri Maspero, *Taoism and Chinese Religion*.

23 See for instance the *Jing Luo Shi Jiang*.

24 Xie Lin, *Nan Jing Zheng Yi* p.50.

25 *Morohashi Encyclopedic Dictionary*, paraphrasing Wang Bing's commentary on the *Su Wen*.

26 Sosen Hirooka, *Nangyo Tekkan* 5:25.

27 Ibid. 6:2.

28 Wang Yi Ren, *Nan Jing Du Ben Mu Lu* p.74.

29 K. Mitsutane, *Kaitai Hatsumou* 3:23-34.

30 We have discussed qi jie extensively in a previous work, *Extraordinary Vessels* pp. 31-34.

31 Zhang Yin An, *Huang Di Nei Jing Su Wen Ji Gua* p.205.

32 Yao Zhi An, *Su Wen Jing Zhu Jie Jie* p.166.

33 Zhang Yin An, *Huang Di Nei Jing Su Wen Ji Gua* p.138.

34 Ibid. Commentary on *Su Wen* 43:168.

35 Warwick and Williams, *Gray's Anatomy* p.902.

36 Xie Lin, *Nan Jing Zheng Yi* p.67.

37 Guo Ai Chun, *Huang Di Nei Jing Su Wen Jiao Zhi Yu Yi* p.212.

38 Zhang Yin An, *Huang Di Nei Jing Su Wen Ji Gua* p.168.

39 From private notes, lectures, and conversations with Dr. Yoshio Manaka.

40 Sun Si-Mo, *Qian Jin Yao Fang* 17:314.

41 K. Shibata, *Ashi No Tsubode Naoru Ken Ko Ho* pp.170-172 passim.

[42] Sosen Hirooka, *Nangyo Tekkan* 5:15.

[43] NanKing Chinese Medical School, *Nan Jing Jiao Shi* p.92.

[44] *Lei Jing* p.266.

[45] See Matsumoto and Birch, *Five Elements and Ten Stems* pp.120-121.

[46] Warwick and Williams, *Gray's Anatomy* p. 972.

[47] This property is implied by the name san jiao, or triple warmer, but not clearly stated in the classical literature, though some modern authors state it quite clearly. See T. Sawada's introduction to *Kaitai Hatsumou* pp.29 and following.

[48] *Guan Zi* book 2, chapter 39 14:2-3.

[49] Chao Yuan Fang, *Zhu Bing Yuan Hou Lun* p.165, with illustrations from Tamba No Yasuyori's *Ishin Po* 982 A.D.; from Teizo Ogawa's *Nihon Igaku Shi Koyo* pp.47-51.

[50] Sun Si-Mo, *Qian Jin Yao Fang* 2:21-24.

[51] Ibid.

Notes to Chapter 8

[1] B.B. Gallaudet, *A Description of the Planes of Fascia of the Human Body* p.2.

[2] Williams and Warwick, *Gray's Anatomy* p.523.

[3] The epidermis is generally 0.07 - 0.12 mm. thick, increasing to 0.8 mm. on the palms and 1.4 mm. on the soles. The dermis is generally 1 to 2 mm. thick, increasing to 3 mm. on the palms and soles, but decreasing to 0.6 mm. on the eyes and prepuce. (W. Bloom and Fawcett, *Textbook of Histology* p.565,577.) Thus, with the exception of the palms and soles, the superficial fascia will lie from just over one to just over two milimeters below the skin surface.

[4] James Oschman, *Natural Science of Healing; a Biology of Whole Systems*. Typescript. We are greatly indebted to Dr. James Oschman of the Woodshole Marine Biological Laboratory for his contributions, suggestions, inspirations, enormous help, encouragement and energy in the writing of this chapter; his presence can be seen throughout.

[5] James Oschman, "The Structure and Properties of Ground Substance, *American Zoologist* 24 no. 1 (1984): 199-215. See also, James Oschman, "The Connective Tissue and Myofascial Systems," paper presented at the 1982 Rolfing conference.

[6] J. Ellison and D.R. Garrod, "Anchoring Filaments of the Amphibian Epidermal-Dermal Junction Traverse the Basal Lamina Entirely from the Plasma Membrane of Hemidesmosomes to the Dermis, *J.Cell.Sci.* 72 (1984): 163-172.

[7] James Oschman, *Natural Science of Healing,* op.cit.

[8] Taken from *Ido no Nippon Magazine* (May 1969).

[9] From the private notes and lectures of Dr. Manaka.

[10] Warrick and Williams, *Gray's Anatomy* p.1389. See also Mark A. Hayes, *The developmental basis for the continuity of the fascial planes of the abdomen and pelvis* PhD diss., 1948, Fig. 40 and 41.

[11] See also, Hua Shou, *Shi Si Jing Fa Hui.*

[12] Inaba Bunrei, *Fuku Sho Kiran* p.250.

[13] Yoshio Manaka, *Shinkyu no Riron to Kangaekata* p.68 passim.

[14] S.B. Oppenheimer and G. Lefevre Jr., *Introduction to Embryonic Development* p.202 passim.

[15] Takeshi Sawada, *Kaitai Hatsumou* p.32-33. In his introduction, Sawada defines clear anatomical relations and function of the three warmers and their qi to the lymphatic system.

[16] Ibid.

[17] See: R. Nuccitelli, "The Involvement of Transcellular Ion Currents and Electric Fields in Pattern Formation," in *Pattern Formation, a Primer*.

[18] Ibid. For another good review article see, L.F. Jaffe and R. Nuccitelli, "Electrical Controls of Development," *Ann. Rev. Biophys. Bioeng.* 6 (1977): 445-476.

[19] Yoshio Manaka, *Shinkyu no Riron to Kangaekata* p.68 passim.

[20] Cited by Y. Nagatomo, *Nagatomo M.P. Shinkyu Kuowa Hachiju Hachi Syu.*

[21] Yoshio Manaka, *Shinkyu no Riron to Kangaekata* p.68 passim.

[22] See for instance, Williams and Warwick, *Gray's Anatomy* p.1365 passim p.1454 passim.

Ibid. p.1366 passim.

[24] Ibid. p.1365 passim.

[25] Lionel F. Jaffe and Claudio D. Stern, "Strong Electrical Currents Leave the Primitive Streak of Chick Embryos, *Nature* 206 (November 2, 1979): 569-571 passim.

[26] See: L. Jaffe, "Developmental Currents, Voltages and Gradients," in A.R. Liss, *Developmental Order; it's Origin and Regulation* p.190. (The rest of his article, pages 183-215 is excellent and interesting reading.)

[27] R.B. Borgens et al, "A Steady Efflux of Ionic Current Predicts Hind Limb Development in the Axolotl," *J. Exper. Zool.* 228 (1983): 491-503.

[28] See L. Hinkle et al, "The Direction of Growth of Differentiating Neurones and Myoblasts from Frog Embryos in an Applied Electric Field," *J. Physiol.* 314 (1981): 121-135. See also, L.F. Jaffe, "Developmental Currents, Voltages and Gradients," in A.R. Liss, *Developmental Order: It's Origin and Regulation* 183-215; S.B. Oppenheimer and G. Lefevre Jr., *Introduction to Embryonic Development* p.247-248.

[29] R.F. Stump and K.R. Robinson, "Xenopus Neural Crest Migration in an Applied Electrical Field," *J. Cell Biol.* 97 (1983): 1226-1233.

[30] See for instance, Harold Saxton Burr, "An Electrodynamic Theory of Development Suggested by the Studies of the Proliferation Rates in the Brain of Ambylstoma," *J. Compar. Neurol.* 56 (1932): 347-371; H.S. Burr and F.S.C. Northrop, "An Electrodynamic Theory of Life," *Quarterly Rev. Biol.* 10, no.3 (Sept. 1935): 322-333; H.S. Burr, *Blueprint for Immortality*; H.S. Burr, *The Nature of Man and the Meaning of Existence*; Lionel Jaffe, "Developmental Currents, Voltages and Gradients" pp.211-215 (very thorough and useful bibliography); E.J. Lund, "Effects of the Electric Current on Regenerating Internodes of Obelia Commissuralis," *Jour. Exp. Zool.* 34 (1921): 471-493; E.J. Lund, "The Normal Electrical Polarity of Obelia; A Proof of its Existence," *Jour. Exp. Zool.* 36 (1922): 477-494; and E.J. Lund, "The Nature of the Control of Organic Polarity by the Electric Current," *Jour. Exp. Zool.* 41 (1925): 155-190.

[31] For instance, **Direct electrical current:** see E.J. Lund's work from the 1920's and 1930's. **Unilateral light; the presence of neighboring eggs; pH gradients; temperature gradients:** see N.J. Berrill, *Developmental Biology* p.242. **The presence of calcium ions:** see for instance, W.R. Jeffery, "Calcium Ionophore Polarizes Ooplasmic Segregation in Ascidian Eggs," *Science* 216 (1982): 545-547. **Gravity:** see for instance, J.C. Gerhart et al., "Control of Polarity in the Amphibian Egg," in A.R. Liss, *Time, Space and Pattern in Embryonic Development* pp.261-286. **Sperm entry point:** see for instance, M. Kirschner et al., "Initiation of the Cell Cycle and Establishment of Bilateral Symmetry in Xenopus Eggs," *Sym. Soc. Dev. Biol.* 38 (1980):187-216; and J.C. Gerhart et al., "A Reinvestigation of the Role of the Gray Crescent in Axis Formation in Xenopus Laevis," *Nature* 292 (1981): 511-516.

[32] N.J. Berrill, *Developmental Biology* p.242.

[33] Ibid. p.239 and following.

[34] Yoshio Manaka, "Shinkyu kenkyu ni oyoshita jiki kotoni sono keiketsu sessyoku koka ni tsuite," pamphlet handed out at his lectures.

[35] Yoshio Manaka, *Shinkyu no Riron to Kangaikata* p.68 passim.

[36] See Matsumoto and Birch, *Extraordinary Vessels* chapter 2, for the pathways of the extraordinary vessels.

[37] L. Hinkle et al., "The Direction of Growth of Differentiating Neurones and Myoblasts from Frog Embryos in an Applied Electric Field," *J. Physiol.* 314 (1981): 121-135.

[38] For a good review article on these gradients and fields, see R. Nuccitelli, "The Involvement of Transcellular Ion Currents and Electric Fields," in G. Malacinski and S.V. Bryant, eds., *Pattern Formation, a Primer* p.23-46.

[39] See volume 2 of the commentary by Wang Shu He on *Nan Jing* 28:14; see Li Shi Zhen, *Qi Jing Ba Mai Kao* 1:2.

[40] Yoshio Manaka, *Shinkyu no Riron to Kangaekata* p.65.

[41] H.S. Burr, *The Fields of Life* p.29.

[42] Ibid. p.41.

[43] Ibid. p.65.

[44] Ibid. p.70.

[45] See for instance, "Current of life," *Science* (June 1959): 164-166.

[46] Ibid.

[47] A.S. Presman, *Electromagnetic Fields and Life* p.6-8 passim; p.235 passim; p.255 passim. See also, S. Krippner and D. Rubin, eds., *Kirlian Aura* p.86-91 passim.

[48] R.O. Becker "The Bioelectric Field Pattern in the Salamander and its Simulation by an Electronic Analog," *IRE Transactions on Medical Electronics* (July 1960): 202-207.

[49] R.O. Becker and A. A. Marino, *Electromagnetism and Life* p.198-199. See also, R.O. Becker "The Basic Biological Transmission and Control System Influenced by Electrical Forces," *Ann N.Y. Acad. Sci.* 238 (1974): 236-241.

[50] S. Hoppenfeld, *Physical Examination of the Spine and Extremities* p.135-136.

[51] Keizo Hashimoto and Y. Kawakami, *Sotai - Balance and Health Through Natural Movement.*

[52] Private notes and discussions of Dr. Manaka.

[53] Ibid.

[54] S. Oppenheimer, and G. Lefevre Jr., *Introduction to Embryonic development* p.113 and following.

[55] J.L. Oschman, *Natural Science of Healing*, op.cit.

[56] H.S. Burr, *Fields of Life.*

[57] D.R. DiBona and M.M. Civan, "Osmotically Induced Conductance Changes in Toad Bladder Under Physiologic Conditions," *Int. Union Pure and Applied Biophysics*, IVth congress, 1972. See also, D.R. DiBona et al., "The Anatomic Site of the Transepithelial Permeability Barriers of Toad Bladder," *J. Cell. Biol.* 40 (1969): 1-7; ———, "The Cellular Specificity of the Effect of Vasopressin on Toad Urinary Bladder," *J. Membrane Biol.* 1 (1969): 79-81.

58 Williams and Warwick, *Gray's Anatomy* pp.1332-1333.

59 Ibid.

60 S.J. Williamson and L. Kaufman, "Biomagnetism," *J. Mag. & Mag. Mater.* 22 (1981): 129-201.

61 Hiroshi Motoyama and R. Brown, *Science and the Evolution of Consciousness* pp.86-88.

62 A.P. Dubrov, *The Geomagnetic Field and Life: Geomagnetobiology* p.138. See also, F.A. Brown and Y.H. Park, "Phase Shifting a Lunar Rhythm in Planarians by Altering the Horizontal Magnetic Vector," *Biol. Bull.* 129, no.1 (1965):79.

63 D.Bensky and J. O'Connor, *Acupuncture a Comprehensive Text* p.8.

64 Wlodzimierz Sedlak, *Bioelektronika 1967-1977.*

65 Ibid. p.83.

66 Ibid.

67 Ibid.

68 See the work of Sedlak who discusses the properties of the body's tissues, including the connective tissues, as capable of producing and emitting laser energy.

69 For good discussions and descriptions of the cleavage lines, see: H. T. Cox, "The Cleavage Lines of the Skin," *Brit.Jour.Surgery* 29:234-240.

70 Ibid.

71 For good articles on this, see: J. H. Gardner and H. E. Raybuck, "Development of Cleavage Line Patterns in the Human Fetus," *Anat.Rec* 118 (1954): 745-754; and C. Hutchinson and C. Everett Koop, "Lines of Cleavage in the Skin of the Newborn Infant," *Anat Rec* 126 (1956): 299-310.

72 Taken from J. H. Gardner and H. E. Raybuck, "Development of Cleavage Line Patterns in the Human Fetus."

73 Ibid.

74 Ibid.

75 Ibid.

76 For good descriptions of this development, see: J. Langman, *Medical Embryology* pp.317-319; W.C. Trier, "Complete Breast Absence," *Plast. and Reconstr. Surg.* 36, no. 4 (1965): 430-439; S. Kon S and A. Cowie, *Milk: the Mammary Gland and its Secretion* 1:3; and K.L. Moore, *The Developing Human* pp.436-438.

77 For good descriptions and examples of this, see: K.L. Moore, *The Developing Human* p.438; L.L. Arey, *Developmental Anatomy* p.452; and Greenhill, *Obstetrics* pp.179-182.

78 A. Presman, *Electromagnetic Fields and Life* p.7 passim.

79 Ibid. p.50.

80 A. P. Dubrov, *The Geomagnetic Field and Life: Geomagnetobiology.*

81 Ibid. p.102 passim; p.116 passim; p.238 passim.

82 R.O. Becker, "The Basic Biological Transmission and Control System Influenced by External Forces," *Ann.N.Y.Acad.Sci.* 238 (1974): 236-241.

83 R.O. Becker, "Electromagnetic Controls Over Biological Growth Processes," *Jour. Bioelect* 3, nos. 1 & 2 (1984): pp.105-118.

[84] Ibid.

[85] Ibid.

[86] Ibid. See also, F.A. Brown, "Biological Clocks, Endogenous Cycles Synchronized by Subtle Geophysical Rhythms," *Biosystems* 8 (1976): 67-81.

[87] See, for example, the treatment systems outlined in **Extraordinary Vessels,** or the Manaka treatments detailed later in this text.

[88] Keiji Yamada, *Konton no Umi E* p.309 passim.

Notes to Chapter 9

[1] Symposia Procedings, National Symposia of Acupuncture and Moxibustion and Acupuncture Anaesthesia, 1-5 June, 1979, p.260 and following. See also, Li Ding Zhong, *Jing Luo Phenomena* 2.

[2] Yoshio Manaka, from private notes and lectures.

[3] Li Ding Zhong, *Jing Luo Phenomena* 1.

[4] See for instance, M. Reichmanis et al, "Electrical Correlates of Acupuncture points," *IEEE, Trans. on Biomed. Eng.* (November 1975): 533-535; M. Reichmanis et al., "Laplace Analysis of Transient Impedance Between Acupuncture Points LI-4 and LI-12," *Bio. Med. Eng.* 24, no.4 (July 1977): 402-405; M. Reichmanis and R.O. Becker, "Physiological Effects of Stimulation at Acupuncture Locii: A Review," *Comp. Med East West* 6 (1978): 67-73; J. Hyvarinen and M. Karlsson, "Low Resistance Skin Points That May Coincide with Acupuncture Locii,;; *Med. Biol.* 55, no.2 (1977): 88-94; M. Reichmanis et al., "DC Skin Conductance Variation at Acupuncture Locii," *Amer. Jour. Chin. Med.* 4, no.1)1976): 69-72; R.O. Becker et al., 'Electrophysiological Correlates of Acupuncture Points and Meridians; *Psychoenergetic Systems* 1 (1976): 105; M. Reichmanis et al, "Laplace Plane Analysis of Impedance Between Acupuncture Points HT-3 and HT-4," *Comp. Med East West* 5 (1977): 289; M. Reichmanis et al, "Laplace Plane Analysis of Impedance on the Heart Meridian," *Amer. Jour. Chin. Med.* 7 (1979): 188.

Also, Tiller describes some Russian research mapping the electrical network of acupoints and meridians. See W.A. Tiller, "Some Physical Network Characteristics of Acupuncture Points and Meridians," Proceding of the Academy of Parapsychology and Medicine, Symposium on Acupuncture, June 1972, at Stanford University.

In Europe the electrical nature of the meridians was also researched and numerous electrical devices were created for diagnostic and therapeutic purposes, based on these electrophysiological findings. For a brief synopsis of this, see: Johannes Bischko, *An Introduction to Acupuncture* p.21 and following. For a good summary of the literature, see: Zhu Zong Xiang, "Research Advances in the Electrical Specificity of Meridians and Acupuncture Points," *Amer. Jour. Acup.* 9, no.3 (1981): pp.203-216.

[5] Becker succinctly describes this phenomenon. See R.O. Becker and G. Selden, *The Body Electric* p.99. Tiller likewise describes changes in response to sleep, mental and emotional states. See W.A. Tiller, "Some Physical Network Characteristics of Acupuncture Points and Meridians," procedings of the Academy of Parapsychology and Medicine, Symposium on Acupuncture, June 1972, at Stanford University.

[6] Zhu Zong Xiang, "Research Advances in the Electrical Specificity of Meridians and Acupuncture Points," *Amer. Jour. Acup.* 9, No.3 (1981): 203-216.

[7] See R.O. Becker and A.A. Marino, *Electromagnetism and Life;* R.O. Becker and G. Selden, *The Body Electric;* R.O. Becker, "The Basic Biological Data Transmission and Control System Influenced by electrical Forces, *Ann. N.Y. Acad. Sci.* 238 (1974): 236. See also James Oschman, "The Connective Tissue and Myofascial Systems," paper presented at the Rolfing Conference, 1981.

□

[8] R.O. Becker and A.A. Marino, *Electromagnetism and Life* pp.198-199.

[9] This is not so dissimilar to Presman's ideas about the properties of the electromagnetic field itself, where it is seen to have various information communication functions. See: A.S. Presman; *Electromagnetic Fields and Life.* See also, S. Krippner and D. Rubin, eds., *The Kirlian Aura* pp.86-91 passim.

[10] R.O. Becker, "The Basic Biological Data transmission and Control System Influenced by Electric Forces, *Ann. N.Y. Acad. Sci.,* 238 (1974): 236.

[11] R.O. Becker and G. Selden, *The Body Electric.*

[12] See for instance: Zhu Zong Xiang, "Research Advances in the Electrical specificity of Meridians and Acupuncture Points," *Amer. Jour. Acup.* 9, no.3 (1981); and R.M. Shenberger, "Acupuncture Meridians Retain Identity After Death; *Amer. Jour. Acup.* 5, no.4 (1977).

[13] Yoshio Nagahama, *Shinkyu no Igaku* p.174 passim.

[14] Ibid. p.142 passim.

[15] Ibid. p.167 passim.

[16] Ibid.

[17] Ibid.

[18] See: Hiroshi Motoyama, "Electrophysiological and Preliminary Biochemical Studies of Skin Properties in Relation to the Acupuncture Meridian," *Research for Religion and Parapsychology* 6, no. 2 (1980). See especially: Hiroshi Motoyama, "A Biophysical Elucidation of the Meridian and Ki Energy: What is Ki Energy and How Does it Flow? *Research for Religion and Parapsychology* 7, no.1 (August 1981).

[19] Ibid. p.15 and following.

[20] Hiroshi Motoyama, "Biophysical Elicidation" p.30 and following.

[21] Yoshio Nagahama, *Shinkyu no Igaku* pp.171-174 passim.

[22] Ibid.

[23] B. Nordenstrom, *Biologically Closed Electric Circuits: Clinical, Experimental and Theoretical Evidence for an Additional Circulatory System* (Published privately by the author). See also: G. Taubes, "An Electrifying Possibility," *Discover* (April 1986): 22-37.

[24] Kazuko Itaya et.al., "Effects of Acupuncture Needle Application Upon the Cutaneous Microcirculation of Rabbit Ear Lobe" (Paper presented at the Symposium on Traditional Oriental Medicine, the Science and Technology Agency, Tokyo, October 1985).
Using rabbits as specimens Drs. Itaya et.al. demonstrated clear effects following the application of one needle for thirty minutes to a point on the back of the animals. These effects were seen to occur strongly for three hours and to a lesser degree for several hours after the insertion, suggesting that the effects are hormonal as well as neural. In some cases, the effects lasted for longer periods. They observed the vascular bed through windows on the rabbits' ears using a technique developed by Dr. Asano, "microphotoelectric plethysmography." Videotapes were made for several hours before and after the application of the needle. The needles used were silver number 32 Chinese needles, inserted shallowly around Thoracic 6-7.

The vascular bed, the arterioles, venules, and capillaries underwent rhythmic contractions and dilations. Over the first two hours after needle application this rhythm increased in amplitude. The frequency of these contractions and dilations was around three to four a minute. These visible changes clearly demonstrate a very large increase in microcirculation. Although only the ears were observed, this phenomenon occurs throughout the body. Test groups were also observed showing that this phenomenon is not a pain response, nor is it related to the heartbeat, which is considerably more rapid than three to four beats per minute.

□

[25] R.O. Becker and D.G. Murray, "The Electrical Control System Regulating Fracture Healing in Amphibians," *Clin. Orthop. Res.* 73 (1970): 169. See also: R.O. Becker and D.G. Murray, "A Method for Producing Cellular Dedifferentiation by Means of Very Small Electrical Currents," *Trans. N.Y. Acad. Sci.* 29 (1967): 606-615; and R.O. Becker and A.A. Marino, *Electromagnetism and Life* pp.49-51.

[26] D.G. Harrington and R.O. Becker, "Electrical Stimulation of R.N.A. and Protein Synthesis in the Frog Erythrocyte," *Exp. Cell Res.* 76 (1973): 95. See also: A.A. Pilla, "Electrochemical Information Transfer at Living Cell Membranes," *Ann. N.Y. Acad. Sci.* 238 (1974): 149.

[27] R.O. Becker and A.A. Pilla, "Electrochemical Mechanisms and the Control of Biological Growth Processes," in J. Bockris and B.E. Conway, *Modern Aspects of Electrochemistry* vol. 10 (New York: Plenum Press, 1975).

[28] R.O. Becker and A.A. Marino, *Electromagnetism and Life* p.51.

[29] A.A. Pilla, "Electrochemical Information Transfer" p.149.

[30] Ibid.

[31] R.O. Becker and G. Selden, *The Body Electric* pp.176-177.

[32] See for instance: W.R. Adey and S.W. Bawin, Brain Interactions with Weak Electric and Magnetic Fields; *Neurosci. Re. Prog. Bull.* 15 (1977): 1-141; W.R. Adey, "Tissue Interactions with Non-ionizing Electromagnetic Fields," *Physiol Rev.* 61, no.2 (1981): 435-514.

[33] L.F. Jaffe, "Developmental Currents Voltages and Gradients," *Developmental Order, It's Origin and Regulation* pp.183-215.

[34] S. McLaughlin and M.M. Poo, "The Role of Electroosmosis in the Electric Field Induced Movement of Charged Macromolecules on the Surface of Cells," *Biophys. Jour.* 34 (1981): 85-93.

[35] A.A. Pilla, "Electrochemical Information Transfer" p.149.

[36] See: James Oschman, "The Structure and Properties of Ground Substance," *Amer. Zool.* 24 (1984): 199-215.

[37] P. Dustin, "Microtubules," *Sci. Amer.* (August 1980): p. 59-68. See also, B. Albert et.al., *Molecular Biology of the Cell* (New York: Garland Publishing, 1983) pp.574 and following.

[38] B. Albert et.al., *Molecular Biology of the Cell* pp.558 and following.

[39] K.R. Porter and J.B. Tucker, "The Ground Substance of the Living Cell," *Sci. Amer.* (March 1981): 57-67.

[40] J. Folkman and A. Moscona, "Roles of Cell Shape in Growth Control," *Nature* 273 (1978): 345-349.

[41] R.O. Becker and G. Selden, *The Body Electric* pp.185-186.

[42] R. Nuccitelli, "The Involvement of Transcellular Ion Currents and Ionic Fields in Pattern Formation," G. Malacinski and S.V. Bryant, eds., *Pattern Formation, a Primer in Developmental Biology* (New York: MacMillan, 1984) pp.23-46. See also: M.M. Poo and K.R. Robinson, "Electrophoresis of Concanavalin-A Receptors along Embryonic Muscle Cell Membrane," *Nature* 265 (1977): pp.602-605.

[43] A.P. Dubrov, *The Geomagnetic Field and Life: Geomagnetobiology* p.236.

[44] Ibid. p.153.

[45] R.O. Becker, "Electromagnetic Controls Over Biological Growth Processes," *Jour. Bioelect.* 3, nos.1&2 (1984): 105-118.

[46] A.T. Barker, L.F. Jaffe, J.W. Vanable, "The Glabrous Epidermis of the Cavies Contains a Powerful Battery," *Amer. Jour. Physiol.* (1981): R358-R366.

⁴⁷ See J. Oschman, "The Connective Tissue and Myofascial Systems;" P.R.C. Gascoyne, R. Pethig, and A. Szent-Gyorgyi, "Water Structure Dependent Charge Transport in Proteins," *Proc. Natl. Acad. Sci.* 78 (1981): 261-265; and R.O. Becker and A.A. Marino, *Electromagnetism and Life* pp.21, 25-26.

⁴⁸ A.R. Liboff and M. Furst, "Pyroelectric Effect in Collagenous Structures," *Ann. N.Y. Acad Sci.* 238 (1974): pp.26-35.

⁴⁹ See: E. Fukada and I. Yasuda, "On the Piezoelectric Effect of Bone," *Journal Phys. Soc. Japan* 12 (1957): 149-154; C.A.L. Bassett and R.O. Becker, "Generation of Electric Potentials by Bone in Response to Mechanical Stress," *Science* 137 (1962): 1063-1064; M. Braden et.al., "Electrical and Piezoelectrical Properties of Dental Hard Tissues," *Nature* 212 (1966): 1565-1566; E. Fukada, "Piezoelectric Properties of Organic Polymer," *Ann. N.Y. Academy of Sciences* 238 (1974): 7-25; E. Fukada and K. Hara, "Piezoelectric Effect in Blood Vessel Walls," *J. Phys. Soc. Japan* 26 (1969): 777-780; E. Fukada and H. Ueda, "Piezoelectric Effect in Blood Vessel Walls," *J. Appl. Phys.* 9 (1970): 844; C.A.L. Bassett, "Biologic Significance of Piezoelectricity," *Calc. Tissue Res.* 1 (1968): 252-272; A.A. Marino et.al, "Piezoelectricity in Collagen Films," *Calcif. Tissue. Int.* 31 (1980): 257-259. See also, J.L. Oschman, "The Connective Tissue and Myofascial Systems;" and R.O. Becker and A.A. Marino, *Electromagnetism and Life* pp.81-84.

⁵⁰ D.E.S. Brown, "The Effect of Rapid Changes in Hydrostatic Pressure Upon the Contraction of Skeletal Muscle, *J. Cell Comp. Physiol.* 4 (1934): 257-281. See also, D.A. Marsland and D.E.S. Brown, "The Effects of Pressure on Sol-Gel Equilibria, with Special Reference to Myosus and Other Protoplasmic Gels, *J. Cell Comp. Physiol. 20 (1942): 295-305; T. Tanaka, "Gels," Scientific American* 244, no.1 (1981): 124-138; N.P. Reddy and G. Van B. Cochran, "Phenomenological Theory Underlying Pressure-Time Relationship in Decubitus Ulcer Formation, Abstract no. 4885, *Fed. Proc.* 38, no.3 (1979): 1153. For a diagrammatic schemata of this see J. Oschman, "The Connective Tissue and Myofascial Systems," fig.10.

⁵¹ See for instance, *Su Wen* 27, *Ling Shu* 1, and *Nan Jing* 76 passim.

⁵² N. Edagawa, *Doctor Nao's Chiryo Jiten* p.30-32 passim.

⁵³ Ibid. p.53.

⁵⁴ He does have a book in English available. N. Edagawa and Lawrence Freidman, *The Treatment of Disordered Function, from Pain to Sexual Complaints - An Introduction to the Edagawa Method* (Pompano Beach, Florida: Exposition Press, 19--).

⁵⁵ See for instance, G.E. Fogg, *The Growth of Plants* pp.229-233.

⁵⁶ See for instance, G.G. Luce, *Biological Rhythms in Human and Animal Physiology* p.121 and following.

⁵⁷ Ibid. p.122.

⁵⁸ Ibid. p.128 and following.

⁵⁹ See for instance: G.E. Fogg, *The Growth of Plants* pp.233-237.

⁶⁰ A.P. Dubrov, *The Geomagnetic Field and Life: Geomagnetobiology* p.138.

⁶¹ Ibid. p.145.

⁶² Ibid. pp.137-138 passim.

⁶³ Ibid. pp.116 and following.

⁶⁴ Ibid. pp.138.

⁶⁵ F.A. Brown and Y.H. Park, "Phase Shifting a Lunar Rhythm in Planarians by Altering the Horizontal Magnetic Vector," *Biol. Bull.* 129, no.1 (1965): 79.

⁶⁶ A.P. Dubrov, *The Geomagnetic Field and Life* p.139.

[67] Ibid. p.12 passim.

[68] Ibid. p.21.

[69] See for instance, G.G. Luce, *Biological Rhythms in Human and Animal Physiology* p.14 passim. See also, A.P. Dubrov, *The Geomagnetic Field and Life* pp.18-25, 27-28.

[70] A.P. Dubrov, *The Geomagnetic Field and Life* p.142.

[71] Ibid.

[72] See for instance, J.C. Gerhart et.al, "Control of Polarity in the Amphibian Egg," in *Time, Space and Pattern in Embryonic Development* (New York: A.R. Liss, 1983) pp.261-286.

[73] A.P. Dubrov, *The Geomagnetic Field and Life* pp.137-138.

[74] M.A. Persinger, "Prenatal Exposure to an ELF Rotating Magnetic Field, Ambulatory Behavior and Lunar Distance at Birth, a Correlation," *Psych. Rep.* 28 (1971): 435-438.

[75] R.O. Becker, "Electromagnetic Controls Over Biological Growth Processes," *Jour. Bioelect.* 3, nos.1&2 (1984): pp.105-118.

[76] See for instance: R.O. Becker, "The Basic Biological Transmission and Control System Influenced by Electrical Forces," *Ann. N.Y. Acad. Sci.* 238 (1974): pp. 236-241.

[77] R.O. Becker and G. Selden, *The Body Electric* p.236.

[78] H. Friedman et.al., "Geomagnetic Parameters and Psychiatric Hospital Admissions," *Nature* 200 (1963): 626-628; H. Friedman et.al., "Psychiatric Ward Behavior and Geophysical Parameters," *Nature* 205 (1965): 1050-1052. See also A.P. Dubrov, *The Geomagnetic Field and Life* pp.184-185.

[79] See for instance, K. Nakagawa, "Magnetic Field Deficiency Syndrome and Magnetic Treatment," *Japan Medical Jour* no.2745 (Decemmber 1976)

[80] See P.R.C. Gascoyne, R. Pethig, and A. Szent Gyorgyi, "Water Structure-Dependent Charge Transport in Proteins," *Proc. Natl. Acad. Sci.* 78 (1981): 261-265.

[81] See A.A. Guyton, *Texbbook of Medical Physiology* (Philadelphia: W. B. Saunders Co, 1976) p.963.

[82] Ibid.

[83] Ibid. p. 957.

[84] Kirlian photography allows us to view these ionized particles. See for instance: S. Krippner and D. Rubin, eds., *The Kirlian Aura, Photographing the Galaxies of Life* (New York: Anchor Books, 1974) pp.51-72, 75-79.

[85] See: I.F. Dumitrescu, *Electrographic Imaging In Medicine and Biology* (London: Neville Spearman, 1983). Also for a brief discussion, as well as an interesting review of the biological effects of electromagnetic fields, see also, J.N. Kenyon, *Modern Techniques of Acupuncture* 2 (Wellingborough, England: Thorsons Publishers, 1983) pp. 145-152.

[86] A.A. Guyton, *Textbook of Medical Physiology* pp.957-958.

[87] Ibid. p.966.

[88] W. Sedlak, *Bioelektronika* 1967-1977, p.84 (with English summaries).

[89] Ibid.

[90] See Maresch, *Deutsche Zeitschrift fur Akupunktur* 2 (1966): p.33.

[91] J. Bischko, *An Introduction to Acupuncture* p.23.

[92] Many references may be found in the literature. The following have brief discussions of the effects of electrical and magnetic fields on the EEG readings:

☐

R.O. Becker and A.A. Marino, *Electromagnetism and Life;* W.R. Adey and S.W. Bawin, "Brain Interactions with Weak Electric and Magnetic Fields," *Neurosci. Res. Prog. Bull.* 15, no.1 (1977) :1-141.

[93] Much research has been done recently with magnetic fields. This has progressed considerably with the development of the SQUID, the "Superconducting Quantum Interference Device." For good, relatively recent reviews of the literature see,

M. Reite and J. Zimmerman, "Magnetic Phenomena of the Central Nervous System," *Ann. Rev. Biophys. Bioeng.* 7 (1978): 167-188; and S.J. Williamson and L. Kaufman, "Biomagnetism," *Jour. Ma. Mag. Mater.* 22 (1981): pp.129-201.

For specific articles on the auditory responses, see: M. Reite et.al., "Magnetic Auditory Evoked Fields: Interhemispheric Asymmetry," *Electroenceph. Clin. Neurophys.* 51 (1981): 388-392; J.T. Zimmerman et.al., "Magnetic Auditory Evoked Fields: Dipole Orientation," *Electroenceph. Clin. Neurophys.* 52 (1981): 151-156; M. Reite et.al., "MEG and EEG Auditory Responses to Tone, Click and White Noise Stimuli," *Electroenceph. Clin. Neurophys.* 53 (1982): 643-651; M. Reite et.al., "Auditory Evoked Magnetic Fields: Response Amplitude Versus Stimulus Intensity," *Electroenceph. Clin. Neurophys.* 54 (1982): 147-152; and J.T. Zimmerman et.al., "Auditory Evoked Magnetic Fields: A Replication with Comments on the P50 Analog," *Il Nuovo Cimento* 2D, no.2 (1983): 460-470.

For specific articles on the visual responses, see: M. Reite et.al., "The Human Magnetoencephalogram: Some EEG and Related Correlations," *Electroenceph. Clin. Neurophys.* 40 (1976): 59-66.

[94] A.A. Marino et.al., "Sensitivity to Change in Electrical Environment, a New bioelectric Effect," *Am. J. Physiol* 239 (1980): R424-427.

[95] See for instance, W.R. Adey and S.W. Bawin, "Brain Interactions with Weak Electric and Magnetic Fields," *Neurosci. Re. Prog. Bull.* 15, no.1 (1977): 1-141; W.R. Adey, "Tissue Interactions with Non-ionizing Electromagnetic Fields," *Physiol. Rev.* 61, no.2 (1981): 435-514. See also, S.W. Bawin and W.R. Adey, "Sensitivity to Calcium Binding in Cerebral Tissue to Weak Environmental Electric Fields Oscillating at Low Frequency," *Proc. Natl. Acad. Sci. USA* 73, no.6 (1976): 1999-2003; S.W. Bawin et.al, "Ionic Factors in Release of 45Ca2+ from Chicken Cerebral Tissue by Electromagnetic Fields," *Proc. Natl. Acad. Sci. USA* 75, no.12 (1978): 6314-6318; and W.R. Adey, "Evidence for Cooperative Mechanisms in the Susceptibility of Cerebral Tissue to Environmental and Intrinsic Electric Fields," in F.O. Schmitt et.al, eds., *Functional Linkage in Biomolecular Systems* (New York: Raven Press, 1975) pp.325-342.

[96] See H. Frohlich, "Bose Condensation of Strongly Excited Longitudinal Electric Modes," *Phys. Lett.* 26A (1968): 402-403; and H. Frohlich, "Evidence for Bose Condensation-Like Excitation of Coherent Modes in Biological Systems," *Phys. Lett.* 51A (1975): 21-22. See also, H.A. Pohl, *Microdielectrophoresis of Dividing Cells*, Research Note 90, Oklahoma State University Department of Physics, June 1979.

[97] See for instance, *Su Wen 4; Su Wen 74; Ling Shu 4; Nan Jing 34; Nan Jing 49; Nan Jing 61.*

[98] From private notes and discussions.

[99] See for instance, *Su Wen 3; Su Wen 10; Su Wen 22; Ling Shu 1; Ling Shu 56; Ling Shu 63.*

[100] See chapter 3 above and also *Su Wen 5; Ling Shu 1; Nan Jing 49.*

[101] S.W. Bawin et.al, "Ionic Factors in Release of 45Ca2+ from Chicken Cerebral Tissues by Electromagnetic Fields" pp.6314-6318.

[102] A.P. Dubrov, *The Geomagnetic Field and Life* pp.116-138.

[103] From private notes of and discussions with Dr. Manaka.

[104] This will be discussed in detail in Manaka's forthcoming book, *Chasing the Dragon's Tail* (Brookline: Paradigm Publications, 1988).

[105] K. Matsumoto and S. Birch, *Extraordinary Vessels* pp.13-15.

[106] Kentaro Takagi, *Seitai no Chosetsukino (The Control Systems of the Biological Organism)* (Tokyo: Chuokoron Pub. Co., 1972).

[107] From lectures and private notes of and discussions with Dr. Manaka.

[108] Williams and Warwick, *Gray's Anatomy* p.798.

[109] M. Birdsong and J.E. Edmunds, "Harlequin Color Change of the Newborn: Report of a Case," *Ob. Gyn.* 7 (1956): 518-521. See also, O. Mortensen and P. Stougard-Andresen, "Harlequin Colour Change in the Newborn," *Acta. Obst. et Gynec. Scandinav.* 36 (1959): 352-359; G.A. Neligan and L.B. Strang, "Harlequin colour change in the newborn," *Lancet* 38 (22 November, 1952): 1005-1007.

[110] R. Hayden and M. Grossman, "Rectal, Ocular and Submaxillary Pain," *Amer. Jour. Diseas. Childhood* 97 (1959): 479-482. See also, R.E. Dugan, "Familial Rectal Pain," *Lancet* (15 April 1972): 854; T.P. Mann, J.E. Cree, "Familial Rectal Pain," *Lancet* (6 May 1972): 1016-1017.

[111] The theory presented here is derived from lecture notes and private discussions with Dr. Manaka.

[112] The terms "explicate" and "implicate" are borrowed from David Bohm. See D. Bohm, *Wholeness and the Implicate Order* (London: Ark Paperbacks, 1980).

[113] R. Sheldrake, *A New Science of Life: The Hypothesis of Formative Causation* (Los Angeles: J.P. Tarcher, 1981).

[114] Good examples can be found in R.G. Brewer and E.L. Hahn, "Atomic Memory," *Sci. Amer.* 251, no.6 (1984): 50-57. See also, D. Bohm, *Wholeness and the Implicate Order* pp.149-150, pp.179-185.

[115] This phrase, "to stand out in relief" is borrowed from D. Bohm, *Wholeness and the Implicate Order* p.152.

[116] See D. Bohm; *Wholeness and the Implicate Order.*

[117] An interesting example of this can be found in S.R. Hameroff, "Ch'i: a Neural Hologram, Microtubules, Bioholography and Acupuncture," *Amer. Jour. Chin. Med.* 2, no.2 (1974): 163-170.

[118] Based on the work of E. Schoffeniels, *Anti-Chance* (New York: Pergamon Press, 1976).

[119] C.C. Conley, in M.F. Barnothy, ed., *Biological Effects of Magnetic Fields* 2 (1969) p.46.

[120] From private correspondence with Dr. Manaka. These ideas are discussed extensively in his book, *Chasing the Dragon's Tail.*

[121] D.C. Lau, trans., *Lao Tzu: Tao Te Ching* (London: Penguin Books, 1963) p.57.

Notes to Chapter 10

[1] From private discussions and notes of Dr. Manaka.

[2] Ibid.

[3] Liu Wan Su, *Su Wen Xuan Ji Yuan Bing Shi* p.109 passim.

[4] Zhang Zhong Jing, *Shang Han Lun.* See *Shang Han Lun Yi Shi* p.127 passim. This passage expresses an understanding of the five phases, which we feel the author was trying to show in contradistinction to his six stages.

[5] See Yoshio Nagahama's commentary on the *Shang Han Lun*, Toyo Igaku Gaisetsu p.65.

[6] *Yixue Rumen,* from by Shohaku Honma, *Shinkyu Byoshu Gaku* p.77 passim.

[7] Ibid.

[8] Ibid.

[9] Todo Yoshimasu, from Sorei Yanagiya, *Kanmei Humon Shinsatsu Ho* p.288.

[10] T. Chikugo, Fukushi Dangi. *Ido No Nippon Magazine* August 1949.

[11] Taken from Sorei Yanagiya, *Kanmei Humon Shinsatsu Ho.*

[12] Mubunryu, from Matsumoto, "Shindo Hiketsushu," *Ido No Nippon Magazine* August 1969, passim.

Notes to Chapter 11

[1] This is a common understanding that comes from passages that can for instance be found in the *Jin Gui Yao Lue Fang Lun.* See *Zhong Yi Zhen Duan Xue* p.129 passim.

[2] T. Ishi, in *Ido No Nippon Magazine* (May, 1969).

[3] *Jinsei to Dairokukan ni Tsuite,* from T. Nagatomo, *Nagatomo M.P. Shinkyu Kuowa Hachiju Hachisyu* p.45 passim.

[4] Sosen Hirooka, *Nangyo Tekkan* 1:28.

Notes to Chapter 12

[1] This information is largely derived from a series of articles in the *Ido No Nippon magazine* that began in October, 1975. Kuzome's own teaching manuals and oral teaching have been included as well.

[2] Editors Note: see Tin Yau So's parallel explanation regarding rib shapes in *The Book of Acupuncture Points.*

[3] The "root" nature of the abdominal findings is clearly described in *Nan Jing* 56 where the abdominal signs become the cause of other symptoms. See chapter 15.

[4] Editors note: This case illustrates one of the real problems of Oriental medicine and cancer treatments. The diagnosis of cancer is a tissue diagnosis, the presence of malignant tissue through biopsy. However, not all cancers are biopsied, and if the lump disappears, there is generally no further tissue testing. This, coupled with misdiagnosis, the availability of spontaneous remission as a facile explanation, and "patient diagnoses" of "cancer," has lead many Oriental healers, like Kuzome, to disclaim cancer cures. For example, the Nagakura Research Clinic in Osaka has ample records of cancer treatment patients who have survived beyond statistical expectations; yet they claim no cures. The same was true of the great Japanese herbalist Otsuka.

[5] According to *Nan Jing* chapter 36, the right kidney is the place where jing and shen stay. After removal of the right kidney, she developed these problems below the sternum, which are often signs of weakened jing and shen.

[6] Perhaps this relates to weak ming men fire.

[7] Kuzome interprets references in the *Shang Han Lun* to mean that when one touches below the rib cage, the muscles are tense. When one presses, it is uncomfortable, tight, or causes a reaction to rise into the chest or elsewhere.

[8] In both cases, we find confirmation of the *Nan Jing* five-phase abdominal palpation theory described in Difficulties 16 and 56. The theory suggests that liver and gallbladder problems reflect to the left side of the umbilicus.

[9] Root qi is related not only to the source or basic qi, it is related to emotional problems like lack of will or determination.

□

[10] In China studies have shown that GB-41 becomes reactive in the presence of gallstones.

[11] In Yoshio Manaka's system, reaction at GB-29 located at the ASIS, may also be indicative of the gallbladder.

Notes to Chapter 13

[1] Shinsai Ota, quoted from Sorei Yanagiya, *Zukai Anma Jutsu* p.91 and following.

[2] Ibid. p.92.

[3] Ibid. pp.95-98.

[4] According to the 1578 text of the *Yi Xue Ru Men* (page 163) there are three pi gen points. One is three and a half divisions lateral to below L1, half a division lateral to BL-46. The second is just below the hua to point of ming men, GV-4. The third is on the stomach meridian, between ST-43 and ST-44 (where the web of the toes meet the flesh of the foot). It is very unlikely that Ota is referring to the point on the toes. Because of the difficulty of holding one's fingers seven divisions apart, it is likely that he is referring to the second pi gen point just below the hua to of ming men. This makes the most sense, since in Ota's view, ming men is a vital point.

[5] I. Fukaya, *Fukaya Kyo Ho* p.198.

[6] Sorei Yanagiya, *Zukai Anma Jutsu* pp.98-103 passim.

[7] Ibid. p.104-105.

[8] Ibid. p.107-108.

Notes to Chapter 14

[1] Sorei Yanagiya, *Kanmei Humon Shinsatsu Ho.*

[2] Sun Si-Mo, *Qian Jin Yao Fang* 27 p.479.

[3] Wang Shu He, commentary on the *Nan Jing* 8(1):12.

[4] A.C. Guyton, *Human Physiology and Mechanisms of Disease* p.191.

[5] The first exercise is derived from the work of Dr. Keizo Hashimoto; the remaining three from Haruchika Noguchi. See: Keizo Hashimoto and Y. Kawakami, *Sotai - Balance and Health Through Natural Movement;* and Haruchika Noguchi, *Noguchi Haruchika Seitai Nyumon.*

[6] We are indebted to our friend Peter Thompson of Mansfield Center, Connecticut, who studied personally with Dr. Hashimoto, and who taught us this exercise and permitted us to describe it in this work. For more information on this exercise system, see Keizo Hashimoto and Y. Kawakami, *Sotai - Balance and Health Through Natural Movement.*

Notes to Chapter 15

[1] The symptoms we have translated as swollen or puffy limbs could be equally interpreted as "lack of flexibility of the limbs." Of the eight commentaries we reviewed, five break the sentence in such a way as to see the latter interpretation; three in the former manner. Again, it is almost impossible to say if it is one or the other we need, instead to be aware of both possibilities.

[2] Honma comments that yawning draws air deep into the body and helps balance the yin. Shohaku Honma, *Nangyo no Kenkyu* p.83.

[3] This is different from the moving qi between the kidneys.

[4] In Wang Shu He's commentary on *Nan Jing* chapter 16, he says that this is diarrhea followed by a heavy feeling in the lower abdomen and a sinking feeling in the lower back.

[5] Chapter 28 of *Su Wen* says cold legs are a symptom of counterflow qi.

[6] Gao Wu, *Zhen Jiu Ju Ying* pp.152-153.

[7] Sosen Hirooka, *Nangyo Tekkan* 7 p.3.

[8] In commenting on this passage, Wang Shu He (56(3):27) says this means "rest and movement." Sosen Hirooka (7:6) says this means "rapid breath like panting."

[9] Wang Shu He (56(3):27) says this last symptom is inability to breathe. Sosen Hirooka (7:6) sees it as "swollen lungs with stagnation from fever."

[10] Sosen Hirooka, *Nangyo Tekkan* 7 p.6.

[11] Kodo Fukushima, *Keiraku Chiryo Yoko* pp.288-289 passim.

[12] Denmei Shudo, *Keiraku Chiryo No Susume* p.86 passim.

[13] Ibid. p.90.

[14] Ibid. p.127-134.

[15] Kodo Fukushima, *Keiraku Chiryo Yoko* p.91.

[16] Lectures in Japan attended by the author.

[17] Denmei Shudo, *Keiraku Chiryo no Susume* p.93. This technique is probably a development of the skin stroking techniques described in *Nan Jing* 13, used to confirm pulse quality observations. See *Five Elements and Ten Stems* p.45.

[18] For more discussions of the patterns of diagnosis by five phases, see *Extraordinary Vessels* pp.249-262. ·For general treatments of five-phase disharmonies see *Five Elements and Ten Stems* pp.169-181, describing the treatments of three famous Japanese acupuncturists, Sorei Yanagiya, Sodo Okabe, and Keiri Inoue. One may select from amongst these sets of treatments according to the principles outlined there. Another useful series of treatment procedures and techniques are described on pp.145-169 of the same volume. Since tonification and dispersion are so fundamental to the effectiveness of five-phase treatments, reviewing the basic tonification and dispersion techniques described therein would be helpful.

[19] Sugiyama here does not specify the use of needles or moxa.

[20] Waichi Sugiyama, *Sugiyama Ryu Sanbusho* p.92 passim.

[21] The author studied with members from this school in the summer of 1986.

Notes to Chapter 16

[1] Yoshio Manaka, *Ika no Tameno Shinjutsu Nyumon Kuoza* p.185.

[2] Yoshio Manaka, *Hukubu Syoken to Hukusyo* p.15 passim.

[3] Ibid. p.16 passim.

[4] Note that the *Shang Han Lun* use of six stages describes the degree of penetration of pathogenic influences into the body and energetic levels of the body, where use of these concepts here involves the energetic inter-meridian relationships.

[5] Tsugio Nagatomo describes the same relationships; see Tsugio Nagatomo, *Nagatomo M.P. Shinkyu Kuowa Hachi Ju Hachi Syu* p.64.

☐

6 Yoshio Manaka, *Shinkyu Rinsho Iten* p.46 passim.

7 Yoshio Manaka, *Ika no Tameno Shinjutsu Nyumon Kuoza* p.354 passim.

8 Ibid.

9 Ibid. p.346.

10 Yoshio Manaka, *Hukubu Syoken to Hukusyo* p.18 passim.

11 Yoshio Manaka, *Ika no Tameno Shinjutsu Nyumon Kuoza* pp.351 passim.

12 Makio Maruyama, *Shinkyu Topology Ron Bunshu* p.39.

13 Yoshio Manaka confided this directly to the author, as did Osamu Ito. This has also been noted by Paul Nogier in his *Theory and Practice of European Ear Acupuncture,* as taken from its Japanese translation, *Obei Jishun Ho no Riron to Rinsho* p.107.

14 Yoshio Manaka, in Y. Seki, *Shinkyu Topology* p.53 passim.

15 *Zhen Jiu Da Quan* pp.128-129 passim.

16 Ibid. pp.131-132.

17 *Zhen Jing Zhi Nan* pp.155-165. Found in the *Zhen Jiu Si Shu (Four Books of Acupuncture and Moxibustion)* compiled by Dou Jie before 1311 A.D. Much of the discussion from the *Zhen Jing Zhi Nan* seems to have been absorbed in large part by the *Zhen Jiu Ju Ying* of 1529 A.D., along with the discussions from the *Zhen Jiu Da Quan.* The *Ju Ying* also influenced the *Zhen Jiu Da Cheng.*

18 *Zhen Jiu Da Cheng* p.43, derived from the earlier text, the *Zhen Jing Zhi Nan* p.146.

19 Yoshio Manaka, *Ika no Tameno Shinjutsu Nyumon Kuoza* p.14-15 passim.

20 Ibid. p.356.

21 Ibid. p.358 passim.

22 Ibid. pp.14-15 passim.

23 See Kiiko Matsumoto and Stephen Birch, *Extraordinary Vessels.*

24 *Zhen Jiu Ju Ying* p.133.

25 These relationships and others similar to them are occasionally described and often ignored. An interesting example can be found in R.A. Dart, "Voluntary Musculature in the Human Body: the Double-Spiral Arrangement," *Brit. Jour. Phys. Med.* 13 no.12 (Dec.1950):265-268.

26 Yoshio Manaka, *Ika no Tameno Shinjutsu Nyumon Kuoza,* p.360 passim.

27 Ibid. p.355 passim.

28 Hirata zones are described more fully in the next chapter. See Yoshio Manaka, *Hiratashi Juni Hannotai Nesshin Shigeki Ryoho* p.93.

29 Yoshio Manaka, *Ika no Tameno Shinjutsu Nyumon Kuoza* p.355 passim.

30 Manaka comments concerning the du mai and the chiropractic idea of treating just the spine (in our terms just the du mai) that this indicates a limitation to the the chiropractic model. The chiropractor's understanding is that all disease relates to dislocations of the spinal vertebrae or subluxations of the spinal nerves. Thus, adjusting the spine will affect symptoms and diseases. Since this model centers entirely on only one dividing line of the body, the du mai, it lacks a full view of the body, in particular the ren mai and the dai mai. How do spinal adjustments treat these lines?

31 Yoshio Manaka, *Hukubu Syoken to Hukusyo* p.17 passim.

³² *Extraordinary Vessels,* pp. 193-248.

³³ *Zhen Jiu Da Cheng* p.191.

³⁴ Ibid.

Notes to Chapter 17

¹ *Zhen Jiu Da Cheng,* page 385 and following.

² Ibid. p.386 passim.

³ Taken from notes and discussions with Dr. Manaka.

⁴ More details of this can be found the forthcoming study of Manaka's work, *Chasing the Dragon's Tail;* and in the works of Tae Woo Yoo (see bibliography).

⁵ *Hiratashi Junihannotai Nesshin Shigekiryoho (Mr. Hirata's twelve dermatomes stimulation therapy with heated needle)* pp.92-93.

⁶ Yoshio Manaka, *Ika no Tameno Shinjutsu Nyumon Kuoza* p.354 passim.

⁷ A more comprehensive systematization can be found in *Chasing the Dragon's Tail.*

⁸ Yukimichi Seki, "How to Use Ion Pumping" p.3.

⁹ Yoshio Manaka, *Bishona Shigeki Moshiku We Eikyo o Mochite Okonau Chiryo Hono Ko Osatsu* p.13 passim.

¹⁰ See for instance Yoshiaki Omura, "The bidigital O-ring Test: Critical Evaluation of it's Abnormal Responses with Laboratory Tests," *Acupuncture and Electro-therapeutics Research* 8, No.1 (1983) pp.37-43.

¹¹ Yoshio Manaka, *Ion-pumping Medical Point Book* pp.102-105 passim.

¹² Yukimichi Seki, *Shinkyu Topology* p.107.

¹³ Reported orally to the author.

¹⁴ Yukimichi Seki, "How to Use Ion Pumping" p.23 passim.

¹⁵ Ibid.

¹⁶ Ibid. p.20.

¹⁷ Makio Maruyama, *Shinkyu Topology Ronbunshu* pp.39-40. Compiled from the clinical experience of many practitioners researching the ion cords.

Notes to Chapter 18

¹ From private notes, lectures, and discussions with Dr. Manaka.

² For more information on the use of magnets on the extraordinary vessels and twelve meridians, see our previous work, *Extraordinary Vessels.* This style is derived from the work of Tsugio Nagatomo.

Notes to Conclusion

³ Robert Sampson, "Healing in the treatment of modern medicine." *Somatics* Autumn (1978):11. Adapted from H. Brody, "The systems view of man: Implications for medicine, science and ethics." *Perspectives in Biology and Medicine* 17 (1973), pp.71-92.

⁴ J.W. Ratcliffe; Notion of validity in qualitative research methodology; *Knowledge, creation, diffusion, utilization* 5, no.2 (Dec. 1983), pp.147-167.

Bibliography

Bibliography

Bibliography of Pre-1900 Books and Articles in Chinese and Japanese

抱朴子
Bao Pu Zi (Book of the Master Who Maintained Solidarity) Ge Hong (A.D. 281-341)). From *Morohashi Encyclopedic Dictionary*.

參同契
Can Tong Qi (The Kinship of the Three). Wei Po-Yang, ed. (ca. A.D. 142). From *Morohashi Encyclopedic Dictionary*.

重广补注黃帝內經素問
Chong Guang Bu Zhu Huang Di Nei Jing Su Wen (Expanded and Annotated Yellow Emperor's Inner Canon, Essential Questions). Wang Bing, 762. Expanded by Lin Yi, Sun Tao, ed. Song, 1057.

春秋
Chun Qiu (Spring and Autumn Annals). Anon. (722-481 B.C.). From *Ki no Shiso*.

春秋緯元命苞
Chun Qiu Wei Yuan Ming Bao (Apocryphal Treatise on the Spring and Autumn Annals). Anon. (ca. 100 B.C.). From *Ki no Shiso*.

丹溪醫學正傳
Dan Xi Yi Xue Zheng Chuan (Verified Records of Dan Xi's Medical Teachings). Yu Bo (1577). Nanking Sanshan Studio. Extant copy in Harvard Yenching Library.

腹證奇覽
Fuku Sho Kiran (Novel Displays of Abdominal Confirmations). Bunrei, Inaba, 1801. Tokyo: Ido no Nippon Sha, 1981.

觀象玩占
Guan Xiang Wan Zhan (Observations on Divinatory Phenomena). ca. A.D. 600. Li Chun-Feng. From *Morohashi Encyclopedic Dictionary*.

管子
Guan Zi (Book of Master Guan). Attrib. Guan Zhong (ca. 300-400 B.C.). Taipei: Taiwan Chinese Publishing Company, 1973.

廣雅
Guang Ya (Enlargement of the *Er Ya*). Anon. (A.D. 230). From *Morohashi Encyclopedic Dictionary*.

漢書

Han Shu (Han Documents). Ban Gu (ca. A.D. 32-92). In Akira Ishihara, *Kanpo.* "Lu Li Zhi" chapter from the *Dao Jiao Da Zi Dian.*

後漢書

Hou Han Shu (Later Han Documents). Fan Ye (ca. A.D. 398-445). From *Ki no Shiso.*

淮南子

Huai Nan Zi (*Book of Master Huai Nan*). Liu An et al. (ca. 122 B.C.). Japanese translation edited by Haruki Kusuyama. Tokyo: Meiji Shyoin Sha, 1979.

黃帝內經靈樞

Huang Di Nei Jing Ling Shu {*Ling Shu*}. Anon. (ca. 100-300 B.C.). From
黃帝內經靈樞譯解
Huang Di Nei Jing Ling Shu Yi Jie (Yellow Emperor's Inner Canon, Spiritual Axis, Interpreted and Explained). Taipei: Chinese Republic Publishing Company, 1978.

黃帝內經素問

Huang Di Nei Jing Su Wen {*Su Wen*} (Yellow Emperor's Inner Cannon, Essential Questions). Anon. Beijing: People's Hygiene Publishing, 1978.

黃帝內經素問集註

Huang Di Nei Jing Su Wen Ji Zhu (Annotated Yellow Emperor's Inner Canon). Zhang Yin-An (1888). Shanghai: Science and Technology Publishing Company, 1980.

黃帝內經太素

Huang Di Nei Jing Tai Su {*Tai Su*} (Yellow Emperor's Inner Cannon, Great Essentials). Yang Shan-Shan (Sui, n.d.). Beijing: People's Hygiene Publishing Company, 1965.

黃帝外景經

Huang Ting Wai Jing Jing (Canon of the External Radiance of the Yellow [Emperor's] Court). Anon. (Song Dynasty). From *Morohashi Encyclopedic Dictionary.*

黃庭經

Huang Ting Jing (Canon of the Yellow [Emperor's] Court). Anon. (1793). From *Ki no Shiso.*

医心方

Ishin Po (The Heart of Medicine). Yasuyori Tambano (A.D. 982). From *Nihon Igaku Shi Koyo.*

集韻

Ji Yun (Collected Rhyming [Dictionary]). Ding Du et al. (ca. 1050). From *Morohashi Encyclopedic Dictionary.*

□

金匱要略方論

Jin Kui Yao Lue Fang Lun (Prescriptions of the Golden Chamber). Zhang Ji (ca. A.D. 220). Quoted from the *Zhong Yi Zhen Duan Xue*.

金闕帝君三元眞一經

Jin Que Di Jun San Yuan Zhen Yi Jing (Canon of the Single Truth of the Three Origins from the Prince's Golden Palace). Anon. (ca. A.D. 700-1600). Found in the *Dao Zang* (Taoist Patrology). Collection of Taoist works. From Henry Maspero, *Taoism and Chinese Religion*.

解体発蒙

Kaitai Hatsumou (Anatomical Elucidations). Misutane, K. (1813). Published privately by T. Sawada, Japan, 1930.

康熙字典

Kang Xi Zi Dian (The [Emperor] Kang Xi Dictionary). Zhang Yu-Shu et al. (1711). From *Morohashi Encyclopedic Dictionary*.

老子　道德經

Lao Zi, Dao De Jing. Attrib. Li Er (ca. 300 B.C.). From Harukai Ogawa, ed., *Lao-Zi Zhuang-Zi*. Tokyo: Chuo Koron Sha, 1978.

類經

Lei Jing (Canon of Categories). Zhang Jie-Bin (1624). Beijing: People's Hygiene Publishing Company, 1965.

类经图翼

Lei Jing Tu Yi (Illustrated Wings to the Canon of Categories). Zhang Jie-Bin (1624). From *Zhong Guo Yi Xue Shi Lue*.

禮記

Li Ji (Records of Rites). Dai Sheng (ca. 50 B.C.) From *Morohashi Encyclopedic Dictionary*.

列子

Lie Zi (Book of Master Lie). Attrib. Lie Yu-Kou (500-100 B.C., with later additions). Japan: Meiji Publishing Company, 1967.

呂氏春秋

Lu Shi Chun Qiu (Mr. Lu's Spring and Autumn Annals). Lu Bu-Wei (d. 235 B.C.). From *Morohashi Encyclopedic Dictionary*.

論衡

Lun Heng (Discourses Weighed in the Balance). Wang Cong (ca. A.D. 82). Sao Ye San Fang Publishing Company, n.d.

脈經

Mai Jing (Canon of the Pulse). Second ed. Wang Shu-He (ca. A.D. 300). Taipei: Shang Wu Shin Shu Publishing Company, 1963.

難經鐵鑑

Nangyo Tekkan (A Firm Scrutinization of the Canon of Perplexities). Hirooka, Sosen (1750). Japan: Harumichi Ogawa Publishing Company, 1971.

難經

Nan Jing (Canon of Perplexities). Attrib. Qin Yue-Ren (ca. 100 B.C.-A.D. 100). Found in Wang Shu-He (ca. A.D. 300), *Tu Zhu Nan Jing Mai Jue.*

難經本義

Nan Jing Ben Yi (Essential Meaning of the Canon of Perplexities). Hua Shou (1361). Taipei: Xuan Feng Publishing Company, 1980.

難經集注

Nan Jing Ji Zhu (Collected Commentaries on the Canon of Perplexities). Wang Jiu-Si, ed. (1505). Taipei Zhong Hua Publishing Company, 1983.

難經正義

Nan Jing Zheng Yi (Verified Meaning of the Canon of Perplexities). Xie Lin (1895). Shanghai: Science and Technology Publishing Company, 1981.

奇經八脈攷

Qi Jing Ba Mai Kao (An Examination of the Extraordinary Vessels). Li Shi-Zhen (ca. 1570). Found in the *Tu Zhu Nan Jing Mai Jue.*

千金要方

Qian Jin Yao Fang (Priceless Prescriptions). Sun Si-Mo (A.D. 652). Taipei: National Chinese Medical Herb Research Center, 1980.

全元起本

Quan Yuan Qi Ben (Quan Yuan-Qi's Writings). Quan Yuan-Qi (ca. A.D. 590). (A commentary on the *Su Wen* by Quan Yuan-Qi.)

三因極一病証方論

San Yin Ji Yi Bing Zheng Fang Lun (A Treatise on the Three Reasons for Disease Having One Cause with Prescriptions). Chen Yan (1174). Quoted from *Wakan Sansai Zue* and *Nan Jing Zheng Yi.*

傷寒論

Shang Han Lun (Treatise on Injury by Cold). Zhang Ji (ca. A.D. 220). From *Toyo Igaku Gaisetsu.*

史記

Shi Ji (Records of History). Si-Ma Qian (ca. 90 B.C.). From *Morohashi Encyclopedic Dictionary.*

釋名

Shi Ming (Explanation of Names). Liu Xi (ca. A.D. 100). From *Morohashi Encyclopedic Dictionary.*

十四経発揮

Shi Si Jing Fa Hui (Elucidation of the Fourteen Meridians). Hua Shou (1341). Yokosuka: Ido no Nippon Sha, 1946.

鍼灸阿是要穴

Shinkyu Azeyoketsu (Essential Acupuncture "Ashi" Points). Okamoto, Ippo (1703). Quoted from Bunshi Shiroda, *Shinkyu Chiryo Kisogaku.*

書経

Shu Jing (Historical Classic). Anon. (ca. Zhou dynasty). From Joseph Needham, *Science and Civilization in China* V, part III.

□

說文解字

Shuo Wen Jie Zi (Explanation of Characters). Xu Shen (ca. A.D. 121). From *Morohashi Encyclopedic Dictionary.*

說文通訓定聲

Shuo Wen Tong Xun Ding Sheng. (Explanation of Characters with Phonetic Verification). Chu Sheng-Chu (ca. 1848). From *Morohashi Encyclopedic Dictionary.*

搜神記

Sou Shen Ji (Records of Spiritual Investigations). Gan Bao (ca. A.D. 348). From *Morohashi Encyclopedic Dictionary.*

素问经注节解

Su Wen Jing Zhu Jie Jie (Annotated and Clarified Essential Questions). Yao Zhi-An (1677). People's Hygiene Publishing Company, 1983.

素問玄機原病式

Su Wen Xuan Ji Yuan Bing Shi (An Investigation into the Profound Truths of Disease Origins in the Essential Questions). Liu Wan-Su (1186). People's Hygiene Publishing Company, 1983.

杉山流三部書

Sugiyama Ryu Sanbusho (Sugiyama's Style of Treatment in Three Parts). Second ed. Sugiyama, Waichi (ca. 1700). Yokosuka: Ido no Nippon Sha, 1978.

太平御覽

Tai Ping Yu Lan (Imperial Readings of the Tai Ping Period). Ed. Li Fang (A.D. 983). From *Ki no Shiso.*

太上道君守元丹上經

Tai Shang Dao Jun Shou Yuan Dan Shang Jing (The Superior Canon of the Heavenly Prince on Preserving the Original Elixir). Anon. (A.D. 700-1600). Found in the *Dao Zang* (Taoist Patrology). Collection of Taoist works. From Henry Maspero, *Taoism and Chinese Religion.*

銅人腧穴鍼灸図経

Tong Ren Shu Xue Zhen Jiu Tu Jing (Illustrated Canon of Bronze Statue Acupuncture Points). Wang Wei-Yi (1027). Compiled and edited by Masao Maruyama. Tokyo: Seiko Bundo Publishing Company, 1970.

和漢三才圖會

Wakan Sansai Zue (Japanese-Chinese Illustrated Essay on the Three Powers). Terashima, Ryoan (1712). Tokyo: Sebundo Publishing Company, 1980.

血証論

Xue Zheng Lun (A Treatise on Blood Patterns). Tang Zong-Hai (1885). Translated by Mikhail Santaro. Unpublished manuscript.

医学入門

Yi Xue Ru Men (Gateway to Medicine). Li Chan (1575). Taipei: Tai Lien Guo Feng Publishing Company, 1977.

雲笈七籤

Yun Ji Qi Qian (Seven Divining Slips from the Cloudy Bamboo Bookcase). Zhang Jun-Fang (1019). From *Morohashi Encyclopedic Dictionary*.

针经指南

Zhen Jing Zhi Nan (Guide to Acupuncture Classics). Dou Jie (ca. 1295). From *Zhen Jiu Si Shu*.

針灸大成

Zhen Jiu Da Cheng (Great Compendium of Acupuncture and Moxibustion). Yang Ji-Zhou (1601). Hong Kong: Nan Guang Publishing Company, n.d.

鍼灸大全

Zhen Jiu Da Quan (Collection of Acupuncture and Moxibustion). Xu Feng (1437). Found in *Bi Chao Zhen Jiu Da Quan*. Anon. (ca. 1600). Taipei: Han Wu Publishing Company, 1974.

针灸甲乙经

Zhen Jiu Jia Yi Jing (Systematized Canon of Acupuncture and Moxibustion). Huang-Fu Mi (A.D. 282). Quoted from *Zhen Jiu Jia Yi Jing Yu Xue Zhong Ji*.

鍼灸聚英

Zhen Jiu Ju Ying (Gathering of Eminent Acupuncturists). Gao Wu (1529). Shanghai: Shanghai Science and Technology Publishing Company, 1961.

针灸四書

Zhen Jiu Si Shu (Four Books of Acupuncture and Moxibustion). Compiled by Dou Gui-Fang (ca. 1311). Beijing: People's Hygiene Publishing Company, 1983.

正字通

Zheng Zi Tong (Rectification of Characters). Zhang Zi-Lie (Ming Dynasty). From *Morohashi Encyclopedic Dictionary*.

周髀算經

Zhou Bi Suan Jing (The Arithmetical Canon of the Gnomon and the Circular Paths [of Heaven]). Anon. (400-100 B.C.). From Joseph Needham, *Science and Civilization in China* 3.

周易

Zhou Yi (Zhou [dynasty version of the Book of] Changes). Anon. (Zhou and Han Dynasties). From *Ki no Shiso*.

諸病源候論

Zhu Bing Yuan Hou Lun (Treatise on the Origin and Outcome of Disease). Chao Yan-Fang (A.D. 610). National Chinese Medical Pharmacology Research Group, 1962.

莊子

Zhuang-Zi (Book of Master Zhuang). Attrib. Zhuang Zhou (ca. 290 B.C.). From Harukai Ogawa, ed. *Lao-Zi Zhuang-Zi* (Master Lao and Master Zhuang). Tokyo: Chuo Koron Sha, 1978.

子午流注针经

Zi Wu Liu Zhu Zhen Jing (Canon of the Noon-Midnight Circulation Needling Method). He Ruo-Yu. From *Zhen Jiu Si Shu*.

□

Bibliography of Post-1900 Books and Articles in Chinese and Japanese

Anon. 道教大字典
Dao Jiao Da Zi Dian (Encyclopedic Dictionary of Taoism). Taipei: Li Shu-Huan Publishing, 1979.

———. 簡明中医辞典
Jing Ming Zhong Yi Ci Dian (Explanatory Dictionary of Chinese Medicine). Hong Kong: Joint Publishing Company, 1979.

———. 圖註難經脈訣
Tu Zhu Nan Jing Mai Jue (Discriminating Pulses from the Canon of Perplexities with Illustrations). Taipei: Shui Cheng Shu Ju Publishing Company, 1970, 2nd ed.

———. 通俗伤寒论
Tong Su Shang Han Lun (Colloquialized Treatise On Injury by Cold), 1916. From the *Zhong Guo Yi Xue Shi Lue*.

———. 內經解剖生理學
Nei Jing Jie Po Sheng Li Xue (Anatomy and Physiology of the Inner Canon). Taipei: National Chinese Medical Herb Research Center Publishing Company, 1977, 2nd ed.

———. 中国医学史略
Zhong Guo Yi Xue Shi Lue (Chinese Medical Studies: An Historical Study). Shanxi: People's Publishing Company, 1979.

Canton Institute of Chinese Medicine. 中医診断学
Zhong Yi Zhen Duan Xue (Chinese Medical Diagnostics). Shanghai: People's Publishing Company, 1964. Japanese translation, Tokyo: Shizensha, 1972.

Chikugo, T. 1949.
"Fukushi Dangi" (Lecture on abdominal diagnosis). *Ido no Nippon Magazine*. August.

Edagawa, N. ドクトルなおさんの治療事典
Doctor Nao's Chiryo Jiten (Dr. Nao's Treatment Dictionary). Tokyo: Giyu Sha, 1983.

Fujido, Akiyasu. 藤堂漢和大字典
Gakuken Kanwadaijiten (Fujido's Etymological Dictionary). Tokyo: Gakushu Kenkyu Sha, 1978.

Fujimoto, R. 弁釈鍼道秘訣集
Bensyoku Shindo Hiketsu Shu (Collected Commentaries on Acupuncture Recipes). Tokyo: Shizensha, 1977.

Fukaya, I. 深谷灸法
Fukaya Kyu Ho (Fukaya's Moxibustion Therapy). Tokyo: Shizensha, 1980.

Fukushima, Kodo. 経絡治療要綱
Keiraku Chiryo Yoko (Principles of Meridian Treatments). Tokyo: Toyohari Igaku Kai Publishing Company, 1960.

Furukawa, R. 1986.
Kukakuseijotai Joho no Sonzai to Sono Teigen. (*A proposal for the existence of an information system across the epithelial systems*). Unpublished manuscript. Kyushu, Japan: Kagoshima University.

Guo, Ai-Chun. 黃帝內經素問校注語譯
Huang Di Nei Jing Su Wen Jiao Zhi Yu Yi (Revised Yellow Emperor's Inner Canon, Essential Questions, in Colloquial Language). Tianjin: Science and Technology Publishing Company, 1981.

Haruchika, Noguchi. 野口晴哉整体入門
Noguchi Haruchika Seitai Nyumon (Seitai Exercises). Tokyo: Kodansha, 1974, 2nd ed.

Hirakoba, Taigi. 気学のすすめ
Kigaku no Susume (Recommended Studies of Qi). Tokyo: Akiyama Publishing Company, 1977.

Hiroko, Yoshino. 隠された神々古代信仰と陰陽五行
Kakusareta Kamigami Kodai Shinko to Yinyo Gogyo (Hidden Spirits, Ancient Religions, and Yin-Yang and the Five Phases). Kyoto: Kodansha, 1975.

Honda, Wataru, ed. 易経
Yi Jing (Canon of Changes). Japan: Heigakuji Publishing Company, 1960.

Honma, Shohaku. 経絡治療講話
Keiraku Chiryo Kuowa (Lectures on Five-Phase Treatment). Yokosuka: Ido no Nippon Sha, 1947.

———. 難経の研究
Nangyo no Kenkyu (Research and Study Book for the Canon of Perplexities). Yokosuka: Ido no Nippon Sha, 1974.

———. 鍼灸病証学
Shinkyu Byosho Gaku (Diseases and Configurations in the Study of Acupuncture and Moxibustion). Yokosuka: Ido no Nippon Sha, 1943.

Ido no Nippon Sha, tr. 経絡十講
Jing Luo Shi Jiang (Ten Lectures on the Meridians). Yokosuka: Ido no Nippon Sha, 1980.

Imamura, S. 1983.
"Zofu Keiraku Oyobi Chukan Keiraku no Ruchu ni Tsuite" (Pathways of the internal meridians). *Ido no Nippon Magazine* June:6-14; July:45-54.

Ishi, T. 1969.
"Juten o Oku Shinsatsu ho" (Where I place emphasis in abdominal diagnosis). *Ido no Nippon Magazine*. May.

Ishihara, Akira. 漢方
Kanpo (Chinese Prescriptions). Tokyo: Chuokoron Publishing Company, 1978, 19th ed.

Kato, Joken, and Katsuni Yamada. 角川字源辞典
Kadokawa Jigen Jiten (Kadokawa Etymological Dictionary). Tokyo: Kadokawa Publishing Company, 1972.

□

Kuzome, Naoichi. 1970,1971.
"Shiatsu no Fukushin to Fukusho" (Shiatsu's abdominal diagnosis and confirmations). *Ido no Nippon Magazine*. October & December (1970); Febru-
ary, March & April (1971).

Li Ding-Zhong.
Jing Luo Phenomena I. Kyoto: Yukonsha, 1984.

———.
Jing Luo Phenomena II Kyoto: Yukonsha, 1985.

Manaka, Yoshio. 1977.
"Bishona Shigeki Moshiku Eikyo o Mochite o Konau Chiryo Hono Ko
Osatsu" (Thoughts about treatment using tiny, tiny stimulation). Seminar
pamphlet. Tokyo: Shizensha.

———. 平田氏十二反応帯熱針刺激療法
Hiratashi Junihannotai Nesshin Shigeki Ryo Ho (Hirata-Style Hot-needle
Therapy). Yokosuka: Ido no Nippon Sha, 1982.

———. 医家のための鍼術入門講座
Ika no Tameno Shinjutsu Nyumon Kuoza (Introductory Lectures on Acupuncture for Medical Doctors). 2d ed. Yokosuka: Ido no Nippon Sha, 1980.

———.
Ion Pumping Medical Point Book. Kyoto: Asahi Butsuryoki Kenkyujo, 1979.

———. n.d.
"Kenkyu ni Oyoshita Jiki Kotoni sono Keiketsu Sessyoku Koka ni Tsuite"
(Research into the effects of magnets and specifically the effects on certain
acupoints). Lecture pamphlet.

———. 針灸の理論と考え方
Shinkyu no Riron to Kangaekata (Thoughts and Theory of Acupuncture and
Moxibustion). Osaka: Sogen Igaku Sha, 1980, 2nd ed.

———. 針灸臨床医典
Shinkyu Rinsho Iten (A Clinical Medical Dictionary of Acumoxa). Yokosuka:
Ido no Nippon Sha, 1970.

Manaka, Yoshio, and Kazuko Itaya. 1986.
"Acupuncture as intervention in the biological informational system."
(Meridian treatment and the x-signal system). Address given at the annual
assembly of the Japan Meridian Treatment Association, Tokyo. March 29-
30.

———. 1983. 腹部所見と腹証
"Hukubu Syoken to Hukusyo" (Abdominal signs and abdominal confirmations). Seminar pamphlet.

Morohashi, ed. 諸橋大漢和辞典
Daikanwa Jiten (Morohashi Encyclopedic Dictionary of Chinese). Tokyo:
Daishukan Sha, 1959).

Maruyama, Masao. 鍼灸医学と古典の研究
Shinkyu Igaku to Koten no Kenkyu (Research Book of Acupuncture and Moxibustion Medicine and the Classics). Osaka: Sogen Sha, 1977.

Maruyama, M. 鍼灸トポロジー論文集
Shinkyu Topology Ronbunshu. (Collected Papers on Acumoxa Topology; Ion Pumping Medical Point.) Kyoto: Asahi Butsuryoki Kenkyujo, 1979.

Matsumoto, M. 1969.
"Shindo Hiketsushu" (Secret recipes of acupuncture). Quoting Mubun Ryu. *Ido no Nippon Magazine*. August.

Ming Han-Chuo, tr. 欧米耳針法の理論と臨床
Obei Jishun Ho no Riron to Rinsho. Translation of Paul Nogier, *Theory and Practice of European Ear Acupuncture*. Yokosuka: Ido no Nippon Sha, 1978.

Nagahama, Y. 針灸の医学
Shinkyu no Igaku (Western Studies of Acupuncture and Moxibustion). Osaka: Sogen Sha, 1956.

———. 東洋医学講座
Toyo Igaku Gaisetsu (Outline of Oriental Medicine). Osaka: Sogen Sha, 1961.

Nagatomo, Tsugio. 長友・ＭＰ鍼灸講話八十八輯
Nagatomo M-P Shinkyu Kuowa Hachiju Hachisyu (Mr. Nagatomo's 88 Lectures on the Minus-Plus Needle Therapy). Kyoto: Shinkyu Shinkuokai Sha, 1976.

Nakano, Miyoko. 中国の妖怪
Chugoku no Yokai (Mythical Creatures of Chinese History). Tokyo: Iwanami Shinsho, 1983.

Nanjing Institute of Chinese Medicine. 难经校释
Nan Jing Jiao Shi (The Canon of Perplexities Revised and Explained). Beijing: People's Hygiene Publishing Company, 1979.

Nanjing Institute of Chinese Medicine Shang Han Research Group.
伤寒论译释
Shang Han Lun Yi Shi (Explanation of the Treatise on Injury by Cold). Shanghai: Science and Technology Publishing Company, 1980.

Ogawa, Harukai. 老子 荘子
Lao-Zi Zhuang-Zi (Master Lao and Master Zhuang). Tokyo: Chuo Koron Sha, 1978.

Ogawa, Teizo. 日本医学史綱要
Nihon Igaku Shi Koyo (Outline of Japanese Medical History). Tokyo: Heibon Publishing Company, 1976, 3rd ed.

Okabe, Sodo. 鍼灸経絡治療
Shinkyu Keiraku Chiryo (Acupuncture and Moxibustion Five-Phase Treatments). Tokyo: Bundo Sha, 1974.

Onozawa, Seiichi et al., eds. 気の思想
Ki no Shiso (Thoughts about Qi). Tokyo: Tokyo University Publishing Company, 1980, 3rd ed.

Sadakatsu, Ooguro, ed. 導引口訣鈔
Do Yin Kuketsu Syo (Collected Oral Traditions of *Do Yin*). Tokyo: Taniguchi Publishing Company, 1986.

□

Sango, Kobayashi. 東洋医学概説
Toyo Igaku Koza (Oriental Medical Lectures) Vol. 8. Tokyo: Kenko Publishing Company, 1980.

Seki, Y. 鍼灸トポロジー
Shinkyu Topology (Acumoxa Topology). Kyoto: Asahi Butsuryoki Kenkyujo, 1981.

———

How to use Ion Pumping. Booklet distributed by the Asahi Company, n.d.

Shanghai Institute of Chinese Medicine. 針灸治療学
Zhen Jiu Zhi Liao Xue (Acupuncture Treatment). Shaohua Cultural Service Society, Hong Kong. n.d.

Shibata, Kazunori. 足のつぼで直る健康法
Ashi no Tsubode Naoru Ken Ko Ho Tokyo: Yamate Publishing, 1974.

Shiroda, Bunshi. 鍼灸治療基礎学
Shinkyu Chiryo Kisogaku (The Basic Study Book of Acupuncture and Moxibustion). Yokosuka: Ido no Nippon Sha, 1978, 7th ed.

———. 鍼灸眞髄
Shinkyu Shin Zui (The True Backbone of Acupuncture and Moxibustion in the Style of Mr. Sawada). Yokosuka: Ido no Nippon Sha, 1977, 11th ed.

Shudo, Denmei. 経絡治療のすすめ
Keiraku Chiryo no Susume (Recommendations for Five-Phase Treatments). Yokosuka: Ido no Nippon Sha, 1984.

Takagi, Kentaro. 生体の調節機能
Seitai no Chosetsukino (The Control Systems of the Biological Organism). Tokyo: Chuokoron Publishing Company, 1972.

Wang, Yi-Ren. 難經讀本目錄
Nan Jing Du Ben Mu Lu (Index to the Study Guide for the Canon of Perplexities). Taipei: Fang Pi Feng Publishing Company, 1973.

Xu, Xi-Nian. 子午針灸療法
Zi Wu Zhen Jiu Liao Fa (Calendrical Acupuncture and Moxibustion Treatments). Hong Kong: Nan Guang Publishing Company, n.d.

Yamada, Keiji. 混沌の海へ
Konton no Umi E (To the Chaotic Ocean). Tokyo: Asahi Shinbun Sha, 1982.

Yanagiya, Sorei. 簡明不問診察法
Kanmei Humon Shinsatsu Ho (Diagnosis of the Body Without Asking). Tokyo: Ishiyama Shinkyu Igaku Publishing Company, 1976.

———. 図解あんま術
Zukai Anma Jutsu (Anma Techniques with Illustrations). Yokosuka: Ido no Nippon Sha, 1973, sixth ed.

Zhang, Shan-Chen and Zhang Deng-Bu. 针灸甲乙经腧穴重辑
Zhen Jiu Jia Yi Jing Shu Xue Zhong Ji (Inductive Points in the Systematized Canon of Acumoxa, Revised Edition). Shandong: Science and Technology Publishing Company, 1982.

□

Bibliography of Books in English

Abercrombie, M. et al. *A Dictionary of Biology*. England: Penguin Books, 1966.

Alberts, B. et al. *Molecular Biology of the Cell*. New York: Garland Publishing Company, 1983.

Alexandroff, P. *Elementary Concepts of Topology*. New York: Dover Publications Inc., 1961.

Anon. *National Symposia of Acupuncture and Moxibustion and Acupuncture Anesthesia*. June 1979, Beijing, China.

Arey, L.B. *Developmental Anatomy*. Philadelphia: W.B. Saunders Company, 1954.

Barnothy, M.F., ed. *Biological Effects of Magnetic Fields*. vol. I. New York: Plenum Press, 1964.

Barnothy, M.F., ed. *Biological Effects of Magnetic Fields*. vol. 2. New York: Plenum Press, 1969.

Becker R.O., and A.A. Marino. *Electromagnetism and Life*. Albany: State University of New York Press, 1982.

Becker R.O., and G. Selden. *The Body Electric*. New York: William Morrow Company, 1985.

Bensky D., and J. O'Connor. *Acupuncture: a Comprehensive Text*. Chicago: Eastland Press, 1981.

Berrill, N.J. *Developmental Biology*. New York: McGraw Hill, 1971.

Bischko, Johannes. *An Introduction to Acupuncture*. Heidelberg: Haug Verlag Publishing Company, 1978.

Bloom, W., and D.W. Fawcett. *Textbook of Histology*. Philadelphia: W.B. Saunders Company, 1975.

Bohm, David. *Wholeness and the Implicate Order*. London: Ark Paperbacks, 1980.

Boileau Grant, J.C. *Grant's Atlas of Anatomy*. Baltimore: Williams and Wilkins Company, 1972.

Burr, Harold Saxton. *The Nature of Man and the Meaning of Existence*. Springfield, IL: Charles C. Thomas, 1962.

———. *Blueprint for Immortality*. London: Neville Spearman, 1972.

———. *The Fields of Life*. New York: Ballantine Books, 1972.

Capra, Fritjof. *The Turning Point*. New York: Bantam Books, 1982.

Children's Hospital Medical Center. *Pregnancy, Birth and the Newborn Baby*. Boston: Delacorte Press, 1972.

□

Chishima, K. *Revolution of Biology and Medicine*. vol. 9. Gifu, Japan: Society of Neo-Haematology, 1972.

Davis, B.D. et al. *Microbiology*. New York: Harper and Row Publishing Company, 1980.

DeGowin, E.L., and R.L. DeGowin. *Bedside Diagnostic Examination*. New York: MacMillan Publishing Company Inc. 1972.

Descartes, Rene. *Discourse on Method and the Meditations*. (First edition ca. 1630.) England: Penguin Books, 1973.

Dubrov, A.P. *The Geomagnetic Field and Life: Geomagnetobiology*. New York: Plenum Press, 1978.

Dumitrescu, I.F. *Electrographic Imaging in Medicine and Biology*. England: Neville Spearman, 1983.

Durkheim, Karlfried. *Hara, the Vital Centre of Man*. England: George Allen and Unwin, 1977.

Fogg, G.E. *The Growth of Plants*. England: Penguin Books, 1970, 2nd ed.

Gallaudet, B.B. *A Description of the Planes of Fascia*. New York: Columbia University Press, 1931.

Gauquelin, M. *The Cosmic Clocks*. San Diego: Astro Computing Services, 1982.

Gray, Henry *Gray's Anatomy: Classic Collectors Edition*. New York: Bounty Books, 1977.

Greenhill, J.P. *Obstetrics*. Philadelphia: W.B. Saunders Company, 1965.

Guyton, A.C. *Human Physiology and Mechanisms of Disease*. Philadelphia: W.B. Saunders Company, 1982.

Hashimoto, Keizo, and Y. Kawakami. *Sotai: Balance and Health through Movement*. Tokyo: Japan Publications Inc., 1983.

Hay, E.D., ed. *Cell Biology of the Extracellular Matrix*. New York: Plenum Press, 1981.

Jeffery, W.R., and R.A. Raff. *Time, Space and Pattern in Embryonic Development*. New York: A.R. Liss Publishing Company, 1983.

Kapit, Wynn, and L.M. Elson. *The Anatomy Coloring Book*. New York: Harper and Row Publishers, 1977.

Kenyon, J.N. *Modern Techniques of Acupuncture*. vol. 2. England: Thorsons Publishers, 1983.

Kervran, Louis. *Biological Transformations*. Brooklyn: New York, Swan House Publishing Company, 1972.

———. *Biological Transmutation* (abridged version). George Ohsawa., ed. Oroville, California: George Ohsawa Macrobiotic Foundation, 1971.

□

Kinoshita, Haruto. *Illustration of Acupoints*. Yokosuka: Ido no Nippon Sha, 1970.

Kon, S., and A. Cowie. *Milk — The Mammary Gland and its Secretion,* vol. 1. London: Academic Press, 1961.

Koryo Sooji Chim Institute. *Treatises in Celebration of the 7th Korea-Japan Koryo Sooji Chim Academic Seminar*. Seoul, Korea: Eum Yang Maek Jin Publishing Company, 1983.

Krippner, Stanley, and D. Rubin, eds. *The Kirlian Aura: Photographing the Galaxies of Life*. New York: Anchor Books, 1974.

Langman, J. *Medical Embryology*. Baltimore: Williams and Wilkins, 1981.

Lau, D.C., trans. *Lao Tzu: Tao Te Ching*. England: Penguin Books, 1963.

Lee, E.W. *Magnetism, an Introductory Survey*. New York: Dover Publications Inc., 1970.

Luce, Gay Gaer. *Biological Rhythms in Human and Animal Physiology*. New York: Dover Publications Inc., 1971.

Malacinski, G., and S.V. Bryant, eds. *Pattern Formation, a Primer in Developmental Biology*. New York: Macmillan and Company, 1984.

Manaka, Yoshio, and I. Urquhart. *Layman's Guide to Acupuncture*. New York: J. Weatherhill Inc., 1972.

Manaka, Yoshio, with S. Birch. *Chasing the Dragon's Tail*. Brookline, MA: Paradigm Publications, 1988.

Mann, W.E. *Orgone, Reich and Eros: Wilhelm Reich's Theory of Life Energy*. New York: Simon and Schuster, 1972.

Maspero, Henry. *Taoism and Chinese Religion*. Amherst: University of Massachusetts Press, 1981.

Matsumoto, Kiiko, and S. Birch. *Five Elements and Ten Stems*. Higganum: Paradigm Publications, 1983.

———. *Extraordinary Vessels*. Brookline, MA: Paradigm Publications, 1986.

Matthews, R.H. *Matthews' Chinese English Dictionary*. Cambridge, Massachusetts: Harvard University Press, 1979.

Meserve, B.E. *Fundamental Concepts of Geometry*. New York: Dover Publications Inc., 1983.

Moore, K.L. *The Developing Human: Clinically Oriented Embryology*. Philadelphia: W.B. Saunders Company, 1982.

Motoyama, Hiroshi, and R. Brown. *Science and the Evolution of Consciousness*. Cambridge, MA: Autumn Press, 1978.

Motoyama, Hiroshi. "PK Influence on the Meridians and Psi-energy." *Research for Religion and Parapsychology*. Tokyo: International Association for Religion and Parapsychology, Vol. 5, No. 2, 1979.

□

———. "Electrophysiological and Preliminary Biochemical Studies of Skin Properties in Relation to the Acupuncture Meridian." *Research for Religion and Parapsychology*. Tokyo: International Association for Religion and Parapsychology, Vol. 6, No.2, 1980.

———. "A Biophysical Elucidation of the Meridian and Ki-energy." *Research for Religion and Parapsychology*. Tokyo: International Association for Religion and Parapsychology, Vol. 7, No. 1, 1981.

Needham, Joseph. *Science and Civilization in China*. vol. 2. Cambridge, England: Cambridge University Press, 1956.

———. *Science and Civilization in China*. vol. 3. Cambridge, England: Cambridge University Press, 1959.

———. *Science and Civilization in China*. vol. 4, part 1. Cambridge, England: Cambridge University Press, 1962.

———. *Science and Civilization in China*. vol. 5, part 3. Cambridge, England: Cambridge University Press, 1976.

Needham, Joseph, and G.D. Lu. *Celestial Lancets*. Cambridge, England: Cambridge University Press, 1980.

Nicolson, I. *The Sun*. New York: Rand McNally and Company, 1982.

Oppenheimer, S.B., and G. Lefevre. *Introduction to Embryonic Development*. Boston: Allyn and Bacon Inc., 1984.

Oschman, James. *The Natural Science of Healing. A Biology of Whole Systems*. Unpublished manuscript, 1985.

Piccardi, G. *The Chemical Basis of Medical Climatology*. Springfield, IL: C.C. Thomas, 1962.

Pohl, H.A. Research note 90: *Microdielectrophoresis of dividing cells*. Stillwater, OK: Quantum Theoretical Research Group, Oklahoma State University, June 1979.

Presman, A.S. *Electromagnetic Fields and Life*. New York: Plenum Press, 1970.

Prigogine, I., and I. Stengers. *Order Out of Chaos*. New York: Bantam Books, 1984.

Requena, Yves. *Terrains and Pathology in Acupuncture*. Brookline, MA: Paradigm Publications, 1986.

Rey, H.A. *The Stars: A New Way to See Them*. Boston: Houghton Mifflin Company, 1976.

Rook, A. et al. *Textbook of Dermatology*. vol 1. Oxford, England: Blackwell Scientific Publications, 1972.

Rucker, R.v.B. *Geometry, Relativity and the Fourth Dimension*. New York: Dover Publications Inc., 1977.

Schmitt, F.O. et al., eds. *Functional Linkage in Biomolecular Systems*. New York: Raven Press, 1975.

□

Schoffeniels, E. *Anti-Chance.* New York: Pergammon Press Inc., 1976.

Sedlak, W. *Bioelektronika 1967-1977,* with English summaries. Poland: Instytut Wyadawniczy Pax, 1979.

Sheldrake, Rupert. *A New Science of Life: The Hypothesis of Formative Causation.* Los Angeles: J.P. Tarcher Inc., 1981.

Singer, E. *Fasciae of the Human Body and Their Relations to the Organs They Envelop.* Baltimore: Williams and Wilkins, 1935.

Slack, J.M.W. *From Egg to Embryo. Determinative Events in Early Development.* Cambridge, England: Cambridge University Press, 1983.

Sobotta. *Atlas of Human Anatomy.* vol. 2. H. Ferner and J. Staubesand, eds. 10th ed., Baltimore: Urban and Schwarzenberg, 1983.

Tompkins, Peter, and Christopher Bird.
 The Secret Life of Plants. England: Penguin Books, 1973.

Upledger, J.E., and J.D. Vredevoogd. *Craniosacral Therapy.* Seattle: Eastland Press, 1983.

Uvarov, E.B. et al. *A Dictionary of Science.* England: Penguin Books, 1971.

Wilber, Ken, ed. *The Holographic Paradigm and Other Paradoxes.* Boulder: Shambala Publications, 1982.

Williams and Warwick. *Gray's Anatomy,* 36th ed. Philadelphia: W.B. Saunders Company, 1980.

Wiseman, Nigel, A. Ellis, and P. Zmiewski. *Fundamentals of Chinese Medicine.* Brookline, MA: Paradigm Publications, 1985.

Yoffey, J., and F. Courtice. *Lymphatics, Lymph and Lymphomyeloid Complex.* London: Academic Press, 1970.

Yoo, Tae Woo. *Lectures on KoRyo Sooji Chim.* Seoul: Eum Yang Maek Jin Publishing Company, 1983.

Bibliography of Articles in English.

Adey, W.R., and S.W. Bawin. 1977. "Brain interaction with weak electric and magnetic fields." *Neurosci. Re. Prog. Bull.* 15:1-141.

Adey, W.R. 1981. "Tissue interactions with nonionizing electromagnetic fields." *Physiol. Rev.* 61(2):435-514.

Barker, A.T., et al. 1982. "The glabrous epidermis of the cavies contains a powerful battery." *Amer. Jour. Physiol.* R358-R366.

Bassett, C.A.L., and R.O. Becker. 1962. "Generation of electric potentials by bone in response to mechanical stress." *Science.* 137:1063-1064.

Bassett, C.A.L. 1968. "Biologic significance of piezoelectricity." *Calc. Tissue Res.* 1:252-272.

Bawin, S.W., and W.R. Adey. 1976. "Sensitivity to calcium binding in cerebral tissue to weak environmental electric fields oscillating at low frequency." *Proc. Natl. Acad. Sci. USA.* 73(6):1999-2003.

Bawin, S.W., et al. 1978. "Ionic factors in release of 45 Ca2+ from chicken cerebral tissue by electromagnetic fields." *Proc. Natl. Acad. Sci. USA.* 75(12):6314-6318.

Becker, R.O. 1960. "The bioelectric field pattern in the salamander and its simulation by an electronic analog." *IRE Transact. Med. Electron.* 202-207.

Becker, R.O., and D.G. Murray. 1967. "A method for producing cellular differentiation by means of very small electrical currents." *Trans. N.Y. Acad. Sci.* 29:606-615.

———. 1970. "The electric control system regulating fracture healing in amphibians." *Clin. Orthop. Res.* 73:169.

Becker, R.O., and A.A. Pilla. 1975. "Electrochemical mechanisms and the control of biological growth processes." In Bockris, J. O'M and B.E. Conway, eds. *Modern Aspects of Biochemistry.* vol. 10. New York: Plenum Press, 1975.

Becker, R.O. 1974. "The basic biological transmission and control system influenced by electrical forces." *Ann. N.Y. Acad. Sci.* 238:236-241.

Becker, R.O. et al. 1976. "Electrophysiological correlates of acupuncture points and meridians." *Psychoenergetic Systems* 1:105.

Becker, R.O. 1984. "Electromagnetic controls over biological growth processes." *Jour. Bioelect.* 3(1+2):105-118.

Birdsong, M., and J.E. Edmunds. 1956. "Harlequin color change of the newborn: Report of a case." *Ob.+Gyn.* 7:518-521.

Borgens, R.B. et al. 1983. "A steady efflux of ionic current predicts hind limb development in the axolotl." *Jour. Exp. Zool.* 228:491-503.

Braden, M. et al. 1966. "Electrical and piezoelectric properties of dental hard tissues." *Nature.* 212:1565-1566.

Brewer, R.G. and E.L. Hahn. 1984. "Atomic memory." *Sci Amer.* 251(6):50-57.

Brown, D.E.S. 1934. "The effect of rapid changes in hydrostatic pressure upon the contraction of skeletal muscle." *Jour. Cell. Comp. Physiol.* 4:257-281.

Brown, F.A. and Y.H. Park. 1965. "Phase shifting a lunar rhythm in planarians by altering the horizontal magnetic vector." *Biol. Bull.* 129(1):79.

Brown, F.A. 1973. "Biological rhythms in integration." *Int. Jour. Chron.* 1:8.

———. 1976. "Biological clocks, endogenous cycles synchronised by subtle geophysical rhythms." *Biosystems.* 8:67-81.

Burr, H.S. 1932. "An electrodynamic theory of development suggested by the studies of the proliferation rates in the brain of ambylstoma." *Jour. Compar. Neur.* 56:347-371.

Burr, H.S. and F.S.C. Northrop. 1935. "An electrodynamic theory of life." *Quart. Rev. Biol.* 10:3. 322-333.

Burr, H.S. 1959. "Current of life." *Science.* June:164-166.

Cox, H.T. 1941. "The cleavage lines of the skin." *Brit. Jour. Surgery.* 29:234-240.

Dart, R.A. 1950. "Voluntary musculature in the human body: The double spiral arrangement." *Brit. Jour. Phys. Med.* 13(12):265-268.

Dibona, D.R. et al. 1969. "The cellular specificity of the effect of vasopressin on toad urinary bladder." *Jour. Membrane Biol.* 1:79-81.

———. 1969. "The anatomic site of transepithelial permeability barriers of toad bladder." *Jour. Cell Biol.* 40:1-7.

Dibona, D.R., and M.M. Civan. 1972. "Osmotically induced conductive changes in toad bladder under physiologic conditions." *Int. Union Pure and Applied Biophysics* 4th Congress.

Dugan, R.E. 1972. "Familial rectal pain." *Lancet.* April 15:854.

Dustin, P. 1980. "Microtubules." *Sci. Amer.* Aug:59-68.

Ellison, J. and D.R. Garrod. 1984. "Anchoring filaments of the amphibian epidermal-dermal junction traverse the basal lamina entirely from the plasma membrane of hemidesmosomes to the dermis." *Jour. Cell Sci.* 72:163-172.

Folkman, J. and A. Moscona. 1978. "Roles of cell shape in growth control." *Nature.* 273:345-349.

Friedman, H. et al. 1963. "Geomagnetic parameters and psychiatric hospital admissions." *Nature.* 200:626-628.

———. 1965. "Psychiatric ward behavior and geophysical parameters." *Nature.* 205:1050-1052.

Frohlich, H. 1968. "Bose condensation of strongly excited longitudinal electric modes." *Phys. Lett.* 26(A):402-403.

———. 1975. "Evidence for bose condensation-like excitation of coherent modes in biological systems." *Phys. Lett.* 51(A):21-22.

Fukada, E. 1974. "Piezoelectric properties of organic polymer." *Ann. N.Y. Acad. Sci.* 238:7-25.

Fukada, E. and I. Yasuda. 1957. "On the piezoelectric effect of bone." *Jour. Phys. Soc. Japan.* 12:149-154.

Fukada, E. and K. Hara. 1969. "Piezoelectric effect in blood vessel walls." *Jour. Phys. Soc. Japan.* 26:777-780.

Fukada, E. and H. Ueda. 1970. Piezoelectric effect in blood vessel walls." *Jour. Appl. Phys.* 9:844.

Gardner, J.H. and H.E. Raybuck. 1954. "Development of cleavage line patterns in the human fetus." *Anat. Rec.* 118:745-754.

☐

Gascoyne, R. et al. 1981. "Water structure dependent charge transport in proteins." *Proc. Nat. Acad. Sci.* 78:261-265.

Gerhart J.C. et al. 1981. "A reinvestigation of the role of the gray crescent in axis formation in xenopus laevis." *Nature.* 292:511-516.

Hameroff, S.R. 1974. "Ch'i: A neural hologram? Microtubules, bioholography and acupuncture." *Amer. Jour. Chin. Med.* 2(2):163-170.

Harrington, D.G. and R.O. Becker. 1973. "Electrical stimulation of RNA and protein synthesis in the frog erythrocyte." *Exp. Cell Res.* 76:95.

Hayden, R. and M. Grossman. 1959. "Rectal, ocular and submaxillary pain." *Amer. Jour. Diseases Childhood* 97:479-482.

Hayes, M.A. 1948. "The developmental basis for the continuity of the fascial planes of the abdomen and pelvis." Ph.D. dissertation, Michigan University.

Hinkle, L. et al. 1981. "The direction of growth of differentiating neurones and myoblasts from frog embryos in an applied electric field." *Jour. Physiol.* 314:121-135.

Hutchinson, C. and Koop C. Everett. 1956. "Lines of cleavage in the skin of the newborn infant." *Anat. Rec.* 126:299-310.

Hyvarinen, J. and M. Karlsson. 1977. "Low resistance skin points that may coincide with acupuncture locii." *Med. Biol.* 55(2):89-94.

Itaya, K. et al. 1985. "Effects of acupuncture needle application on the cutaneous microcirculation of rabbit ear lobe." Paper presented at the Symposium on Traditional Oriental Medicine, Science and Technology Agency, Tokyo.

Jaffe, L.F. 1966. "Electric currents through the developing fucus eggs." *Proc. Nat. Acad. Sci.* 56:1103.

———. 1982. "Developmental Currents, Voltages and Gradients." In Subtelny S., Green P.B., eds. *Developmental Order: Its Origin and Regulation.* New York: A.R. Liss Publishing Company, 1982.

Jaffe, L.F. and R. Nuccitelli. 1977. "Electrical controls of development." *Ann. Rev. Biophys. Bioeng.* 6:445-476.

Jaffe, L.F. and C.D. Stern. 1979. "Strong electrical currents leave the primitive streak of chick embryos." *Nature.* 206(2):569-571.

Jeffery, W.R. 1982. "Calcium ionophore polarizes ooplasmic segregation in ascidian eggs." *Science.* 216:545-547.

Kirschner, M. et al. 1980. "Initiation of the cell cycle and establishment of bilateral symmetry in xenopus eggs." *Sym. Soc. Dev. Biol.* 38:187-216.

Lemonick, M.D. 1985. "Chaotic body rhythms." *Science Digest.* Sept:20.

Liboff, A.R. and M. Furst. 1974. "Pyroelectric effects in collagenous structures." *Ann. N.Y. Acad. Sci.* 238:26-35.

□

Lund, E.J. 1921. "Effects of the electric current on regenerating internodes of obelia commissuralis." *Jour. Exp. Zool.* 34:471-493.

———. 1922. "The normal electrical polarity of obelia. A proof of its existence." *Jour. Exp. Zool.* 36:477-494.

———. 1925. "The nature of the control of organic polarity by the electric current." *Jour. Exp. Zool.* 41:155-190.

Manaka, Y. et al. 1985. "Abdominal diagnosis and indications in traditional chinese medicine." *Amer. Jour. Acup.* July-Sept. 13:3, 223-234.

Manaka, Y. 1985, 1986. "Acupuncture as intervention in the biological information system." Seminar pamphlet. San Francisco, Boston.

Mann, T.P. and J.E. Cree. 1972. "Familial rectal pain." *Lancet.* May 6:1016-1017.

Marino, A.A. et al. 1980. "Piezoelectricity in collagen films." *Calc. Tissue Res.* 31:257-259.

———. 1980. "Sensitivity to change in electrical environment, a new bioelectric effect." *Am. Jour. Physiol.* 239:R424-427.

Marsland, D.A. and D.E.S. Brown. 1942. "The effects of pressure on sol-gel equilibria with special reference to myosus and other protoplasmic gels." *Jour. Cell Comp. Physiol.* 20:295-305.

McLaughlin, S. and M.m. Poo. 1981. "The role of electroosmosis in the electric field induced movement of charged macromolecules on the surface of cells." *Biophys. Jour.* 34:85-93.

Mortensen, O. and P. Stougard-Andresen. 1959. "Harlequin colour change in the newborn." *Acta. Obst. et Gynec. Scandinav.* 38:352-359.

Nakagawa, K. 1976. "Magnetic field deficiency syndrome and magnetic treatment." *Japan Medical Jour.* No. 2745. Dec.

Neligan, G.A. and L.B. Strang. 1952. "A 'harlequin' colour change in the newborn." *Lancet.* Nov. 22:1005-1007.

Omura, Y. 1983. "The bidigital o-ring test: Critical evaluation of its abnormal responses with laboratory tests including 'Blood pressure and blood flow method', 'Blood chemistry' and 'Neurological method'." *Acup. and Electro-Thera. Res.* 8(1):37-43.

Oschman, J.L. 1981. "The connective tissue and myofascial systems." *Rolfing '81.* Los Angeles: Aspen Research Institute.

———. 1984. "The structure and properties of ground substance." *Amer. Zool.* 24(1):199-215.

Persinger, M.A. 1971. "Prenatal exposure to an ELF rotating magnetic field, ambulatory behavior and lunar wistance at birth, a correlation." *Psych. Rep.* 28:435-438.

Pilla, A.A. 1974. "Electrochemical information transfer at living cell membranes." *Ann. N.Y. Acad. Sci.* 238:149.

☐

Poo, M.m. and K.R. Robinson. 1977. "Electrophoresis of concanavalin a receptors along embryonic muscle cell membrane." *Nature.* 265:602-605.

Porter, K.R. and J.B. Tucker. 1981. "The ground substance of the living cell." *Sci. Amer.* March:57-67.

Reddy, N.P., B. Van, and G. Cochran. 1979. "Phenomenological theory underlying pressure-time relationships in decubitus ulcer formation." *Fed. Proc.* 38(3):1153 (abstract no. 4885).

Reichmanis, M. et al. 1975. "Electrical correlates of acupuncture points." *IREE Trans. on Biomed. Eng.* 533-535.

———. 1976. "DC skin conductance variation at acupuncture locii." *Amer. Jour. Chin. Med.* 4(1):69-72.

———. 1977. "Laplace analysis of transient impedance between acupuncture points LI-4 and LI-12." *Bio. Med. Eng.-24.* 4:402-405.

———. 1977. "Laplace plane analysis of impedance between acupuncture points HT-3 and HT-4." *Comp. Med. East West.* 5:289.

———. 1979. "Laplace plane analysis of impedance on the heart meridian." *Amer. Jour.•Chin. Med.* 7:188.

Reichmanis, M. and R.O. Becker. 1978. "Physiological effects of stimulation at acupuncture locii: A review." *Comp. Med. East West.* 6:67-73.

Reite, M. et al. 1976. "The human magnetoencephalogram. Some EEG and related correlations." *Electroenceph. Clin. Neurophys.* 40:59-66.

———. 1981. "Magnetic auditory evoked fields: Interhemispheric asymmetry." *Electroenceph. Clin. Neurophys.* 51: 388-392.

———. 1982. "MEG and EEG auditory responses to tone, click and white noise stimuli." *Electroenceph. Clin. Neurophys.* 53:643-651.

———. 1982. "Auditory evoked magnetic fields: Response amplitude versus stimulus intensity." *Electroenceph. Clin. Neurophys.* 54:147-152.

Reite, M. and J. Zimmerman. 1978. "Magnetic phenomena of the central nervous system." *Ann. Rev. Biophys. Bioeng.* 7:167-188.

Shenberger, R.M. 1977. "Acupuncture meridians retain identity after death." *Amer. Jour. Acup.* 5(4): 357-361.

Stump, R.F. and K.R. Robinson. 1983. "Xenopus neural crest migration in an applied electrical field." *Jour. Cell Biol.* 97:1226-1233.

Tanaka, T. 1981. "Gels." *Sci. Amer.* 244(1):124-138.

Taubes, G. 1986. "An electrifying possibilty." *Discover.* April:22-37.

Tiller, W.A. 1972. "Some physical network characteristics of acupuncture points and meridians." *Proc. Acad. Parapsych. and Med. Symp.* Stanford University.

Trier, W.C. 1965. "Complete breast absence. Case report and review of the literature." *Plast. Reconstr. Surg.* 36(4):430-439.

Williamson, S.J. and L. Kaufman. 1981. "Biomagnetism." *Jour. Mag. and Mag. Mater.* 22:129-201.

Zhu, Zong-Xiang. 1981. "Research advances in the electrical specificity of meridians and acupuncture points." *Amer. Jour. Acup.* 9(3):203-216.

Zimmerman, J.T. et al. 1981. "Magnetic auditory evoked fields. Dipole orientation." *Electroenceph. Clin. Neurophys.* 52:151-156.

———. 1983. "Auditory Evoked Magnetic Fields: A Replication with Comments on the P50 Analog." *Il Nuovo Climento.* 2D(2):460-470.

Index

Index

fibronectin: 163, 211
field signatures: 227
finger pressure: 214-215
fire jing: 155
fire yang: 398
fire yin: 398
five mansions (*wu cheng*): 76, 124
five phases: 82, 112, 123-124, 140, 200, 226, 228, 235, 241, 385; [abdominal correspondences]: 28; [areas]: 342, 389; [correspondences]: 153-154, 160, 334; [cycle]: 199, 339, 357; [diagnosis]: 168, 187, 344, 346; [jing]: 155; [points]: 74, 112, 349; [relationship]: 352, 369-370; [theory]: 24, 228-229, 347; [treatment]: 336, 402
five sapors: 226
five yin organs: 39; [insecurity of]: 39
flaccidity, muscles below umbilicus: 326
flesh, weak and soft: 24
fluid accumulation: [abdominal indication]: 27, 252; [differential diagnosis]: 264; [significant reactions]: 286
fluid stagnation: 272; [in stomach]: 293-294, 305, 309
food: [& water metabolism]: 97; [lumps]: 316; [poisoning]: 368;
foot reflexology: 149
four limbs, diseases of: 288
fright: 42
frigid limbs: 284, 305
front of neck, diseases of: 290, 294
fu: 143-145, 151, 173; [of no form]: 140; [of the great muscles]: 143; [of the kidneys]: 143; [yang organs]: 155
Fukushima, Kodo: 342-344
fullness in the epigastrium: 281
Fujido's Etymological Dictionary: 33, 116
Fuku Sho Kiran: 26, 171
fundamental qi: 112

— G —

gallbladder: 40, 64, 355, 366, 398, 405; [inflammation]: 289, 293; [meridian, pressure pain]: 368; [problems]: 291, 374, 389
gallstone pain: 279, 308, 403
gan (liver): 103
gao: 99-103, 105-108, 135, 140, 149-151, 153-155; [membranes]: 149; [source]: 145
gao huang shu: 148
gao mo (greasy membrane): 146
Gao Wu: 28
gas with occasional cramping: 258
gastritis and swelling of the stomach: 283
gastroptosis: 394
gathering lump: 338
geomagnetic field: 212, 217-221, 227, 234, 236
geomancers: 20
geotropism: 217
gold needle: 29, 386
gonads: 171
gong xue: 20
gout, neuralgia, and walking problems: 288
gravitation: 217-218
gravitational field of moon: 218
great middle pole: 124
greater omentum: 51, 139, 311
grief: 38-39, 338
gu: 154
gu qi: 27, 78-79; [counterflow, abdominal indication]: 27
Guan Xiang Wan Zhan: 70
guan yuan (lower regulator): 83
Guan Zi: 153-154
guang ming (broad brightness): 126
Guang Ya: 140, 154

Guo Ai Chun: 147
gut tube: 183-185
gynecologic problems: 286, 291, 297, 305-306, 374, 394, 408

— H —

hai (ocean): 79
Han Dynasty: 12, 70, 103, 107, 133, 135, 141, 146, 205; [Former]: 133
Han Shu: 133-134
hands red and warm: 388
hara: [breathing]: 321; [healthy]: 243-244, 325; [infants]: 278; [infirm]: 274; [lump on]: 244, 271; [palpitation]: 244; [pulsing of]: 244, 301; [root of all disease]: 28; [shiatsu]: 243, 271, 276-277; [shiatsu treatment for lumps]: 277; [swollen]: 307; [temperature of]: 244; [tightness on]: 271; [vacant]: 278; [weak]: 30; [woman's, characteristics of]: 245
hardness & tightness, CV-13 to CV-10: 258
harlequin color change: 230
Hashimoto, Keizo: 187, 330, 381
he point: 112, 114, 123, 173, 228, 375, 399
head, diseases of: 301
head tilted to one side: 288
headache: 40, 279, 281, 284, 286, 288, 291, 293, 298, 303, 367, 374, 394; [migraine]: 288, 291
healing crisis: 273
hearing, hardness of: 40
heart: 398, 405; [and shen, overwork]: 84; [attack]: 361; [diseases of]: 364; [electromagnetic field of]: 191; [function]: 88; [lump]: 345; [meridian]: 50, 54-55; [pain]: 337; [problem]: 262, 361, 368, 374; [pulse]: 337; [stopping, fears of]: 300; [suffering of]: 300; [suffering of]: 40, 285, 337; [symptoms]: 288
heart qi: [cannot pass down]: 54; [repletion]: 38-39; [vacancy]: 38-39
heartbeat, visible on hara: 244
heart-shen: 137
heart-wrapping luo: 61, 104, 124, 138, 369
heat: [effect on biomagnetic field]: 223; [in stomach]: 379; [of the lower limbs]: 305; [overexposure to]: 84; [therapy]: 385
heaven qi: 72, 111
heaven's pond: 83
heaviness: 360; [of the head]: 286, 293
hemidesmosome system: 164
hemiplegia: 282, 295-296
hemorrhage, cerebral: 177
hemorrhoids: 284, 298, 374
heng (star calibrator): 75
hepatic portal vein: 105
hepatitis: 386, 388; sun exposure effect: 388
hepatorenal ligament: 169
herbal medicine: 156, 336, 385
hernia: 297; [abdominal indication]: 27
hiccoughs: 279, 284
high blood pressure: 291-292, 391, 407
hip joint or lower limb diseases: 308
Hirata zones: 369, 380, 369
Hirooka, Sosen: 97, 111, 113, 120, 122, 150, 267, 339, 341
Honma, Shohaku: 82
hua (alchemical transformation): 89, 91-92
Hua Shou: 50, 53, 122, 137
hua to points: 278, 368
Huai Nan Zi: 20, 71, 76-77, 85, 87, 90-92, 97, 100, 107, 144, 153-154
huang: 101-103, 105-108, 135, 140, 146-147, 151, 172; [source]: 105, 145
Huang Di Nei Jing Ling Shu: 11
Huang Di Nei Jing Su Wen Ji Gua: 145-146
Huang Di Nei Jing Su Wen: 11
Huang Di Nei Jing Tai Su: 125
Huang Di Wai Jing Jing: 77